Springer

36th Hemophilia Symposium

Hamburg 2005

Editors: I. Scharrer, W. Schramm

Presentation:

Epidemiology
Hemophilia Therapy – Management of Bleedings and Inhibitors
Orthopedic Treatment in Hemophiliacs
Hemostaseologic Diagnostics
Pediatric Hemostaseology
Free Lectures

Scientific Board:
I. Scharrer, Mainz
W. Schramm, Munich

Chairmen:
G. Auerswald (Bremen); L. Gürtler (Greifswald);
A. Kurth (Frankfurt/Main); U. Nowak-Göttl (Münster);
J. Oldenburg (Bonn); B. Pötzsch (Bonn); I. Scharrer (Mainz);
W. Schramm (Munich); M. Spannagl (Munich);
B. Zieger (Freiburg); R. Zimmermann (Heidelberg)

Springer

Professor Dr. med. **Inge Scharrer**
III. Med. Clinic
University Hospital
Langenbeckstr. 1
D-55131 Mainz
Germany

Professor Dr. med. **Wolfgang Schramm**
Dept. of Hemostaseology
University Hospital
Ziemssenstr. 1a
D-80336 München
Germany

ISBN-10 3-540-36714-4 Springer Berlin Heidelberg New York
ISBN-13 978-3-540-36714-7 Springer Berlin Heidelberg New York

Library of Congress Control Number: 2006929905

A catalog record for this book is available from Library of Congress.

Bibliographic information published by Die Deutsche Bibliothek.
Die Deutsche Bibliothek lists this publication in the Deutsche Nationalbibliografie; detailed bibliographic data is available in the Internet at http://dnb.ddb.de

Springer is a part of Springer Science+Business Media

springeronline.com

Printed in Germany

Editor: Dr. Ute Heilmann, Heidelberg, Germany
Desk editor: Meike Stoeck, Heidelberg, Germany
Production: Goldener Schnitt, Sinzheim, Germany
Typesetting: cicero Lasersatz GmbH & Co. KG, Dinkelscherben, Germany
Print: Druckerei Stürtz, Würzburg, Germany

Printed on acid-free paper 21/3151 Di - 5 4 3 2 1 0

Contents

I. Epidemiology

II. Hemophilia Therapy – Management of Bleedings and Inhibitors

III. Orthopedic Treatment in Hemophiliacs

VI. Free Lectures

VII. Poster

List of Participants

Akbulut, A, Dr.

Andresik, G., Frau
Universitätsklinik für Innere Medizin I, A-Wien

Andritschke, K., Frau
Universitätskliniken Frankfurt/M., Kinderklinik, D-Frankfurt

Arends, P., Dr.
Ordination, A-Güssing

Aspöck, G., Dr.
Krankenhaus der Barmherzigen Schwestern vom heiligen Kreuz, A-Wels

Auerswald, G., Dr.
Klinikum Bremen Mitte gGmbH, Prof. Hess-Kinderklinik, D-Bremen

Aumann, V., Dr.
Otto-von-Guericke-Universität Magdeburg, D-Magdeburg

Avoledo, Pierino, Dr.
Arztpraxis, CH Riehen

Bach, Jürgen, Dr.
Klinikum Ludwigshafen, Hämostaseologie, D-Ludwigshafen

Balleisen, L., Prof.
Evangelisches Krankenhaus Hamm, D-Hamm

Bartels, S., Frau
Medizinische Hochschule Hannover, D-Hannover

Barthels, M., Frau Prof.
D-Hannover

Baumgartner, Ch., Dr.
Arztpraxis, CH-Gossau SG

Bechter, M.

Beck, Ch., Frau
D-Berlin

Beck, K.-H.
Med. Dienst der Krankenkassen, D-Lahr

Becker, Th., Dr.
Interessengemeinschaft Hämophiler, D-Trier

Becker, D., Frau
Universitätsklinik Hamburg-Eppendorf, Päd. Hämatologie/Onkologie, D-Hamburg

Beeser, H., Prof.
D-Nimburg

Beha, L.-M., Frau
Praxis Dr. Wolfgang Mondorf, D-Frankfurt/Main

Behnisch, W., Dr.
Universitätskinderklinik Heidelberg, D-Heidelberg

Belkaidi, R., Frau
Medizinische Hochschule Hannover, D-Hannover

Berger, St.
D-Hannover

Berthold, B., Dr.
Dietrich-Bonhoeffer-Klinikum, Klinik f. Innere Medizin 1, D-Neubrandenburg

Beutel, K., Frau Dr.
Universitätsklinikum Hamburg-Eppendorf, D-Hamburg

Bidlingmaier, Ch., Dr.
Dr. von Haunersches Kinderspital, D-München

Binder, A., Dr.
Universitätsklinik für Kinder- und Jugendheilkunde, A-Graz

BINDER, FL., Dr.
DHG, D-Salz

BLATNY, J., Dr.
Faculty Hospital Brno, CS-Brno

BLICKHEUSER, R., Dr.
DRK Kinderklinik, Siegen, D-Siegen

BODA, Z., Dr.
DEOEC, I. Clinic of Internal Medicine, H-Debrecen

BOGDANOVA, N., Frau Dr.
W.W. Universität Münster, Institut für Humangenetik, D-Münster

BÖKER, M.,
Annastift Hannover, Klinik I, D-Hannover

BOLDT, K., Frau
DAK Zentrale, D-Hamburg

BRACKMANN, H.-H., Dr.
D-Bonn

BRAND, B., Frau Dr.
Universitätsspital Zürich, Gerinnungslabor D-LAB 28, CH-Zürich

BRAZZOLA, P., Dr.
Ospedale Civico Lugano, CH-Lugano

BROCKHAUS, W., Dr.
D-Nürnberg

BRUHN, P., Frau Dr.
D-Rostock

BRÜNNICH, H., Frau
D-Rostock

BUDDE, U., Prof.
AK Laborbetriebsgesellschaft mbH, D-Hamburg

BURKART, C., Frau Dr.
Universitätsspital Zürich, CH-Zürich

Calatzis, A., Dr.
Ludwig-Maximilians-Universitätsklinik, Hämostaseologie und Transfusionsmedizin, D-München

Camacho, J.

Caster, Ch., Frau
Universitätsklinikum des Saarlandes, D-Homburg/Saar

Cicigoi, B., Frau
Kispex Kinderspitex Kt. Zürich, CH-Zürich

Cimenti, Ch., Frau Dr.
Universitätsklinik Graz, A-Graz

Crea, R.

Cvirn, G., Dr.
Universitätsklinik Graz, A-Graz

Daniels, G., Frau
Medizinische Hochschule Hannover, D-Hannover

Delev, D.
DRK Blutspendedienst Baden-Württemberg – Hessen, Institut für Transfusionsmedizin und Immunhämatologie Frankfurt, D-Frankfurt

Dingeldein, E., Frau
Praxis Dr. Wolfgang Mondorf, D-Frankfurt/Main

Dockter, G., Prof.
Universitätsklinik für Kinder-und Jugendmedizin Homburg-Saar, D-Homburg-Saar

Dörges, I., Frau Dr.
Universitätsklinikum Lübeck, D-Gross Grönau

Dwenger, A., Frau Dr.
D-Bonn

Ebenebe, Ch., Dr.
D-Göttingen

Eberl, W., Dr.
Klinikum Braunschweig, D-Braunschweig

EICHERT-NAUMANN, A., Frau
DHG, D-Hamburg

EICKHOFF, H., Dr.
Orthopädische Klinik St. Josef-Hospital, D-Troisdorf

ESCURIOLA-ETTINGSHAUSEN, C., Frau Dr.
J.W. Goethe Universität, Kinderklinik, D-Frankfurt am Main

ESSERS, E., Frau Dr.
D-Berlin

FAESSLER, H., Dr.
Arztpraxis, CH-Chiasso

FENGLER, V., Frau
Praxis Dr. Nimtz-Talaska, D-Frankfurt/Oder

FISCHER, B., Frau
Universitätskrankenhaus Hamburg-Eppendorf,
Abt. f. päd. Hämatologie/Onkologie, D-Hamburg

FÖRSTER, T., Frau
Universität Würzburg, Institut für Humangenetik, D-Thüngersheim

FRANKE, D., Dr.
Praxis für Blutgerinnungsstörungen und Gefäßkrankheiten, D-Magdeburg

FRANKE, ST., Frau
D-Frankfurt/Main

FREGIN, A., Dr.
Universität Würzburg, Institut für Humangenetik, D-Randersacker

FREUNEK, G., Dr.
Universitätsklinik Regensburg, Hämatologie und Onkologie, D-Wenzenbach

FRITSCH, P., Dr.
Universitätsklinik Graz, A-Graz

FUCHS, A., Frau Dr.
Universitätsklinik für Innere Medizin I, A-Wien

GAJEK, K., Frau
A-Wien

GALLISTL, S., Prof.
Universitätsklinik für Kinder- und Jugendheilkunde, D-Graz

GAMPER, A., Frau Dr.
St. Johanns Spital – Landeskliniken Salzburg, A-Salzburg

GANSCHOW, A., Frau Dr.
Blutzentrale Linz, A-Linz

GARVE, D., Frau
D-Hannover

GEISEN, U., Dr.
Medizinische Universitätsklinik, Abt. Klinische Chemie, D-Freiburg

GEISEN, CH., Dr.
DRK-Blutspendedienst BW – Hessen, D-Frankfurt am Main

GERBER, A., Frau
Baxter Deutschland GmbH, D-Berlin

GERHARDT, A., Frau Dr.
Universitätsklinikum Düsseldorf, D-Düsseldorf

GIANGRANDE, P., Prof.
Churchill Hospital, Oxford Hemophilia Center, GB-Oxford

GIEBL, A., Dr.
Klinikum Innenstadt, D-München

GIERSDORF, G., Frau
Kurpfalzkrankenhaus Heidelberg, D-Ketsch

GILDBERG, P.
Praxis, D-Flensburg

GIRISCH, M., Frau Dr.
Universitätsklinik für Kinder und Jugendliche, D-Tübingen

GÖHAUSEN, M., Frau
Praxis Dr. Pollmann, D-Münster

GOTTSTEIN, S., Frau Dr.
Hämophiliezentrum am Vivantes-Klinikum im Friedrichshain, D-Berlin

Gross, J., Dr.
Institut für Klinische Hämostaseologie und Transfusionsmedizin, D-Homburg

Grossmann, R., Dr.
Universitätsklinik Frankfurt/M., Hämostaseologie, D-Frankfurt

Güldenring, H., Dr.
Städtisches Krankenhaus Dresden Neustadt, Kinderklinik, D-Dresden

Gürtler, L., Prof.
Ernst-Moritz-Arndt-Universität – Loeffler-Institut für Medizinische Mikrobiologie, D-Greifswald

Habermann, B., Dr.
Orthopädische Universitätsklinik Frankfurt, D-Frankfurt am Main

Hähling, D., Dr.
Helios Kliniken Schwerin, Zentrum für Innere Medizin, Abt. Hämatologie und Onkologie, D-Schwerin

Haidl, H., Dr.
Universitätsklinik Graz, A-Graz

Halbmayer, M., Dr.
Krankenhaus Lainz, A-Wien

Halimeh, S., Frau Dr.
Praxis f. Laboratoriums- und Transfusionsmedizin, D-Duisburg

Hartmann, S., Frau
Hämophilieregister Schweiz, CH-Chur

Haschberger, B., Frau
Paul-Ehrlich-Institut, D-Langen

Hawlina-Hess, N., Frau
D-Wipperfürth

Heide, D., Frau
Universitätskinderklinik Düsseldorf, D-Düsseldorf

Heine, S., Frau Dr.
Universitätskinderklinik Homburg Saar, D-Homburg

Heistinger, M.L., Dr.
Landeskrankehaus Klagenfurt, A-Klagenfurt

Hellstern, P., Prof.
Klinikum Ludwigshafen, IHT, D-Ludwigshafen

Hennewig, U., Frau Dr.
Universität Düsseldorf, Klinik für Kinderonkologie und Hämatologie, D-Düsseldorf

Henseler, D., Frau
Institut für Experimentelle Hämatologie u. Transfusionsmedizin, D-Bonn

Herrmann, F. H., Prof.
D-Neuenkirchen

Herwig, R., Prof.
Universitätsklinik für Urologie, A-Innsbruck

Herzig, D.
AOK Schleswig Holstein, D-Kiel

Hesse, J., Frau
Paul-Ehrlich-Institut, D-Langen

Hilger, A., Frau Dr.
Paul-Ehrlich-Institut, D-Langen

Hlusi, A., Dr.
Faculty Hospital Olomouc, CS-Olomouc

Hofmann, H., Prof.
D-Werder (Havel)

Hofmann, M., Dr.
Klinikum der Friedrich-Schiller-Universität, D-Jena

Hofmann, K., Dr.
Klinikum Chemnitz gGmbH, D-Chemnitz

Holstein, K., Frau Dr.
D-Hamburg

Horneff, S., Frau
Martin-Luther-Universität Halle-Wittenberg, Kinderklinik, D-Halle

Horvathova, D., Frau Dr.
Clinic of Hematology and Transfusion Med., University, SW-Bratislava

Hünerberg, M., Frau
Universität Würzburg, Institut für Humangenetik, D-Würzburg

Huth-Kühne, A., Frau Dr.
Kurpfalzkrankenhaus, D-Heidelberg

Imahorn, P., Dr.
Kinderspital Luzern, CH-Luzern

Ingerslev, J., Dr.
DK-Hojbjerg

Ivaskevicius, V., Dr.
Universitätsklinik Bonn, Institut f. Experimentelle Hämatologie und Transfusionsmedizin, D-Bonn

Jankovicova, D., Frau Dr.
University of Bratislava, Clinic of Hematology and Transfusion Med., SW-Bratislava

Jenkins, S., Frau
Klinikum der Universität München, Hämostaseologie, D-München

Jones, R., Frau Dr.
St. Johanns Spital - Landeskliniken Salzburg, A-Salzburg

Julen, E., Dr.
CH-Zermatt

Kadar, J., Dr.
Praxis-Labor für Transfusionsmedizin, D-Köln

Kalnins, W.
DHG, D Hamburg

Kalus, U., Dr.
Universitätsmedizin Berlin Charité Campus Mitte, D-Berlin

Kätzel, R., Prof.
Städtisches Klinikum St.Georg, D-Leipzig

Kauke, T., Frau Dr.
Klinikum Innenstadt, D-München

KEHREL, B., Frau Prof.
Universitätsklinik Münster, Experimentelle und Klinische Hämostaseologie, D-Münster

KEISKER, A., Dr.
Kinderspital Zürich, Medizinische Klinik, CH-Zürich

KEMKES-MATTHES, B., Frau Prof.
Zentrum Innere Medzin, D-Gießen

KIESEWETTER, H., Prof.
D-Berlin

KIRCHMAIER, C. M., Dr.
Deutsche Klinik für Diagnostik, D-Wiesbaden

KLAMROTH, R., Dr.
Vivantes Klinikum im Friedrichshain, D-Berlin

KLARE, M., Dr.
Helios-Klinikum Berlin-Buch, D-Berlin

KLUGE, A., Frau
Praxis für Innere Medizin und Gefäßkrankheiten, D-Magdeburg

KNÖBL, P., Prof.
Universitätsklinik für Innere Medizin I, A-Wien

KNÖFLER, R., Dr.
Universitätskinderklinik Dresden, D-Dresden

KÖHLER-VAJTA, K., Frau Dr.
Kinder- und Jugendarztpraxis, D-Grünwald

KOMRSKA, V., Dr.
Faculty Hospital Motol, CS-Praha 5

KÖNIGS, CH., Dr.
JW Goethe Universität, Kinderklinik, D-Frankfurt am Main

KOSCIELNY, J., Dr.
Universitätsklinik, Charité, Institut für Transfusionsmedizin, D-Berlin

KÖSTERING, H., Prof.
D-Lemgo

Krause, M., Frau Dr.
Klinikum der J.W. Goethe Universität, Hämostaseologie, D-Frankfurt/Main

Krcova, V., Frau Dr.
Faculty Hospital Olomouc, CS-Olomouc

Krebs, H., Dr.
Klinikum der Ludwig-Maximilians-Universität München,
Abt. für Transfusionsmedizin und Hämostaseologie, D-München

Kremer, D., Frau
Institut für Experimentelle Hämatologie u. Transfusionsmedizin, D-Bonn

Kurme, A., Dr.
D Hamburg

Kurnik, K., Frau Dr.
Ludwig-Maximilians-Universität, Dr. von Haunersches Kinderspital,
D-München

Kurth, A., Prof.
Orthopädische Universitätsklinik Stiftung Friedrichsheim, D-Frankfurt/Main

Küting, A., Frau
Uniklinikum Homburg/Saar, Hämostaseologie, D-Schönenberg-Kübelberg

Lages, P., Dr.
Kurpfalzkrankenhaus Heidelberg, D-Heidelberg

Lang, A., Dr.
Landeskrankenhaus Feldkirch, D-Feldkirch

Lang, R.
Österreichische Hämophiliegesellschaft, A-Wien

Lauer, E., Frau
D-Homburg

Lehmann, I., Frau
Universität Leipzig, Med. Klinik I, Hämostaseologie, D-Leipzig

Lenk, H., Prof.
Universitäts- und Poliklinik für Kinder und Jugendliche, D-Leipzig

Lestin, H.-G., Prof.
Helios-Kliniken Schwerin, Institut für Laboratoriumsmedizin, D-Schwerin

NAGY, A., Frau Dr.
PTE, I. Clinic of Internal Medicine, H-Pecs

NEMES, L., Dr.
National Hemophilia Center OGYK, H-Budapest

NEUMANN, S., Frau
D-Martfeld

NEUNER, H., Frau Dr.
Tiroler Gebietskrankenkasse, A-Innsbruck

NIEKRENS, C., Frau Dr.
Klinikum Delmenhorst, D-Delmenhorst

NIEMANN, B., Frau Dr.
Hämophilie-Zentrum Bonn, D-Bonn

NIMTZ-TALASKA, A., Frau Dr.
Praxis, D-Frankfurt/Oder

NOWAK-GÖTTL, U., Frau Prof.
Universitätsklinik, Pädiatrische Hämatologie und Onkologie, D-Münster

OLDENBURG, J., Prof.
Universitätsklinikum Bonn, Institut für Experimentelle Hämatologie und Transfusionsmedizin, D-Bonn

ORLOVIC, A.-M., Frau
Klinikum Friedrichshain, Hämostaseologie, D-Berlin

OTT, K., Frau
D-Magdeburg

PARENTI, M., Frau Dr.

PAVLOVA, A., Frau Dr.
DRK Blutspendedienst Baden-Württemberg-Hessen, Institut für Transfusionsmedizin und Immunohämatologie, D-Frankfurt/Main

PEETZ, D., Dr.
Klinikum der Johannes Gutenberg-Universität Mainz, Institut für Klinische Chemie und Laboratoriumsmedizin, D-Mainz

PENKA, M., Prof.
Faculty Hospital Brno, CS-Brno

Peter-Salonen, K., Frau Dr.
Inselspital Bern, Hämatologisches Zentrallabor, CH-Bern

Petrini, P., Frau Dr.
Karolinska University Hospital, SE-Stockholm

Petros, S., Dr.
Universität Leipzig, Hämophiliezentrum, D-Leipzig

Pindur, G., Prof.
Universitätsklinikum, D-Homburg

Pötzsch, B., Prof.
Universitätsklinikum Bonn, Institut für Experimentelle Hämatologie und Transfusionsmedizin, D-Bonn

Ptoszkova, H., Frau Dr.
Faculty Hospital Ostrava, CS-Ostrava

Rabenstein, C., Frau
Klinikum der J.W. Goethe Universität, Hämostaseologie, D-Frankfurt/Main

Raddatz, P., Frau Dr.
Kantonsspital Luzern, CH-Luzern

Rehberger, G., Dr.
Ordination, A-Frastanz

Reif, Ch.
Universitätsklinik für Kinder- und Jugendheilkunde, A-Innsbruck

Reinhard, H., Dr.
Universitätskinderklinik, Pädiatrische Hämatologie und Onkologie, D-Homburg/Saar

Reiter, W., Dr.
Facharzt für Innere Medizin, D-Viersen

Rieke, M.
Interessengemeinschaft Hämophiler e.V., D-Bergisch Gladbach

Ringkamp, H., Frau
Praxis Dr. Pollmann, D-Münster

Roschitz, B., Frau Dr.
Universitätsklinik Graz, A-Graz

ROSENLECHNER, S., Frau
Salzburger Landeskliniken, Universitätsklinik f. Innere Medizin III, A-Salzburg

ROST, S., Frau
Universität Würzburg, Institut für Humangenetik, D-Würzburg

ROTHE, B., Frau
Klinikum im Friedrichshain, Hämophiliezentrum, D-Berlin

ROTT, H., Frau Dr.
Gemeinschaftspraxis Prof. Trobisch/Dr. Rott, D-Duisburg

ROWOLD, CH., Frau
Städtisches Klinikum Braunschweig gGmbH, Klinik für Kinder- und Jugendmedizin, D-Braunschweig

RUIZ, SOLEDAD, Frau

SAENKO, E., Dr.
University of Maryland School of Medicine, Center for Vascular and Inflammatory Diseases, USA-Maryland

SAILE, S., Frau Dr.
D-Halle

SANIO, G., Frau
Universitätsklinik für Innere Medizin III, A-Salzburg

SCHÄFER, CH., Frau
Klinik für Kinder- und Jugendmedizin, Abt. Hämatologie/Onkologie, D-Homburg

SCHARRER, I., Frau Prof.
Universitätsklinik Mainz, III. Med. Klinik, D-Mainz

SCHELLE, G.
Interessengemeinschaft Hämophiler e.V., D-Bonn

SCHLENKRICH, U., Dr.
DHG, D-Hamburg

SCHLOMM, A., Frau
Klinikum Braunschweig, D-Braunschweig

SCHMID, L., Dr.
Kantonsspital St. Gallen, CH-St. Gallen

Schmidt, O., Dr.
Praxis für Gefäßkrankheiten, D-Magdeburg

Schmitt, K., Prof.
Landeskinderklinik Linz, A-Linz

Schobess, R., Frau
M.L.-Universität Halle, Klinik für Kinder- und Jugendmedizin, D-Halle

Schoenauer, M.-L., Frau
Universitätsspital Basel, CH-Basel

Scholz, U., Frau Dr.
Praxis für Gerinnungstörungen/Hämophilie, D-Leipzig

Schramm, W., Prof.
Klinikum Innenstadt, Abt. Hämostaseologie, D-München

Schröder, J., Dr.
Universitätsklinik Bonn, Institut für Experimentelle Hämatologie und Transfusionsmedizin, D-Bonn

Schröder, W., Frau
Ernst-Moritz-Arndt-Univerisätsklinik Greifswald, Institut für Humangenetik, D-Greifswald

Schrum, J., Frau
D-Hamburg

Schubert, Ch., Frau Dr.
Helios-Klinik Erfurt, D-Erfurt

Schubiger, G., Prof.
Kinderspital Luzern, CH-Luzern

Schulze, S., Frau
Universitätsklinik, Zentrum für Kinderheilkunde, Hämatologie/Onkologie, D-Magdeburg

Schulzki, Th., Dr.
Blutspendezentrum SRK, CH-Thur

Schumacher, R., Dipl.-Med.
D-Schwerin

SCHÜTZE, B., Frau Dr.
Universität Ulm, Abteilung Innere III, D-Ulm

SEDLAK, W., Dr.
Ordination, A-Linz

SEIFRIED, E., Prof.
Blutspendedienst Baden Württemberg – Hessen, D-Frankfurt/Main

SELLENG, K., Frau Dr.
Ernst-Moritz-Arndt-Universität, Institut für Immunologie und Transfusionsmedizin, D-Greifswald

SERBAN, M., Frau Prof.
RO-Timisoara

SEUSER, A., Dr.
Kaiser-Karl-Klinik, D-Bonn

SIEGEMUND, TH.
Universität Leipzig, D-Leipzig

SIEGEMUND, A., Frau Dr.
Universität Leipzig, D-Leipzig

SIEGERT, G., Frau Prof.
Universitätsklinikum Dresden, Institut für Klinische Chemie und Laboratoriumsmedizin, D-Dresden

SIGUTOVA, P., Frau Dr.
Faculty Hospital Plzen, CS-Plzen

SPANNAGL, M., Dr.
Klinikum Innenstadt, D-München

STEIGERWALD, U., Dr.
Universitätsklinik Würzburg, Zentrallabor, Gerinnungsambulanz, D-Würzburg

STEIN, G.
AOK Baden-Württemberg, D-Lahr

STEINER-KRAMMER, B., Frau Dr.
Südstadtklinikum, D-Rostock

STOLL, H., Frau
Universitätkinderklinik Frankfurt, D-Frankfurt/Main

Strauch, P., Frau
Universitätsklinikum Gießen, D-Ranstadt

Streif, W., Prof.
Universitätsklinik für Kinder- und Jugendheilkunde, D-Innsbruck

Strey, R.,
Universität Greifswald, Institut für Humangenetik, D-Karlshagen

Stumpe, Ch., Frau
Klinikum im Friedrichshain, Hämophiliezentrum, D-Berlin

Sturm, A.
Universitätskinderklinik, Zentrallabor, D-Würzburg

Svorcova, V., Frau Dr.
UHKT, CS-Praha

Syrbe, G., Dr.
Asklepios-Fachklinikum Stadtroda, D-Stadtroda

Thom, K., Frau Dr.
Universitätsklinik für Kinder- und Jugendheilkunde, A-Wien

Thürmel, K.
Klinikum der Ludwig-Maximilians-Universität, Klinik für Anästhesiologie, D-München

Thuysbaert, C., Frau

Tiede, A., Dr.
Medizinische Hochschule Hannover, D-Hannover

Timelthaler, H., Dr.
Ordination, A-Uttendorf

Tomasits, J., Dr.
Allgemeines Österreichisches. Krankenhaus Linz, Zentrallabor, A-Lin

Tregel, M., Dr.
Klinikum Frankfurt/Oder GmbH, D-Berlin

Trummer, A., Dr.
Medizinische Hochschule Hannover, D-Hannover

Tsakiris, D., Dr.
Universitätsspital Basel, Hämostaselabor, CH-Basel

Türk-Kraetzer, B., Frau Dr.
D-Oldenburg

Udvardy, M., Dr.
DEOEC, I-II Clinic of Internal Medicine, H-Debrecen

Unger, J., Dr.
Landesklinik Salzburg, Institut für Labordiagnostik, A-Salzburg

Veldman, A., Dr.
Kinderherzzentrum, Universitätsklinik, D-Gießen

Verbruggen, B., Dr.
Radboud University Nijmegen Medical Centre Dept CHL, NL-Nijmegen

Vidovic, N., Frau
Hämophilie-Zentrum Bonn, D-Bonn

Vigh, Th.
Johannes Gutenberg Universität Mainz, Klinikum, D-Mainz

Voerkel, W., Dr.
Labor Reising-Ackermann & Partner Leipzig, D-Leipzig

Vogel, G., Prof.
D-Erfurt

Vogt, B., Frau
Universitäts-Kinderpoliklinik Leipzig, D-Leipzig

von Auer, Ch., Frau Dr.
Universitätsklinikum Mainz, D-Mainz

von Depka Prondzinski, M., Dr.
Werlhoff-Institut, D-Hannover

von der Weid, N., Dr.
CHUV Lausanne, CH-Lausanne

von Pape, K.-W., Dr.
Klinikum Fulda gAG, Institut f. Labormedizin, D-Fulda

Vondryska, F.
Czech Hemophilia Society, CS-Klatovy IV

Waclawiczek, E., Frau
Universitätsklinik Graz, A-Graz

Wagner, B., Frau Dr.
Klinikum Großhadern, D-München

Wallny, Th., Dr.
St. Bernhard-Hospital, Orthopädie I, D-Kamp-Lintfort

Wank, H., Dr.
St. Anna Kinderspital, A-Wien

Weidenhammer, A., Frau
Prof.-Hess-Kinderklinik, D-Bremen

Weinstock, N., Dr.
Labor Wagner und Partner, D-Göttingen

Weiss, J.
Österreichische Hämophiliegesellschaft, A-Wien

Wendisch, J., Dr.
Kinderzentrum Dresden, D-Dresden

Wendisch, E., Frau Dr.
D-Dresden

Wermes, C., Frau Dr.
Medizinische Hochschule Hannover, D-Hannover

Wickmann, R., Frau
Vivantes Klinikum Friedrichshain, D-Berlin

Wieding, J. U., Dr.
D-Göttingen

Wieland, I., Frau Dr.
Medizinische Hochschule Hannover, Pädiatrische Hämatologie und Onkologie, D-Hannover

Wilken, G., Frau
Gerinnungsambulanz Dr. Auerswald Bremen, D-Bremen

Winkelmann, Th.
Städtisches Klinikum Heinrich-Braun, Klinik für Kinder- und Jugendmedizin, D-Zwickau

Wissmann, E., Frau
Universitätsklinik für Kinder- und Jugendheilkunde, A-Wien

Witt, E., Frau
Universitätsklinikum Giessen, D-Gießen

Wohlleben, M., Frau

Wolf, H.-H., Dr.
Universitätskliniken Halle, D-Halle

Wulff, K., Frau
Institut für Humangenetik, D-Greifswald

Zähres, J., Frau
D-Bonn

Zeller, W., Dr.
D-Hamburg

Zellhofer, J.
Österreichische Hämophiliegesellschaft, A-Wien

Zieger, B., Frau PD Dr.
Universitätskliniken Freiburg, Kinderklinik, D-Freiburg

Ziemer, S., Frau
Charité-Universitätsmedizin Berlin, ILP, CCM, D-Berlin

Zimmermann, R., Prof.
Kurpfalzkrankenhaus, D-Heidelberg

Zöhrer, I., Frau
Universitätsklinik für Kinder- und Jugendheilkunde, A-Wien

Zotz, R., Dr.
Institut für Hämostaseologie und Transfusionsmedizin, D-Düsseldorf

Zwiauer, K., Prof.
Landesklinikum St. Pölten, A-St. Pölten

I. Epidemiology

Chairmen:

L. Gürtler (Greifswald)
W. Schramm (Munich)

HIV Infection and Causes of Death in Patients with Hemophilia in Germany (Year 2004/2005 Survey)

H. KREBS, and W. SCHRAMM on Behalf of the Participating German Hemophilia centers

Introduction

The annually survey »HIV Infection and Causes of Death in Patients with Hemophilia in Germany« already goes along with a fine tradition. Already in the late 1970s Professor Landbeck began to survey annually hemophiliacs in West Germany for causes of death and the prevalence of diseases. This was carried on till today, so that our actual considerations rest upon a broad database which allows us a deep insight into the long-term health state development of people with bleeding disorders.

Patients and Methods

Established paper based questionnaires called „Todesursachenstatistik 2004/2005" were sent to all known facilities treating hemophilia patients in Germany. Prompted was information about patients with hemophilia A, B and von Willebrand disease. In particular anonymous data concerning the last 12 months about number of treated patients, type and severity of illness, HIV-status and detailed information about causes of death were inquired. This data were merged with existing data returning to 1982 and analyzed statistically. In the 2004/2005 survey, a total number of 8359 patients with bleeding disorders have been reported from 71 participating centers.

Results

In the last five year's surveys the number of reporting hemophilia centers persisted relatively constant. The assignment of reporting centers and number of patients to regions in Germany are given in Figures 1a, b. In this year 71 centers contributed data (Table 1). Thereby the total number of patients (including patients with von Willebrand disease) reported from all centers added up to 8359 patients compared to 8445 patients in the last year's survey. The trend of reported patients with hemophilia A/B and von Willebrand disease since 1998 is shown in Figure 2.

I. Scharrer/W. Schramm (Ed.)
36th Hemophilia Symposium Hamburg 2005

Participating centers

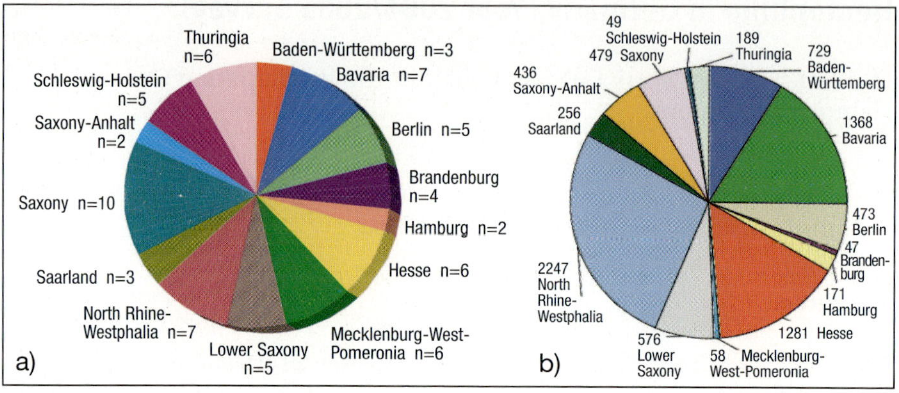

Fig. 1. Numbers of participating hemophilia centers, reported patients and regions

Table 1. Numbers of participating hemophilia centers

	1991	1992	1993	1994	1995	1996	1997	1998	1999	2000	2001	2002	2003	2004	2005
East	47	62	79												
West	18	18	24												
Totals	65	80	103	111	119	119	71	75	93	87	72	75	71	70	71

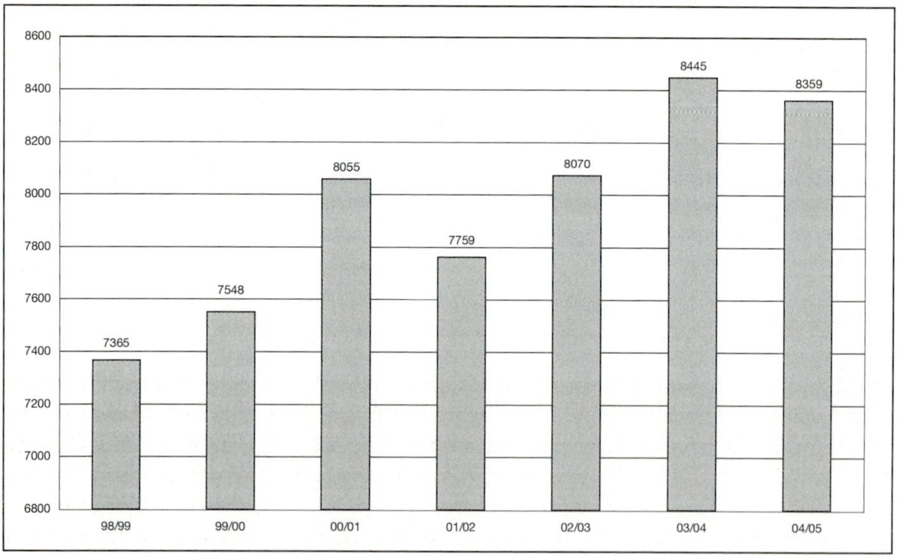

Fig. 2. Number of reported patients since 1998

Patients

The distribution of patients with hemophilia A (43.5%), B (8,0%) and patients with von Willebrand disease (48.5%) is given in Table 2. Compared to the data of previous surveys these are relative consistent findings. Analyzing severity of disease with a cut-off of 2% factor activity, the distribution between the two subgroups, i.e. below 2% and above 2%, is similar in patients with hemophilia A (55.0/45.0%) and B (48.1/51.9%) as shown in Table 2. 21.7% of patients with von Willebrand disease showed Ristocetin cofactor levels below 30% as demonstrated in Table 2.

Table 2. Cumulative data from 71 centers as of 2004/2005

	Hemophilia A		Hemophilia B		von Willebrand disease		Σ	
	N	%*	N	%	N	%	N	%
Total	3635	43.5 (–)	666	8.0 (–)	4058	48.5 (–)	8359	100.0
Factor activity ≤ 2%	1998	23.9 (54.9)	320	3.8 (48.0)	–	–	2318	27.7
Factor activity > 2%	1637	19.5 (45.0)	346	4.1 (51.9)	–	–	1983	23.7
Ristocetin Cofactor = 30%	–	–	–	–	879	10.5 (21.6)	879	10.5
Ristocetin Cofactor > 30%	–	–	–	–	3176	37.9 (78.2)	3176	37.9
Inhibitor (low responders)	31	0.3 (0.8)	9	0.1 (1.3)	–	–	40	0.4
Inhibitor (high responders)	84	1.0 (2.3)	10	0.1 (1.5)	–	–	94	1.1
HIV negative	3086	36.9 (84.8)	591	7.0 (88.7)	4050	48.4 (99.8)	7727	92.4
HIV positive	549	6.5 (15.1)	75	0.8 (11.2)	8	0.1 (0.1)	632	7.5

* percentage of all patients; in brackets: percentage of row

Inhibitors

In 3.2% (115) of the patients with hemophilia A and in 2.9% (19) of the patients with hemophilia B an inhibitor was found (see Table 2). These findings correspond to international large-scale prevalence studies and registry data indicating that the prevalence of inhibitors in the hemophiliac A population overall is up to 5% [6]. Regarding data back to 1999 the inhibitor prevalence observed in our cohort is slightly declining as depicted in Figure 3. Combining these data with further data of other authors and surveys presented at the Hamburg Hemophilia-Symposium since 1978 (see Fig. 4) implying an approximated rate of 0.5 % successful immune tole-

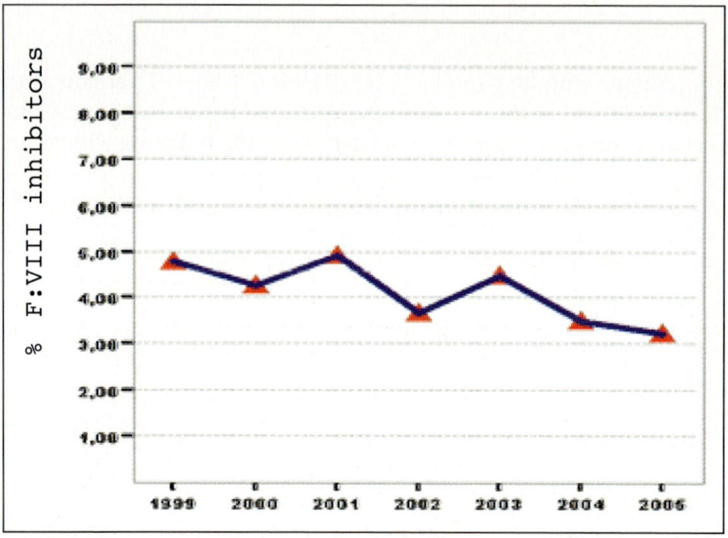

Fig. 3. Prevalence of patients with hemophilia A and inhibitors since 1999

rance therapies per year there is also no indication of an increasing prevalence of inhibitors in patients with hemophilia A.

HIV Status

Of all reported patients a total of 632 (7.5%) were infected with HIV. Analyzed for HIV distribution in subgroups 15.1% of all patients with hemophilia A, 11.2% of all patients with hemophilia B, and 0.1% of all patients with von Willebrand disease were HIV-infected (Table 3). A total of 33 patients (5.6% of all HIV positive patients)

Table 3. HIV-status

	Hemophilia A		Hemophilia B		von Willebrand disease		Σ	
	N	%*	N	%	N	%	N	%
HIV positive, no AIDS	250	39.5 (45.3)	37	5.8 (49.3)	6	0.9 (75.0)	293	46.3
HIV positive, CD4<200 cell/µl	48	7.5 (8.7)	6	0.9 (8.0)	0	0.0 (0.0)	54	8.5
HIV positive, full blown AIDS	34	5.3 (6.1)	2	0.3 (2.6)	0	0.0 (0.0)	36	5.6
HIV positive, no comment	217	34.3 (39.5)	30	4.7 (40.0)	2	0.3 (25.0)	249	39.3
Σ	549	86.8	75	11.8	8	1.2	632	100.0

* percentage of all patients; in brackets: percentage of row

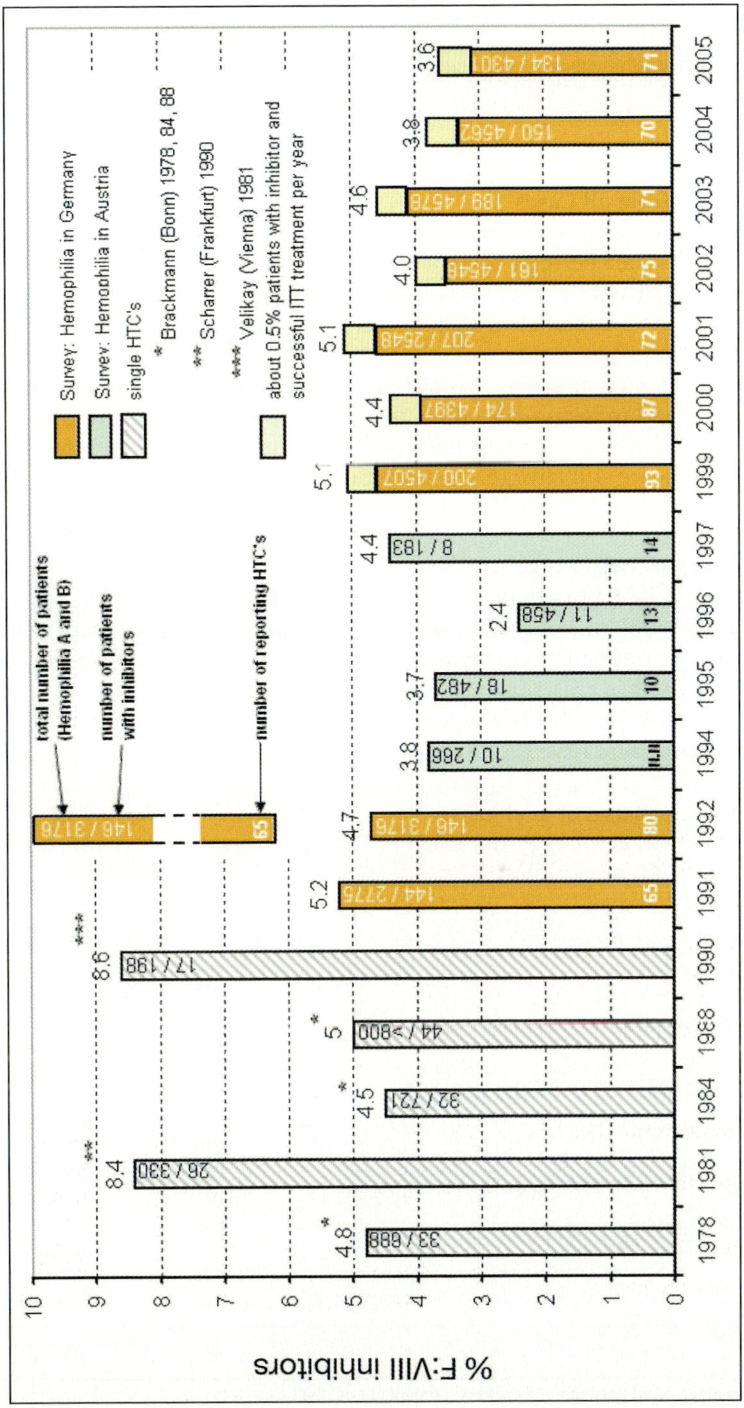

Fig. 4. Prevalence of patients with hemophilia A and inhibitors since 1978 (Presented at the Hamburg Hemophilia-Symposium)

has reached the stage of full-blown AIDS, compared to 293 patients (46.3% of all HIV positive patients) that have up to now not shown severe symptoms (Table 3). 249 HIV positive patients with no further details concerning stadium were reported.

Mortality from all Cases

In the 2004/2005 period a total of 28 patients (19 HIV-, 9 HIV+) were reported dead with the distribution of causes of death given in Table 4. Since the beginning of the survey in 1982 a total of nearly 800 patients have been reported dead (Fig. 9). The development of mortality and causes of death since 82/83 are depicted in Figures 6 and 7. In this year's survey liver disease (25.0%) again has been the main cause of death. After a todiac in 1995 the number of AIDS-related deaths is declining continuously. As at present more than half of the primary HIV-infected patients with hemophilia are still alive (632), the main reason for this development can probably be attributed to improved antiretroviral therapies as described by many authors [1, 2, 3]. In contrast liver disease (25.0%) and cancer (21.4%) as a cause of death have been increasing again (see Fig. 5 (c), (e)), pulled oneself together now liable for 45.5 % of all reported death cases. Three patients (10.7%) died of a bleeding. Overall annual mortality in patients with bleeding disorders in the 2004/2005 survey adds up to 0.33% per year. Five patients (21.4%) died of other diseases not distinguished in this survey. No indications for Creutzfeldt-Jakob disease in our patient collective has been reported since. Only two dead patients (7.1%) with no further comment have been reported.

Table 4. Distribution of death causes

Cause of death	HIV–		HIV+ no AIDS		HIV+ CD4+ < 200		AIDS		Σ	
	N	%*	N	%	N	%	N	%	N	%
Died of AIDS	–	–	1	3.6 (33.3)	0	0.0 (0.0)	2	7.1 (66.7)	3	10.7
Died of liver disease	4	14.3 (21.1)	0	0.0 (0.0)	3	10.7 (100)	0	0.0 (0.0)	7	25.0
Died of bleeding	3	10.7 (15.8)	0	0.0 (0.0)	0	0.0 (0.0)	0	0.0 (0.0)	3	10.7
Died of cancer	5	17.9 (26.3)	0	0.0 (0.0)	0	0.0 (0.0)	1	3.6 (33.3)	6	21.4
Died of other diseases	5	17.9 (26.3)	1	3.6 (33.3)	0	0.0 (0.0)	0	0.0 (0.0)	6	21.4
Died of accident. suicide, drugs, murder	1	3.6 (5.3)	0	0.0 (0.0)	0	0.0 (0.0)	0	0.0 (0.0)	1	3.6
Died, no comment	1	3.6 (5.3)	1	3.6 (33.3)	0	0.0 (0.0)	0	0.0 (0.0)	2	7.1
Σ	19	67.9	3	10.7	3	10.7	3	10.7	28	100

* percentage of all patients; in brackets: percentage of row

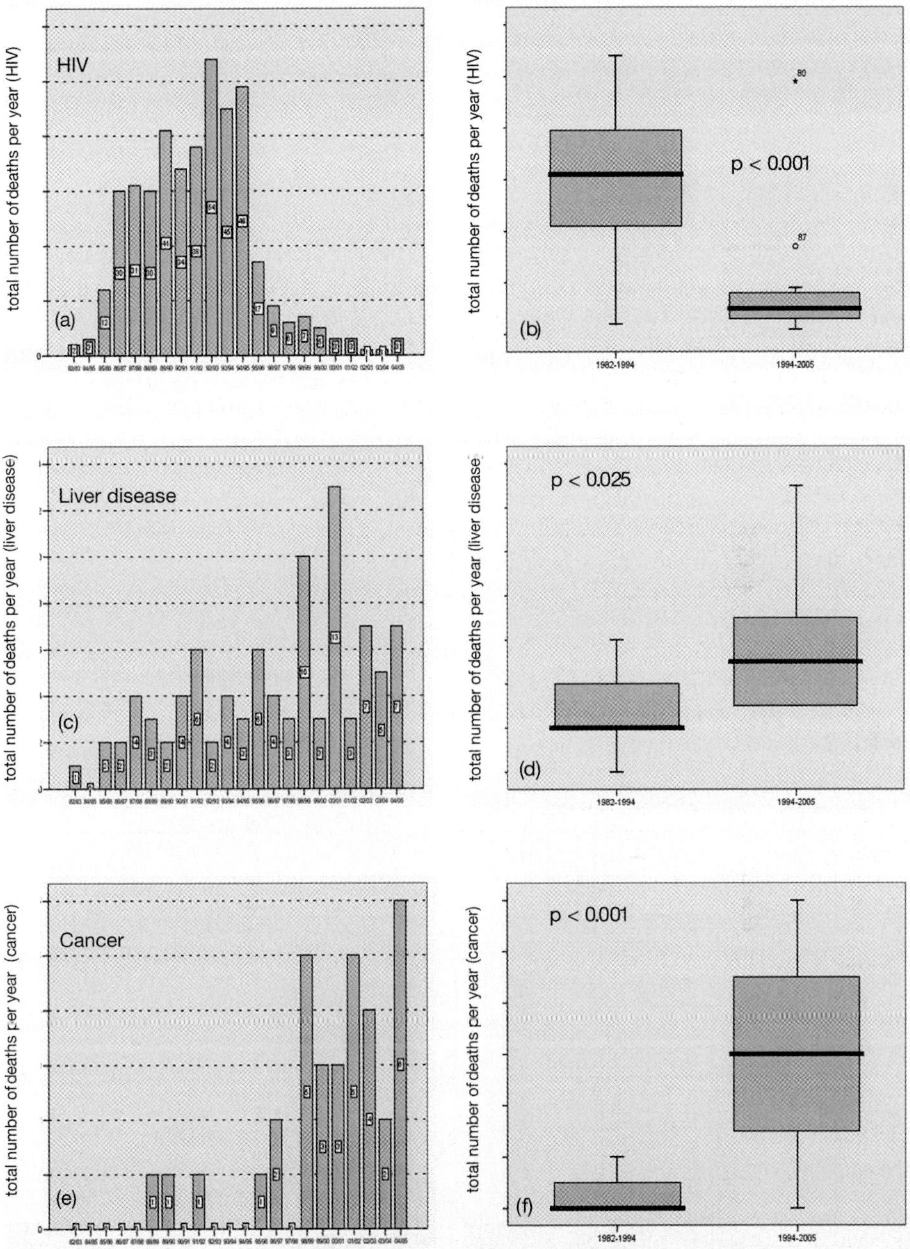

Fig. 5a-f. Comparison total number of deaths of HIV, liver disease and cancer

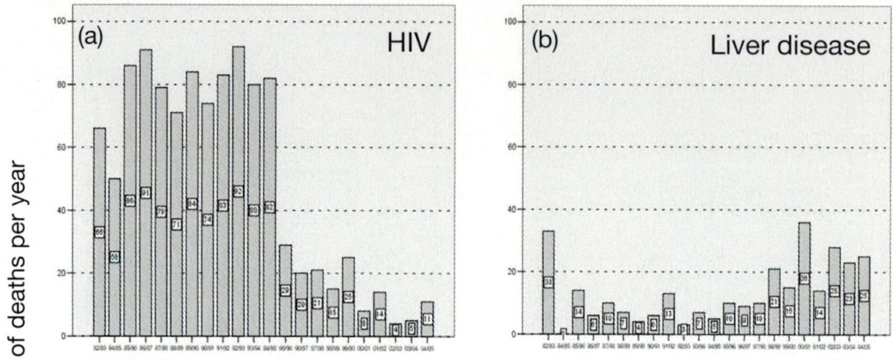

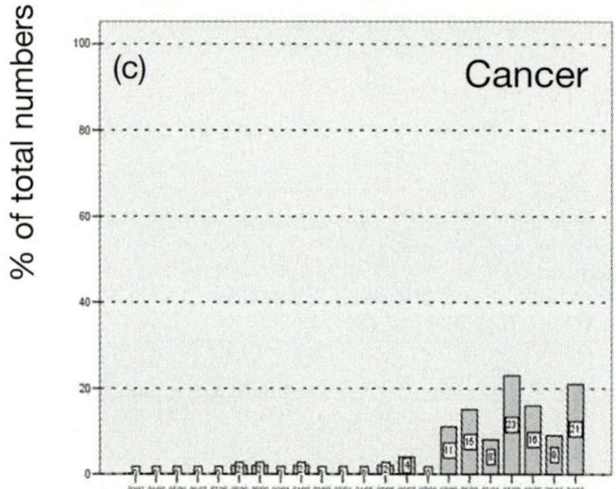

Fig. 6a-c. Comparison % of total number of deaths of HIV, liver disease and cancer

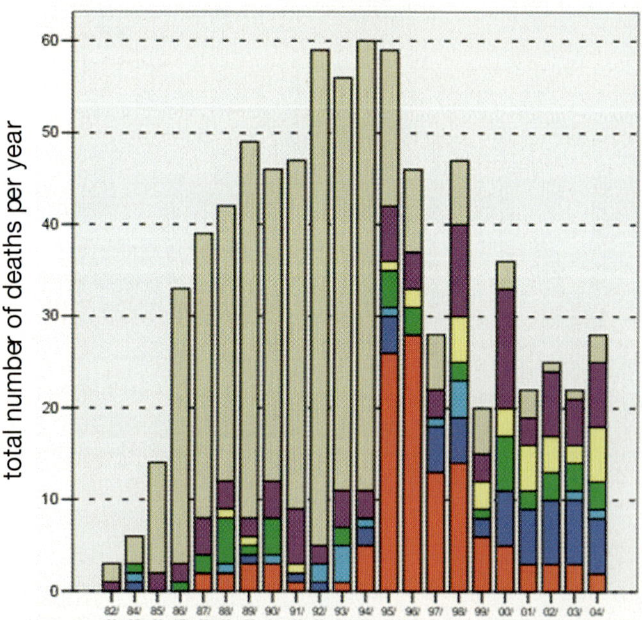

Fig. 7. Causes of death since the beginning of the survey

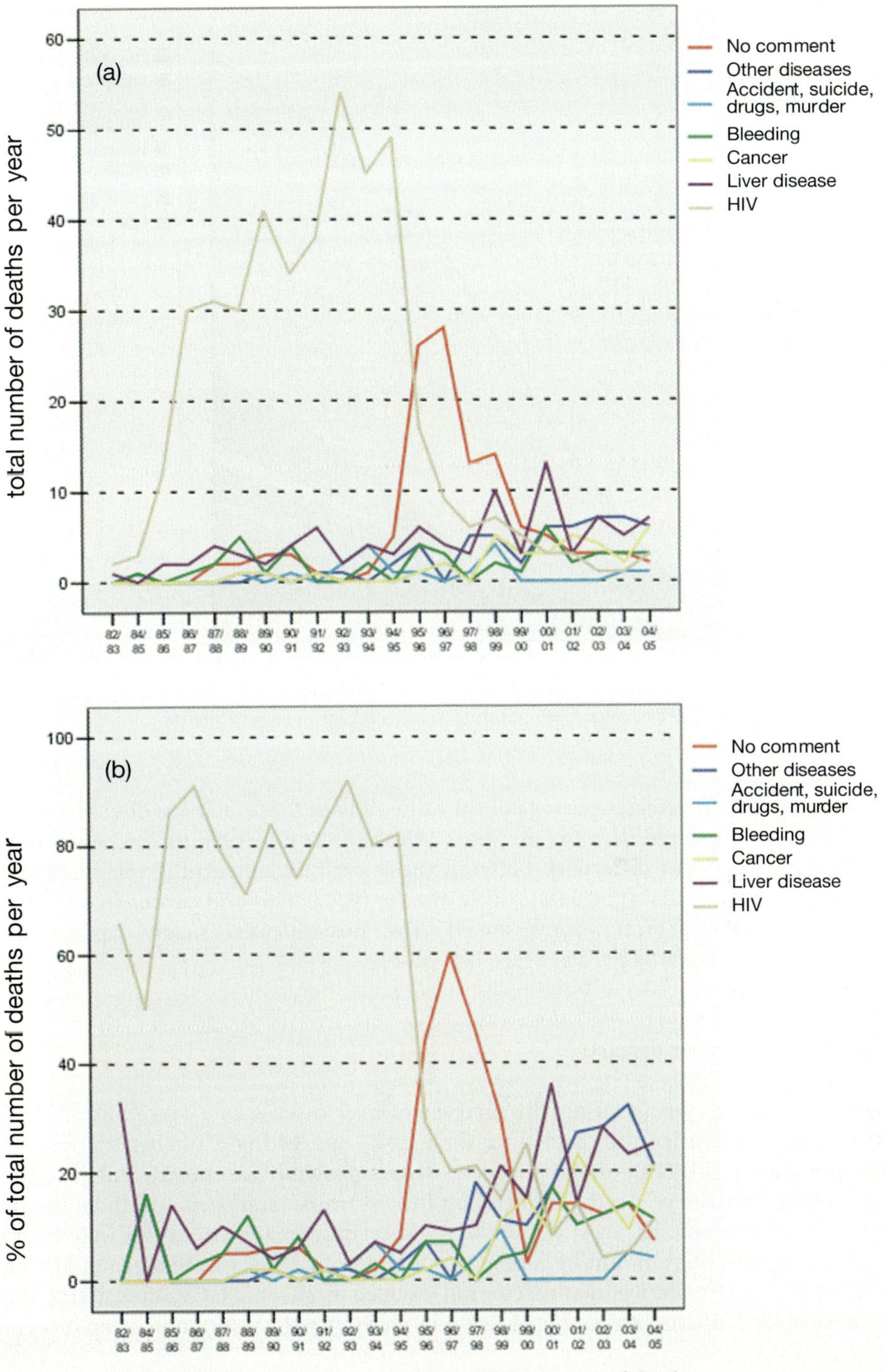

Fig. 8. Chart of deceased patients per year, separated for causes of death

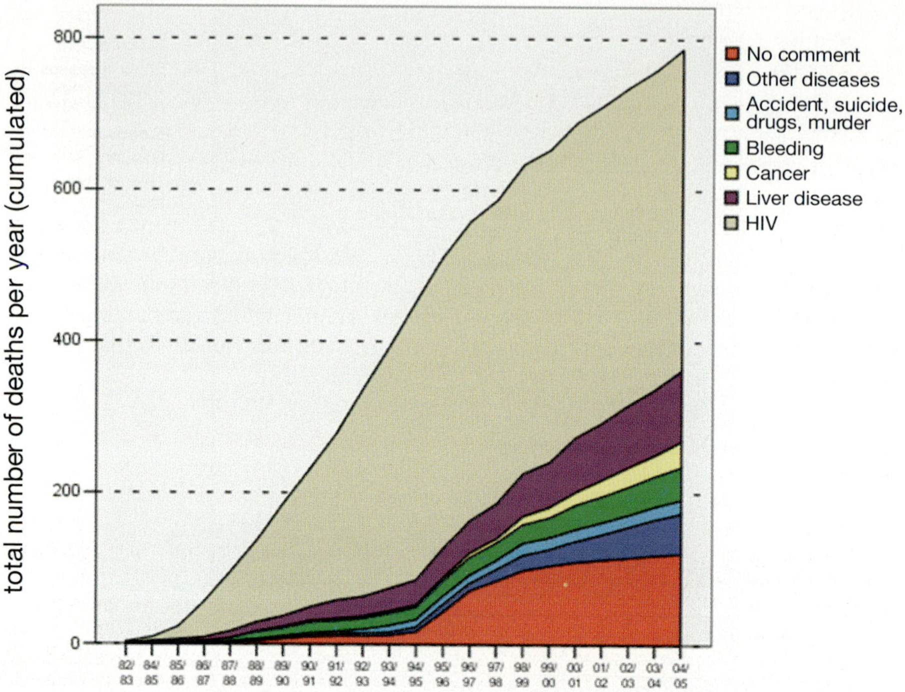

Fig. 9. Cumulative chart of deceased patients, separated for causes of death

Arranging data for greater periods of time one can see these changes obviously (see Fig. 5b, d, f). Clustered data for the years 1982 to 1994 and 1994 to 2005 gives us a statistical significant difference between these periods concerning all important causes of death as HIV ($p < 0.001$), liver disease ($p < 0.025$) and cancer ($p < 0.001$). The same numerical picture shows the HIV/liver disease/cancer deaths expressed as percentage of all deaths per year (see Fig. 6a–c).

Mortality from liver disease

Therewith in this year's survey the increase of liver disease as a cause has reached statistical significance the third time since 2002, suggesting a further increase in future (see Fig. 5d). The obvious reason for this probably can be attributed to the increasing number of deaths induced by liver cirrhosis and hepatocellular carcinoma due to chronic HCV [4]. As we did not discriminate type of cancer in our surveys up to now, there might be a relevant portion of patients in this group having died of primary hepatocellular carcinoma induced by chronic HCV intensifying the impact of liver disease on causes of death in patients with hemophilia even more.

Conclusion

Comparing actual data to those of the previous surveys we again got very consistent findings indicating fairly good data quality. In addition our data are comparable to that of international large-scale prevalence studies and registry data. Despite mortality from HIV in patients with hemophilia is keeping on decreasing, HIV still remains an important factor as an HIV/HCV coinfection seems to increase risk of progression of liver disease to cirrhosis and hepatocellular carcinoma [5, 7]. In addition our findings stress the hypothesis that a relevant portion of patients reported dead of cancer might have died of primary hepatocellular carcinoma induced by chronic HCV. The fact that our data does not show an increasing number of patients with inhibitors over the last three decades does not support the thesis that recombinant factor VIII products induce a higher inhibitor risk.

References

1. Chorba TL, Holman RC, Clarke MJ, Evatt BL: Effects of HIV infection on age and cause of death for persons with hemophilia A in the United States. Am J Hematol. 2001 Apr;66(4): 229–40
2. Darby SC, Kan SW, Spooner RJ, Giangrande PL, Lee CA, Makris M, Sabin CA, Watson HG, Wilde JT, Winter M; UK Haemophilia Centre Doctors' Organisation: The impact of HIV on mortality rates in the complete UK haemophilia population. AIDS. 2004 Feb 20;18(3):525–33
3. Quintana M, del Amo J, Barrasa A, Perez-Hoyos S, Ferreros I, Hernandez F, Villar A, Jimenez V, Bolumar F: Progression of HIV infection and mortality by hepatitis C infection in patients with haemophilia over 20 years. Haemophilia. 2003 Sep;9(5):605–12
4. Ragni MV, Belle SH: Impact of human immunodeficiency virus infection on progression to end-stage liver disease in individuals with hemophilia and hepatitis C virus infection. J Infect Dis. 2001 Apr 1;183(7):1112–5. Epub 2001 Mar 01
5. Santagostino E, Colombo M, Rivi M, Rumi MG, Rocino A, Linari S, Mannucci PM; Study Group of the Association of Italian Hemophilia Centers: A 6-month versus a 12-month surveillance for hepatocellular carcinoma in 559 hemophiliacs infected with the hepatitis C virus. Blood. 2003 Jul 1;102(1):78–82. Epub 2003 Mar 20
6. Wight J, Paisley S: The epidemiology of inhibitors in haemophilia A: a systematic review. Haemophilia. 2003 Jul;9(4):418–35
7. Yee TT, Griffioen A, Sabin CA, Dusheiko G, Lee CA: The natural history of HCV in a cohort of haemophilic patients infected between 1961 and 1985. Gut. 2000 Dec;47(6):845–51

Acknowledgment

Ammon
Anstadt
Auerswald
Aumann
Balleisen
Beck
Beneke
Berthold
Beutel
Böhmann
Bokemeyer
Breuer
Brockhaus
Bruhn
Döhner
Eberl
Edelmann
Eifrig
Eisert
Eleni
Erdlenbruch
Erler
Feickert
Ficke
Franke
Gansen
Geib
Gerhardt
Gildberg
Graf
Güldenring
Günther

Haberland
Hafften
Hähling
Hallek
Heine
Herold
Hesse
Höffken
Hofmann
Holfeld
Holstein
Horneff
Horst
Kabus
Karl
Kemkes-Matthes
Kentouche
Kiesewetter
Kirchmaier
Klamroth
Klare
Klinge
Knöfler
Köhler-Vajta
Körholz
Koscielny
Kosterij
Krebs
Kreibich
Kretschmer
Kreuz
Kurnik
Lenk
Lentz
Loreth
Maak
Meyer
Mittler
Möller
Mondorf
Mößeler
Niekrens
Nimtz-Talaska
Notheis
Nowak-Göttl
Oldenburg
Pindur
Pollmann
Pralle
Reiter
Ries
Scharf
Scharrer
Schilling
Schmeltzer
Schneppenheim
Schobeß
Schramm
Schubert
Schumacher
Siemens
Sirb
Stuckert
Suttorp
Syrbe
Wedemeyer
Weigel
Weippert
Weisser
Wendisch
Winkelmann
Zimmermann
Zintl

Development of the German Hemophilia Register

B. Haschberger, J. Hesse, M. Heiden, and R. Seitz

The aim of the German Hemophilia Register (»*Deutsches Hämophilieregister*«, DHR) is to provide a national database for medical investigation and scientific evaluation in order to optimize hemophilia treatment. A broad database is a prerequisite for assuring an optimal supply of clotting factor in Germany. Separate reporting of the demanded data according to Section 21 TFG (German Transfusion Act) will not be required as long as the DHR is used by the treaters.

In December 2004 it was decided to establish the DHR at the Paul-Ehrlich-Institut (PEI) financed through initial funding by the BMGS *(Bundesministerium für Gesundheit und Soziale Sicherung* [Federal Ministry for Health and Social Security]). Together with an external IT company, the PEI developed the draft for the DHR databank. This draft was discussed and accepted together with representatives of the patient organizations DHG and IGH as well as with the GTH hemophilia commission in a wide circle of hemophilia treaters in March 2005.

The draft was then transmitted to the federal representative for data protection and all the 16 *Länder* (states) representatives for data protection for assessment. The *Länder* representatives were involved because public hemophilia centers are usually under their supervision, and the Länder have their own data protection laws. The PEI is currently still in contact with the data protection representatives. Programming can only start after a positive opinion on the DHR draft has been obtained from all data protection officials.

In addition, the PEI authorized an external law firm to prepare a co-operation contract in order to create a legal basis between the parties involved in the DHR.

The DHR is a register in which no identity features such as personal data of the patients are stored. The database assigns pseudonyms to observe the development of diseases. These are only known to the database itself. However, a treater shall have access to the treatment data of his own patients (but only of those) at any time.

The DHR is run as an online database. Authentification occurs by the use of register software, user ID and password. Before the DHR is put into operation, it is defined which user will receive the appropriate access rights.

Initially only the so-called basic data has to be enrolled in the DHR as treatment data. These are data on the primary disorder, inhibitors, immunetolerance therapy, consumption, and peculiarities. The DHR has been drafted with regard to the future. It therefore offers the possibility to integrate additional query modules, e.g. infections or cause of death etc. at any time.

I. Scharrer/W. Schramm (Ed.)
36th Hemophilia Symposium Hamburg 2005

National Hemophilia Registry – Source of Information about the Quality of Hemophilia Medical Care in a Developing Country

D. Lighezan, F. Vladareanu, V. Uscatescu, C. Petrescu, C. Jinca, D. Mihailov, M. Bătăneant, L. Pop, W. Schramm, and M. Serban

Introduction

Descriptive epidemiology can provide useful information concerning the quality of medical assistance in the case of genetic diseases, notorious for their equal and homogeneous distribution and independence from race, ethnicity and geographic belonging. Hemophilia is part of this group.

National Hemophilia Registry (NHR) is a collection of records of people with hemophilia or inherited bleeding disorders which contains information on personal details, such as age, sex, type of bleeding disorder, severity, type and amount of substitutive therapy, complications (inhibitors, infections, etc.). A national registry centralizes this data for an entire country to avoid duplication of names. Its performing is an important and indispensable resource allocation tool for hemophilia.

These aspects are particularly important in a country like Romania, which has some specific issues. Being a big country (surface = 238.4 sq km), with a population of 20.7 million inhabitants, the expected number of hemophilia patients is high, in contrast with the low socio-economic level, reflected in a low total health expenditure (total health expenditure/capita = 117$; total health expenditure = 4.2%) and in one of the highest infant mortality in Europe (20 ‰).

There are also some particular aspects of hemophilia treatment in Romania. One of them is that only 75% of estimated hemophilia patients are diagnosed in present. Substitution with clotting factor concentrates began in 1990, the whole quantity being assured from donations. Purchased clotting factor concentrates from Health Ministry and Health Insurance Programs was possible starting from 1997,

Table 1. Mean FVIII and FIX consumption in Romania, compared to EU countries

		F VIII	F IX
Romania	IU/patient/year	2 228.25	8 856.92
	IU/kg/year	74.26	~177.13
	IU/capita/year	0.1	0.02
EU	IU/patient/year	20 000–30 000	
	IU/kg/year	520–7800	
	IU/capita/year	2–5	

I. Scharrer/W. Schramm (Ed.)
36th Hemophilia Symposium Hamburg 2005

but the insufficient financial resources allocated for hemophilia treatment allow a FVIII consumption of only 0.1 IU/capita/year, which is very low, compared to both European Union countries and to other European countries, including Romania's neighbors (Table 1, 2). Blood donor screening using Elisa was introduced in 1990 for HBV and HIV, and in 1993 for HCV.

Table 2. Factor VIII consumption in Europe

Country	FVIII (IU/capita)
Albania	0.28
Serbia	0.5
Macedonia	0.6
Bulgaria	1.1
Slovakia	2.9
Hungary	5.1

Objectives

Starting from these aspects, the aim of this study was to achieve an analysis of reliable information within the NHR, from the point of view of diagnostic efficiency and of the consequences of therapeutic approach in patients with hemophilia, as well as the identification of the most important means by which epidemiological data can reflect the quality of care in patients with hemophilia.

Methods

The initiative of NHR belonged to the Romanian Hemophilia Association, the IIIrd Pediatric Clinic Timişoara and the Clinical Center for Evaluation and Rehabilitation of Children and Adolescents »Cristian Serban«–Buziaş.

A questionnaire was administered to all County Directions for Public Health, to Hemophilia Treatment Centers, Transfusiology Centers, and the National Insurance Houses.

This questionnaire comprised questions referred to demographic data, type and severity of disease, treatment modalities, treatment complications (inhibitor status, infectious complications) and death causes.

Results

After data collection, NHR comprises in present 1585 patients, 1088 of them being HA, 122 HB and the rest of them, von Willebrand disease patients.

The prevalence of hemophilia is 6.05/100 000 subjects, varying between below 5 and 20 in the different counties of Romania (Fig. 1).

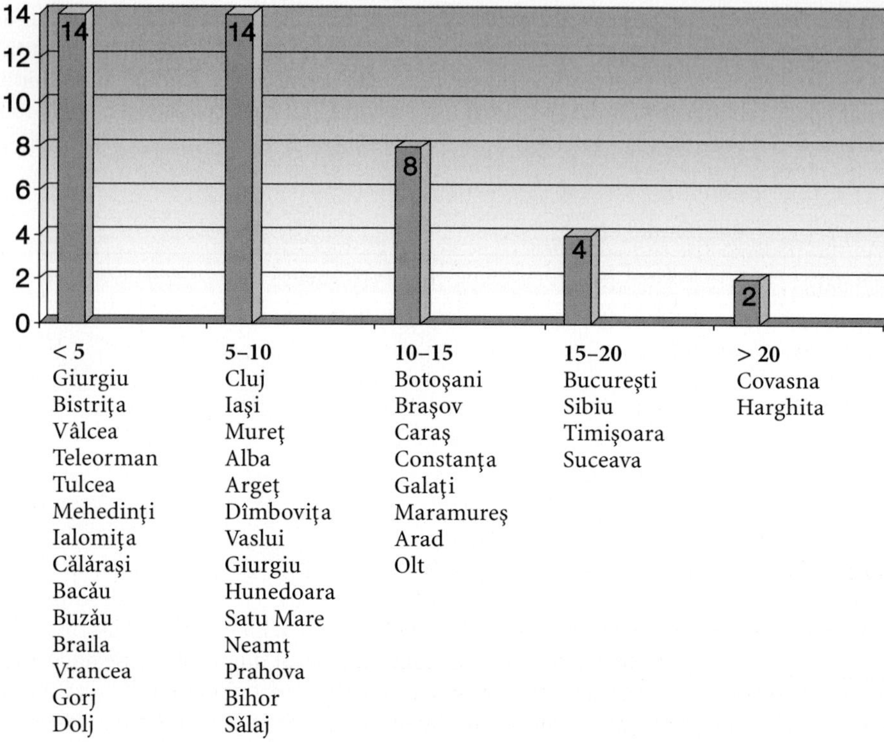

Fig. 1. Prevalence of hemophilia – territorial distribution

The explanation of this large variation is that the disease is insufficiently recognized in different parts of the country, especially in non-university centers. The high prevalence in a non-university center (Suceava) is due to a special demographic status, namely an area of families with many children, explaining the prevalence of hemophilia in these large phratries.

Having only 2 comprehensive centers, the number of hemophilia patients per center is very high (Table 3). The great distance to a laboratory service capable of carrying out all tests necessary for the definitive diagnosis of hemophilia is another explanation for the underestimation of prevalence of the disease.

Compared to other countries, the high hemophilia A/B incidence ratio (Fig. 2) in our country might be either due to the underdiagnosis of hemophilia B, or to the inclusion of von Willebrand disease patients among hemophilia A ones.

Proportion of severity forms, compared to other countries (Table 4), suggests that in Romania the mild forms are often not recognized.

Substitutive therapy is a decisive prognostic factor. In our patients, hospital treatment is the main treatment modality, being achieved in 90.48% of cases, which means that patients have to travel long home-hospital distances, leading to a delay of substitution administration. Travel costs represent an important factor of poor treatment compliance, favourizing complications appearance.

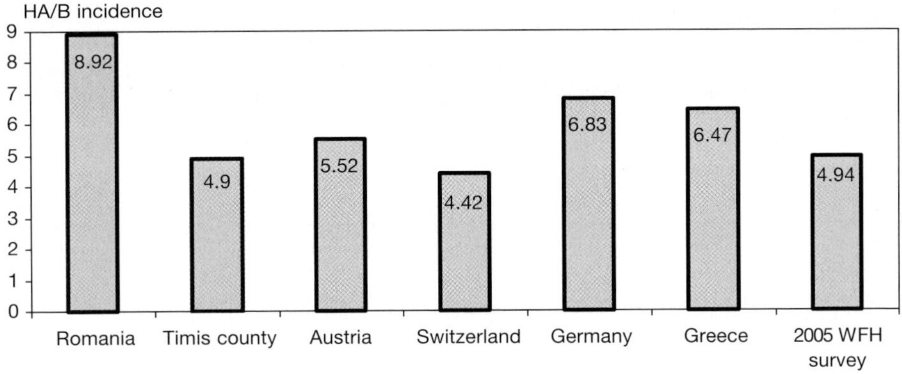

Fig. 2. Hemophilia A/B incidence ratio

Table 3. Comprehensive care centers (CCC)

Country	No of CCC	No of hemophiliacs	CCC patients
Netherlands	16	1500	1:94
Ireland	5	495	1:99
Italy	47	5000	1:106
Denmark	3	417	1:139
Slovenia	1	175	1:175
Greece	4	804	1:201
France	20	5000	1:250
United Kingdom	24	6109	1:255
Sweden	3	830	1:277
Germany	13	4723	1:363
Poland	2	2227	1:1114
Romania	***2***	***1210***	***1:605***

Table 4. Proportion of clinical severity forms

Country	Hemophilia severity forms ratio (severe/moderate/mild)
Romania	1.2 / 1 / 0.8
Timiş	2.35 / 1 / 3.5
Greece	2.3 / 1 / 2.5
Switzerland	1.57 / 1 / 2.92
Austria	4.77 / 1 / 4.45

Inhibitors were found in 19.23% of patients, only 5.13% being in high titer (>5BU) and 14.1% in low titer (<5BU).

The high mortality among the young hemophiliacs is suggested by the low proportion of patients below 30 years (34.4% in Romania and 40.65% in Timiş county). We observe a reverse ratio of Romanian hemophiliacs belonging to these two age groups compared to hemophiliacs from Switzerland (Table 5).

Table 5. Age distribution of hemophilia patients

COUNTRY	AGE GROUP < 10	11–20	21–30	31–40	41–50	51–60	> 60
Romania		~ 65.6%				~34.4%	
Timis	5.76%	30.18%	21.49%	20.19%	20.46%		
Greece	6.59%	18.26%		16.94%	22.78%	14.50%	20.71%
Austria	14.4%	19.1%	18.1%	17.5%	10.9%	7.2%	11.11%
Switzerland		~35.7%				~64.3%	

In Romania, 90% of death causes are represented by hemorrhagic complications, AIDS represented 5%, and the rest were other causes, suggesting the treatment deficiencies of our country. Poor access of Romanian hemophiliacs to clotting factor concentrates lead to a very low proportion of HIV-infected patients, but, in the absence of substitutive therapy, bleeding represents an important cause of death.

Results

These data demonstrate the deficiencies in diagnosis and treatment of hemophilia patients in Romania. Because our goal is to optimize life expectancy and quality of life, we consider that the NHR is an important instrument for improving the quality of care of hemophiliacs. It allows the identification of people with hemophilia, and monitoring of their health. It is an important tool for policy makers, care givers and patient organizations in planning health-care resources for the treatment of hemophilia, and it is one of the first steps in establishing an effective hemophilia program. Comparing information among different countries can be helpful for improving patients' care.

References

1. Skinner MW. Increasing The Worldwide Supply Of Safe, Affordable Factor Replacement Therapy. 26 September 2005 – Fourth WFH Global Forum – Montreal, Canada
2. Evatt B. Guide to Developing a National Patient Registry. WFH 2005
3. Evatt BL, Black C, Batorova A, Street A, Srivastava A. Comprehensive care for hemophilia around the world. Hemophilia 2004;10 (Suppl 4):9–13.
4. Krebs H, Domsch C, Adelhard K, Brackmann HH, Graw J, Oldenburg J, Schwaab R, Schramm W. The national GTH hemophilia registry as database within the scope of the German human genome project. Hämostaseologie. 2003; 23(1):18–23

II. Hemophilia Therapy – Management of Bleedings and Inhibitors

Chairmen:

W. Schramm (Munich)
J. Oldenburg (Bonn)

Regulation of Factor VIII Life-Cycle by Receptors from LDL Receptor Superfamily

E. L. Saenko

Summary

The present review discusses the current concept of receptor-mediated clearance of coagulation factor VIII (FVIII) from the circulation in vivo, which is one of the mechanisms regulating FVIII level in plasma. Several lines of experimental evidence suggest that two receptors from the LDL receptor family, low-density lipoprotein receptor-related protein (LRP) and LDL receptor, cooperate in this process. Administration of receptor-associated protein, a classical antagonist of these receptors, leads to prolongation of FVIII half-life in mice. The elevation of FVIII level and prolongation of its mean residence time, recorded in conditional LRP-deficient mice, directly confirm the physiological role of LRP in mediating clearance of FVIII. Mice with combined LRP and low-density lipoprotein receptor (LDLR) deficiency show a further increase of FVIII level and more impressive, ~5-fold, prolongation of FVIII residence time in the circulation. Receptor-mediated clearance of FVIII is facilitated by heparan sulfate proteoglycans of extracellular matrix, which provide the initial binding of FVIII to the cell surface. We discuss the mapping of the major high-affinity LRP-binding sites to the regions 484-509 and 1811-1818 of A2 and A3 domains of FVIII, respectively; LDLR-binding sites are yet to be identified. Mutagenesis of these sites may result in disruption/reduction of FVIII/receptor interaction and consequently lead to clinically-significant prolongation of FVIII lifetime in the circulation. We demonstrate the feasibility of this approach by the results of Ala-scanning mutagenesis of the A2 LRP-binding site. Generation of a novel recombinant FVIII with prolonged lifetime would meet the demands, improve the efficacy and reduce the cost of FVIII replacement therapy of Hemophilia A.

Coagulation factor VIII (FVIII) [1] serves its function in the intrinsic coagulation pathway as a cofactor for the serine protease FIXa in activation of FX to FXa [1, 2]. Genetic or functional deficiency in FVIII phenotypically results in the bleeding disorder Hemophilia A, as the intrinsic pathway is responsible for normal spatial propagation of the clotting process from the surface of tissue factor-bearing cells.

The FVIII molecule (~300 kDa, 2332 amino acid residues) consists of three homologous A domains, two homologous C domains and the unique B domain (A1-A2-B-A3-C1-C2). In plasma, FVIII circulates as a metal ion-linked heterodimer consisting of the heavy chain (HCh), which is comprised of the A1 (1-336), A2 (373-719) and B domains (741-1648), and the light chain (LCh), which includes the A3 (1690-2019), C1 (2020-2172) and C2 (2173-2332) domains.

I. Scharrer/W. Schramm (Ed.)
36th Hemophilia Symposium Hamburg 2005

In the circulation, FVIII is tightly non-covalently associated with its carrier protein von Willebrand factor ($K_d \sim 0.4$ nM), which prevents premature assembly of the Xase complex and protects FVIII from proteolytic inactivation [2, 3]. Limited proteolysis by physiological activators, thrombin or FXa, at Arg^{372} and Arg^{740} within FVIII HCh and at Arg^{1689} within LCh converts FVIII into its active form. In heterotrimeric activated FVIII, the A1 and A3 domains retain the metal ion bridge, and the relatively stable A1/A3-C1-C2 dimer is weakly associated with the A2 subunit through electrostatic interactions [1, 2].

The cofactor activity of FVIIIa in the assembled intrinsic Xase complex is provided by three essential interactions of FVIIIa: with the phospholipid membrane, with the enzyme FIXa and the substrate FX. The high-affinity interaction ($K_d \sim 15$ nM) between FVIIIa and FIXa is provided by residues 1811-1818 of the A3 domain of LCh [4]. Binding of the A2 domain to FIXa, although with low-affinity (K_d~300 nM), modulates the active site of FIXa and in this way amplifies the enzymatic activity of FIXa by 100-fold [5]. Specifically, the A2 residues 484-509 were shown to be involved in this interaction [6]. The FX-binding site was localized to *A*1 residues 349-372 of FVIII.

Current Knowledge on Receptor-Mediated Catabolism of Factor VIII

While the structure and role of FVIII in the functional Xase complex are well characterized, the mechanisms of FVIII turnover remained unknown less than a decade ago. In 1999, two groups established that catabolism of FVIII is mediated by low-density lipoprotein receptor-related protein (LRP), a member of low-density lipoprotein receptor superfamily [7–11]. LRP is predominantly expressed in the liver on hepatocytes and is also present in the lung, placenta, and brain [12].

The role of LRP as a catabolic receptor for FVIII was established based on the following findings:

1. FVIII was able to bind to LRP [7, 8] in a purified system, and this process was inhibited by 39-kDa receptor-associated protein (RAP), a classical antagonist of LRP;
2. *in vitro*, FVIII was efficiently internalized and degraded by various LRP-expressing cell lines, and these processes were also RAP-sensitive;
3. *in vivo*, in clearance experiments in mice, FVIII half-life in the circulation could be significantly prolonged (3.3-fold) by co-injection of RAP [7].

We further demonstrated that, as with many other LRP ligands, LRP-mediated clearance of FVIII is facilitated by cell-surface heparan sulfate proteoglycans (HSPGs), one of the major glycoprotein components of the extracellular matrix [13]. The role of HSPGs in the initial surface binding of FVIII was suggested *in vitro* from the strong inhibitory effects of heparin (a competitive inhibitor of HSPGs) and heparinase (which removes carbohydrate portions of HSPGs from the cell surface) on the surface binding of ^{125}I-FVIII/vWf complex to LRP-expressing cells. The role of HSPGs in FVIII clearance *in vivo* was further confirmed in clearance studies in mice in the presence of RAP or/and protamine, which prevents HSPGs from interaction with their ligands. The simultaneous blocking of these two receptors led to a more significant prolongation of FVIII half-life in mice (5.5-fold) than the blocking of LRP alone (3.3-fold) [13] reflecting that HSPGs substantially facilitate LRP-mediated clearance of FVIII *in vivo*. We proposed a model of FVIII catabolism: HSPGs provide the initial binding of the FVIII/vWF complex to the cell surface; this leads to an increase of the local FVIII concentration and is followed by LRP-mediated endocytosis and degradation of FVIII. Since vWF did not follow FVIII in the endocytic pathway in cell culture [7], the present concept postulates that vWF dissociates prior to FVIII internalization.

The discovery of FVIII interaction with LRP [7–11] led further to accumulation of direct experimental evidence, which convincingly confirmed the physiological role of LRP in regulating plasma levels of FVIII *in vivo* [14]. It was demonstrated that inactivation of the LRP gene in cre/loxP-mediated conditional LRP-deficient mice (MX1cre^{+}LRP$^{flox/flox}$) led to a 2-fold increase in plasma FVIII level compared to that in control mice. In clearance experiments, MX1cre^{+}LRP$^{flox/flox}$ mice displayed a 1.5-fold prolongation of FVIII mean residence time. Adenovirus-mediated overexpression of RAP in normal mice resulted in a 3.5-fold increase of plasma FVIII level thus confirming that its regulation *in vivo* is mediated by RAP-sensitive receptor(s). Additional evidence of LRP involvement in regulation of FVIII level is provided by clinical observations that liver cirrhosis is associated with markedly elevated plasma FVIII levels and with a decreased expression of LRP [15].

While the role of LRP in catabolism of FVIII has been unequivocally confirmed, the recent evidence indicated possible involvement of other member(s) of the LDL receptor family in regulation of plasma FVIII levels and its clearance. Adenovirus-mediated overexpression of RAP in conditional LRP-deficient mice unexpectedly resulted in a 2-fold increase in plasma FVIII level [14], suggesting that other member(s) of the LDL receptor family may be involved in FVIII clearance. Indeed, Bovenschen *et al.* demonstrated that FVIII interacts with LDL receptor (LDLR) *in vitro* and assessed the relevance of this interaction *in vivo* in LDLR-/- mice, cre/loxP-mediated conditional LRP-deficient mice and in mice with combined receptor deficiency [16]. While plasma FVIII levels in LDLR-deficient mice remained normal, mice with combined deficiency displayed much higher FVIII levels (~4-5-fold) than mice lacking LRP alone. In clearance studies, the mean residence time of FVIII in LDLR-/- mice was comparable to that in normal mice; was increased 1.6-fold in LRP-/- mice; and, strikingly, was dramatically prolonged (~5-fold) in mice with combined receptor deficiency.

These findings suggest that LRP and LDLR act in concert in regulating FVIII level and clearance *in vivo*. LDLR is ubiquitously expressed and, similar to LRP, is most prominent in the liver that supports the concept of their cooperation. While LRP has more than 30 structurally and functionally distinct ligands, LDLR has restricted specificity and represents a classical receptor for the binding and cellular uptake of ApoB- and ApoE-containing lipoproteins [12]. Importantly, significantly elevated plasma FVIII levels in LDLR-/-LRP- double-knockout mice were not secondary to an increase in the levels of ApoE and ApoB, but were directly attributed to LDLR deficiency, thus further supporting the role of LDLR in modulating hemostasis.

Our group and others found that FVIII also interacts with high affinity *in vitro* with very-low-density lipoprotein receptor (VLDLR) [17], abundantly expressed on endothelial cells, and with megalin (gp330) [18], which is predominantly expressed in the kidney on epithelial cells lining the proximal tubules. The binding sites within the A2 domain for LRP, VLDLR and megalin probably overlap [19]. While the physiologic relevance of these interactions is yet to be explored, experiments in knockout mouse models demonstrated that VLDLR does not act in concert with LRP or LDLR in FVIII clearance *in vivo* [20].

Thus, based on accumulated experimental evidence, the current concept states that receptor-mediated FVIII catabolism *in vivo* involves cooperation of two members of the LDL receptor superfamily, LRP and LDLR, and is facilitated by HSPGs.

LRP-Binding Sites Within FVIII Molecule

At present, we know that interaction of FVIII with LRP involves multiple, at least three, FVIII binding sites: within the A2 domain of HCh [7] and the A3 and C2 domains of LCh [8, 21]. Our group localized the *high-affinity* LRP-binding site of HCh within *the A2 domain* ($K_d = 25.8 \pm 1.3$ nM) and mapped it to the region R484-F509 based on the ability of a monoclonal antibody 413, which epitope encompasses this region, and the synthetic peptide 484-509 to inhibit FVIII binding to LRP [7]. To identify residues within HCh, critical for FVIII/LRP interaction, we have further accomplished a comprehensive site-directed mutagenesis of the A2 region 484-509 and residues spatially close to this region suggested by a three dimensional structure (3D) model of A2 [22]. In competition and surface plasmon resonance (SPR) assays, affinities of A2 mutants K466A, R471A, R484A, S488A, R489A, R490A, H497A and K499A for LRP were found decreased by several fold [23]. This correlated with a decrease in LRP-mediated internalization of the mutants in cell culture. Importantly, combining these mutations into pairs led to accumulative effects, i.e. ~10-fold decrease in the affinity for LRP of A2 double-point mutants and ~2-fold decrease in their LRP-mediated internalization in cell culture. Based on these results, the A2 residues K466, R471, R484, S488, R489, R490, H497 and K499 were identified as major determinants in the formation of the A2 binding site for LRP.

The *high-affinity* LRP-binding site within LCh has been recently localized to *the A3 domain* based on the similarity of the binding parameters of LCh (K_d 18 and 59 nM for two classes of binding sites), *a3*-A3-C1 (K_d 26 and 74 nM) and A3-C1-C2 fragments (K_d 22 and 60 nM) for LRP in SPR analysis [21]. The site was mapped to the residues E1811-K1818 based on the following observations:

1. Competition studies using a panel of synthetic peptides showed that the K1804-K1818 and Y1815-A1834 peptides efficiently inhibited interaction of LCh and immobilized LRP;
2. A recombinant antibody fragment that specifically binds to the FVIII sequence E1811-K1818 produced a marked inhibitory effect on the binding of LCh to full-length LRP and LRP cluster II; and

3. A FVIII/FV chimera, in which the region E1811-K1818 was replaced with the corresponding sequence of FV, demonstrated a 5-fold lower affinity to immobilized LRP cluster II thus confirming the role of the E1811-K1818 region [21]. In contrast to the A2 and A3 domains, the isolated recombinant C2 domain was reported to exhibit a *low-affinity* interaction with LRP, K_d~3.6 μM [8, 21]. This is in line with the observation that deletion of the C2 domain did not affect the affinity of FVIII LCh for LRP [21].

Thus, the A2 and A3 sites seem to be the major contributors to the FVIII/LRP interaction. Noteworthy, the fact that the FVIII-(1811-1818)/FV LCh showed residual binding to the LRP cluster II suggests that besides the identified region Glu1811-Lys1818, other surface-exposed structural elements within the A3-C1 fragment may also contribute to the binding to LRP.

The Role of vWF and Activation in FVIII/LRP Interaction

Which of the LRP-binding sites is exposed within the FVIII/vWF complex, the form in which FVIII is normally present in the circulation, and governs clearance of FVIII remains an open question. The fact that LRP-binding sites within the A3 and C2 domain of LCh are in close proximity or overlap with vWF-binding sites [3, 8, 13] suggests that these sites may be blocked by vWF in FVIII/vWF complex. The observation that FVIII can be effectively internalized by LRP-expressing cells from its complex with vWF is consistent with the hypothesis that the A2 binding site may remain available [7].

On the other site, in cell culture experiments isolated FVIII was internalized and degraded more efficiently than FVIII from the complex with vWF [7]; the inhibitory effect of vWF on FVIII degradation was registered in a similar study with the use of different cell lines and experimental conditions [8]. These *in vitro* findings correlate with *in vivo* reports that the half-life of infused FVIII in patients with severe von Willebrand disease, who lack plasma vWF, is approximately 3-fold shorter [24] in comparison with normal individuals [25] and Hemophilia A patients, who have normal levels of vWF [26]. Noteworthy, the half-life of infused FVIII in patients with von Willebrand disease can be reverted to the normal level (12–14 hours) by co-infusion of vWF [24]. In vWF-knockout mice, representing an experimental model of vWF disease, clearance of FVIII is faster than in normal mice and can be inhibited by pre-administration of RAP thus confirming that the accelerated clearance of FVIII in the absence of vWF is mediated by LRP [9–11]. Among patients with Hemophilia A, a considerable inter-individual variation in half-life of infused FVIII (range of 6–28.8 h [27]; 7.4–20.4 h [28]) is observed; patients with shorter FVIII half-life require more clotting factor to prevent joint bleeds and subsequent arthropathy [28]. Importantly, it was revealed that the half-life of infused FVIII correlates with pre-infusion VWF:Ag levels [27, 29, 30]. Together, these data further support the role of LRP-binding sites within LCh in clearance of FVIII, when not involved in interaction with vWF. As judged from the 3D model of intact FVIII [22], both LRP-interactive regions within A2 and A3 domains are positioned at the same flank of the FVIII molecule. This implies that when exposed, both regions of FVIII might cooperate in the high-affinity interaction with LRP.

Physiological condition leading to dissociation of vWF from FVIII is *activation*, when the binding sites within LCh become fully exposed and available for interaction with LRP [3, 8]. Interestingly, the recent study demonstrated that activation also increases the affinity of FVIII HCh for LRP as evidenced by SPR and solid-phase binding methods [31]. Indeed, isolated A2 domain from thrombin-activated FVIII proved to be more effective in the interaction with LRP as compared to intact HCh. Competition experiments using a recombinant antibody fragment against the region 484-509 suggested that the cleavage of HCh by thrombin induces conformational rearrangement of the region 484-509 into a high-affinity LRP-interactive site and does not generate additional LRP-interactive sites [31]. Thus, full exposure and optimal conformation of LRP-binding sites both in heavy and light chains are acquired only upon activation of FVIII into heterotrimeric FVIIIa (A1/A2/A3-C1-C2) that may be important for LRP-mediated regulation of the level of activated FVIII.

On the other side, FVIIIa is an unstable molecule which rapidly dissociates into A2 and A1/A3-C1-C2 [1, 2]. The findings that the isolated A2 domain has a shorter half-life in mice in comparison with full-length FVIII [23] and that A3-C1-C2 subunit of FVIII can be efficiently catabolized by LRP-expressing cells [32] may reflect existence of LRP-dependent pathway for clearance of the two constituents of activated FVIII *in vivo*, driven via the A2 and A3 LRP-binding sites.

LRP Regions Responsible for Interaction with FVIII

All members of the LDL receptor family are structurally similar and consist of intracellular, transmembrane and extracellular domains. The structure of LRP and LDLR involved in clearance of FVIII, as well as the structure of two other receptors, gp330 and VLDLR, which interact with FVIII, are shown in Figure 1. The structure of these receptors is similar. All of them contain homologous cysteine-rich complement type repeats of class A (CR), involved in ligand binding. LRP and GP330 contain four, whereas VLDLR and LDLR contain only one cluster of CRs (Fig. 1).

The extracellular subunit of LRP contains 31 homologous CRs of about 40 residues each, arranged in four clusters (I-IV) of 2, 8, 10 and 11 CRs, respectively. CRs represent the ligand-binding elements in LRP: they contain a highly conserved cluster of negatively charged amino acids interacting with positively charged residues of ligands [12]. LDLR is a much shorter protein containing only one cluster (homologue of LRP cluster II) formed of 7 CRs [12]. It appears that clusters II and IV contain the binding sites of most LRP ligands [33, 34]. Clusters II and IV can be considered duplicated domains in LRP as they bind the identical repertoire of ligands with similar binding parameters. To this end, no binding of any LRP ligand to cluster I has been reported. The ability of RAP to bind to clusters II, III and IV with high affinity is its unique feature which evidently provides the ability of RAP to antagonize the binding of all other LPR ligands.

A deeper insight into mechanisms of FVIII/LRP interaction can be gained through mapping respective binding sites within receptor molecule. In particular,

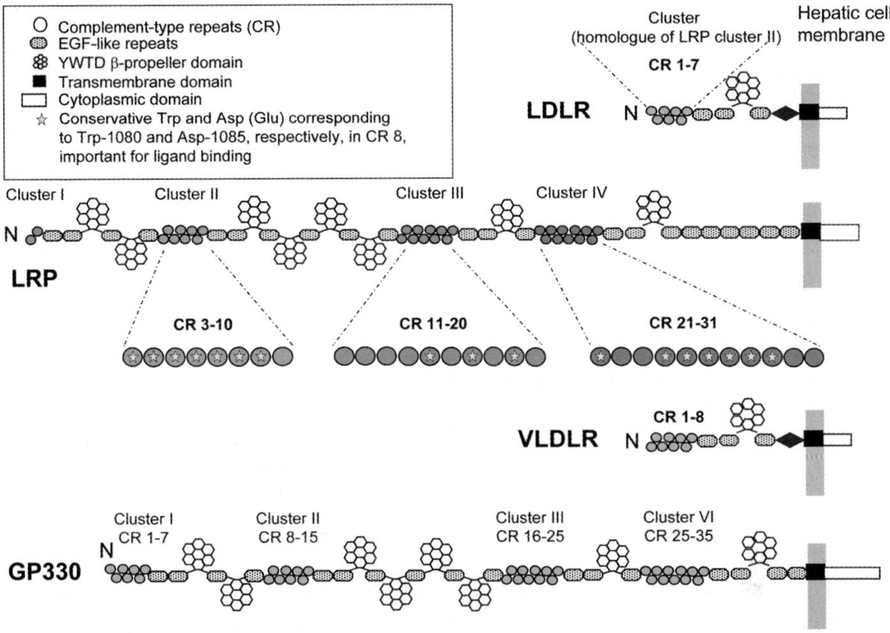

Fig. 1. Domain structure of the members of the mammalian LDL receptor family, LDLR and LRP, gp330 and VLDLR, interacting with FVIII. Receptors contain various numbers of ligand-binding CRs, organized in four clusters of 2, 8, 10 and 11 in LRP and in four clusters of 7, 8, 10 and 11 in gp330. The LDLR and VLDLR contains one cluster of 7 and 8 CRs, respectively. In LRP, the binding sites for the A2 domain of HCh and LCh of FVIII are located within clusters II and IV. While CRs of the extracellular subunit are mainly responsible for ligand binding, the transmembrane domain anchors receptor in the cell membrane, and the cytoplasmic domain contains motifs which serve as a signal for receptor endocytosis. Other domains present in all receptors include epidermal-growth factor (EGF)-like repeats and YWTD β-propeller domains. While LRP and LDLR proved to be involved in clearance and regulation of FVIII, the function of gp330 and VLDLR, which bind FVIII, is not yet known

immobilized FVIII LCh was shown to interact with recombinant cluster II (K_d=121.4 nM) and cluster IV (K_d=87.8 nM) as studied by SPR [34]. Interestingly, the A3 region 1811-1818 of LCh is positioned in close proximity to the membrane surface [22] so that a slightly higher affinity of LCh to cluster IV is consistent with location of cluster IV closest to the cell surface. Our group studied interaction of isolated A2 domain of HCh with recombinant clusters II, III and IV. We demonstrated that A2 was also able to bind to immobilized cluster II and cluster IV (K_d 20-50 nM) in a RAP-sensitive manner in SPR-based assay, but not to cluster III [35]. Further mapping of FVIII-binding sites within LRP can be accomplished by studying interaction of FVIII fragments with shorter fragments of clusters II and IV.

A new and yet unexplored field in the LRP biology, which may provide important information, is analysis of the relationship between coding polymorphisms of the LRP gene and the level of FVIII, variability of which is a well-recognized fact.

For example, association of the LRP D2080N genotype with elevated plasma FVIII activity levels in normal individuals is being discussed [36, 37]. Such data could be another line of evidence of involvement of LRP to regulation of FVIII level.

Implications for Treatment of Hemophilia A

Mutagenesis of LRP- (and LDLR-) binding sites, besides identification of residues, critical for FVIII/receptor interaction, is also important from clinical standpoint. The mainstay in treatment of Hemophilia A is replacement therapy with repeated infusions of expensive FVIII products with the trend towards the use of recombinant products [38]. While the earlier bioengineering efforts were directed towards increasing expression and secretion levels of rFVIII, lately, special attention has been given to improving the properties of rFVIII, including development of a novel rFVIII with a prolonged lifetime in the circulation. In this respect, establishment of the role of LRP as the major clearance receptor of FVIII and identification of LRP-binding sites within the A2 and A3 domains, together with the new evidence of involvement of LDLR in regulating FVIII removal suggests a direction for *clinically-significant* prolongation of FVIII lifetime in the circulation. This can be achieved by disrupting/reducing FVIII interactions with its clearance receptors via mutagenesis of respective binding sites. Considering that the A3 region E1811-K1818 represents a high-affinity FIXa-binding site [4] and the A2 region 484-509 contributes to FVIIIa cofactor activity [5, 6], the challenge is to select mutations which will maximally reduce interaction of FVIII with LRP but will not affect the functional properties of FVIII.

While site-directed mutagenesis within the A3 LRP-binding site has not yet been performed, our experimental data on the generated A2 mutants suggest certain mutations that may be promising for generation of the improved FVIII. These mutations yielded proteins with reduced affinity for LRP yet retaining the cofactor activity in FVIIIa molecules reconstituted from the A2 mutants and A1/A3-C1-C2 heterodimer [23]. Based on our findings that the A2 residues critical for the binding to LRP, VLDLR and megalin are identical [19], one may expect that this A2 site may be also shared with LDLR.

It is possible that introduction of mutations within LRP-binding sites may also have a favorable effect on FVIII immunogenicity, which is a serious and well-recognized problem in treatment of Hemophilia A. Indeed, since the LRP-binding regions 484-509 and 1804-1834 constitute the major determinants of the A2 and A3 epitopes of inhibitory antibodies (for review, see [39]), the introduced mutations may disrupt these epitopes. It has been recently reported that immunogenicity of FVIII was reduced by mutations within B cell epitope: inhibitor titers in Hemophilia A mice receiving the R484A/R489A/P492A human FVIII mutant were significantly lower than in mice receiving control wt-human FVIII [40].

On a final run, generation of a novel rFVIII with prolonged lifetime in the circulation may improve the efficacy and reduce the cost of FVIII replacement therapy of Hemophilia A.

References

1. Fay PJ. Regulation of Factor VIIIa in the Intrinsic Factor Xase. Thromb Haemost 1999; 82: 193–200.
2. Saenko EL, Ananyeva NM, Tuddenham EG, Kemball-Cook G. Factor VIII – novel insights into form and function. Br J Haematol 2002; 119: 323–31.
3. Saenko EL, Scandella D. The acidic region of the light chain and the C2 domain together form a high affinity binding site for von Willebrand factor. J Biol Chem 1997; 272: 18007–14.
4. Lenting PJ, van de Loo JW, Donath MJ, van Mourik JA, Mertens K. The sequence Glu1811-Lys1818 of human blood coagulation factor VIII comprises a binding site for activated factor IX. J Biol Chem 1996; 271: 1935–40.
5. Fay PJ, Koshibu K. The A2 subunit of factor VIIIa modulates the active site of factor IXa. J Biol Chem 1998; 273: 19049–54.
6. Fay PJ, Scandella D. Human inhibitor antibodies specific for the factor VIII A2 domain disrupt the interaction between the subunit and factor IXa. J Biol Chem 1999; 274: 29826–30.
7. Saenko EL, Yakhyaev AV, Mikhailenko I, Strickland DK, Sarafanov AG. Role of the low density lipoprotein-related protein receptor in mediation of factor VIII catabolism. J Biol Chem 1999; 274: 37685–92.
8. Lenting P, Neels JG, van den Berg BM, Clijsters PFM, Meijerman DWE, Pannekoek H, van Mourik JA, Mertens K, Zonneveld A-J. The light chain of factor VIII comprises a binding site for low density lipoprotein receptor-related protein. J Biol Chem 1999; 274: 23734–9.
9. Schwarz HP, Lenting PJ, Binder B, Mihaly J, Denis C, Dorner F, Turecek PL. Involvement of low-density lipoprotein receptor-related protein (LRP) in the clearance of factor VIII in von Willebrand factor-deficient mice. Blood 2000; 95: 1703–8.
10. Turecek PL, Lenting PJ, van Mourik JA, Binder B, Mihaly J, Denis C, Wagner D, Dorner F, Schwarz HP. Low density lipoprotein receptor-related protein (LRP) mediates the clearance of factor VIII in vWF-deficient mice. Blood 1999; 94: 647a.
11. Turecek PL, Schwarz HP, Binder BR. In vivo inhibition of low density lipoprotein receptor-related protein improves survival of factor VIII in the absence of von Willebrand factor. Blood 2000; 95: 3637–8.
12. Neels JG, Horn IR, van den Berg BMM, Pannekoek H, van Zonneveld A-J. Ligand-receptor interactions of the low density lipoprotein receptor-related protein, a multi-ligand endocytic receptor. Fibrinolysis and Proteolysis 1998; 12: 219–40.
13. Sarafanov AG, Ananyeva NM, Shima M, Saenko EL. Cell surface heparan sulfate proteoglycans participate in factor VIII catabolism mediated by low density lipoprotein receptor-related protein. J Biol Chem 2001; 276: 11970–9.
14. Bovenschen N, Herz J, Grimbergen JM, Lenting PJ, Havekes LM, Mertens K, van Vlijmen BJ. Elevated plasma factor VIII in a mouse model of low-density lipoprotein receptor-related protein deficiency. Blood 2003; 101: 3933–9.
15. Hollestelle MJ, Geertzen HG, Straatsburg IH, van Gulik TM, van Mourik JA. Factor VIII expression in liver disease. Thromb Haemost 2004; 91: 267–75.
16. Bovenschen N, Mertens K, Hu L, Havekes LM, van Vlijmen BJ. LDL receptor cooperates with LDL receptor-related protein in regulating plasma levels of coagulation factor VIII in vivo. Blood 2005; 106: 906–12.
17. Kouiavskaia DV, Ruiz JF, Strickand DK, Saenko EL. Very low density lipoprotein receptor interacts with coagulation factor VIII. Blood 2003; 102: 88a.
18. Mertens K, Bovenschen N, Voorberg J, Meijer AB. The endocytic receptors megalin and low-density lipoprotein receptor-related protein share binding to coagulation factor VIII. Blood 2003; 102: 89a.
19. Makogonenko E, Sarafanov A, Pechik I, Andersen O, Ananyeva N, Radtke K-P, Strickland D, Saenko E. The A2 domain of coagulation factor VIII shares residues critical for interaction with three members of LDL receptor superfamily – LRP, VLDL and megalin receptors. J Thromb Haemost 2005; 3(Suppl 1): P0646.

20. Bovenschen N, van Dijk KW, Havekes LM, Mertens K, van Vlijmen BJ. Clearance of coagulation factor VIII in very low-density lipoprotein receptor knockout mice. Br J Haematol 2004; 126: 722–5.
21. Bovenschen N, Boertjes RC, van Stempvoort G, Voorberg J, Lenting PJ, Meijer AB, Mertens K. Low density lipoprotein receptor-related protein and factor IXa share structural requirements for binding to the A3 domain of coagulation factor VIII. J Biol Chem 2003; 278: 9370–7.
22. Stoilova-McPhie S, Villoutreix BO, Mertens K, Kemball-Cook G, Holzenburg A. Three-dimensional structure of membrane-bound coagulation factor VIII: modeling of the factor VIII heterodimer within a three-dimensional density map derived by electron crystallography. Blood 2002; 99: 1215–23.
23. Sarafanov A.G., Makogonenko E, Pechik I.V., Radtke K-P, Khrenov A.V., Ananyeva N.M., Strickland D.K., Saenko E.L. Identification of coagulation factor VIII A2 domain residues forming the binding epitope for low-density lipoprotein receptor-related protein. Biochemistry 2006; 45: 1829–1840.
24. Lethagen S, Berntorp E, Nilsson IM. Pharmacokinetics and hemostatic effect of different factor VIII/von Willebrand factor concentrates in von Willebrand's disease type III. Ann Hematol 1992; 65: 253–9.
25. Over J, Sixma JJ, Bruine MH, Trieschnigg MC, Vlooswijk RA, Bieser-Visser NH, Bouma BN. Survival of 125iodine-labeled factor VIII in normals and patients with classic hemophilia. Observations on the heterogeneity of human factor VIII. J Clin Invest 1978; 62: 223–34.
26. Fijnvandraat K, Berntorp E, Ten Cate JW, Johnsson H, Peters M, Savidge G, Tengborn L, Spira J, Stahl C. Recombinant, B-domain deleted factor VIII (r-VIII SQ): pharmacokinetics and initial safety aspects in hemophilia A patients. Thromb Haemost 1997; 77: 298–302.
27. Fijnvandraat K, Peters M, Ten Cate JW. Inter-individual variation in half-life of infused recombinant factor VIII is related to pre-infusion von Willebrand factor antigen levels. Br J Haematology 1995; 91: 474–6.
28. Van DK, van der Bom JG, Lenting PJ, de Groot PG, Mauser-Bunschoten EP, Roosendaal G, Grobbee DE, van den Berg HM. Factor VIII half-life and clinical phenotype of severe hemophilia A. Haematologica 2005; 90: 494–8.
29. Vlot AJ, Mauser-Bunschoten EP, Zarkova AG, Haan E, Kruitwagen CL, Sixma JJ, van den Berg HM. The half-life of infused factor VIII is shorter in hemophilic patients with blood group O than in those with blood group A. Thromb Haemost 2000; 83: 65–9.
30. Bjorkman S, Berntorp E. Pharmacokinetics of coagulation factors: clinical relevance for patients with haemophilia. Clin Pharmacokinet 2001; 40: 815–32.
31. Bovenschen N, van Stempvoort G, Voorberg J, Mertens K, Meijer AB. Cleavage of factor VIII heavy chain by thrombin increases the affinity for low-density lipoprotein receptor-related protein (LRP). J Thromb Haemost 2003; Suppl July: OC095.
32. Neels JG, Bovenschen N, Zonneveld A-J, Lenting P. Interaction between factor VIII and LDL receptor-related protein. Trends Cardiovasc Med 2000; 10: 8–14.
33. Herz J, Strickland DK. LRP: a multifunctional scavenger and signaling receptor. J Clin Invest 2001; 108: 779–84.
34. Neels JG, Berg BMM, Looken A, Olivecrona G, Pannekoek H, Zonneveld A-J. The second and fourth cluster of class A cysteine-rich repeats of the low density lipoprotein receptor-related protein share ligand-binding properties. J Biol Chem 1999; 274: 31305–11.
35. Sarafanov A, Makogonenko E, Andersen O, Khrenov A, Mikhailenko I, Strickland D, Saenko E. Identification of regions in low-density lipoprotein receptor-related protein responsible for interaction with A2 and A1/A3-C1-C2 portions of coagulation factor VIII. J Thromb Haemost 2005; 3(Suppl 1): OR248.
36. Morange PE, Tregouet DA, Frere C, Saut N, Pellegrina L, Alessi MC, Visvikis S, Tiret L, Juhan-Vague I. Biological and genetic factors influencing plasma factor VIII levels in a healthy family population: results from the Stanislas cohort. Br J Haematol 2005; 128: 91–9.
37. Cunningham N, Laffan MA, Manning RA, O'Donnell JS. Low-density lipoprotein receptor-related protein polymorphisms in patients with elevated factor VIII coagulant activity and venous thrombosis. Blood Coagul Fibrinolysis 2005; 16: 465–8.

38. Ananyeva N, Khrenov A, Darr F, Summers R, Sarafanov A, Saenko E. Treating haemophilia A with recombinant blood factors: a comparison. Expert Opin Pharmacother 2004; 5: 1061–70.
39. Ananyeva NM, Lacroix-Desmazes S, Hauser CA, Shima M, Ovanesov MV, Khrenov AV, Saenko EL. Inhibitors in hemophilia A: mechanisms of inhibition, management and perspectives. Blood Coagul Fibrinolysis 2004; 15: 109–24.
40. Parker ET, Healey JF, Barrow RT, Craddock HN, Lollar P. Reduction of the inhibitory antibody response to human factor VIII in hemophilia A mice by mutagenesis of the A2 domain B-cell epitope. Blood 2004; 104: 704–10.

Update of the Inhibitor-Immunology-Study

I. Wieland, C. Wermes, B. Eifrig, K. Holstein, H. Pollmann, B. Siegmund, A. Nimtz-Talaska, C. Niekrens, R. Eisert, A. Tiede, K. Welte, and K.-W. Sykora

Abstract

We are presenting an update of our study in which risk factors for the development of inhibitors in patients with hemophilia are to be explored. The ultimate goal is to find out why some children suffering from severe or moderate hemophilia develop inhibitory antibodies during replacement therapy and others do not, and to define genetic and immunological risk factors.

The development of inhibitors is one of the most important complications of the replacement therapy in hemophilia affecting mortality and morbidity. The development of inhibitory antigens is based on complex immunological factors, and to date, too little is known about the basic mechanisms of inhibitor development. Risk factors are presumably derived from the immune system. Inhibitory antibodies are mostly IgG-type immunoglobulins, especially subclass 4, rarely subclass 1. During inhibitor formation, CD4+ T cells are directed in a cytokine-dependent manner to the Th1 or Th2 pathway. The development of inhibitors is very likely to be a Th-2 mediated event where cytokines and their receptors, T-cell receptors, and the Major Histocompatibility Complex may also play important roles. One examples of the cytokine connection is a mouse model, in which the development of inhibitors is prevented by the blockade of the co-stimulating factor B7/CD28.

Within the scope of our study we want to compare genetic polymorphisms in immune-response associated genes between patients with and without inhibitors and between patients and the normal population: The characterization of genetic polymorphisms including for instance TLR, TNF-α, CD40, IL-10 and IL-1β are emphasized. The correlation between some genotypes or polymorphisms in cytokines and the development of inhibitory antigens is to be studied.

Up to now 15 centers agreed to take place in our study. 5 of these already sent samples, amounting to 46 samples of hemophiliacs. We evaluated 10 polymorphisms in different genes in the first 40 patients with Taq-Man-PCR, restriction fragment length polymorphisms (RFLP), ARMS and direct sequence analyzing. Promising results were seen in some polymorphisms, but in most of them so far the number of samples is too small to get significant results.

I. Scharrer/W. Schramm (Ed.)
36th Hemophilia Symposium Hamburg 2005

Introduction

About 31% of the patients with a factor VIII replacement therapy develop a factor VIII inhibitor. From these are 23% low-responder (< 5BE) and 77% high-responder (> 5BE) [8]. In the case of severe hemophilia B, about 10.5% of the patients develop inhibitory antibodies [9]. Anti-factor VIII-antibodies are also seen in 15–78% healthy people without hemophilia [7, 17, 19]. Lacroix-Desmazes et al. [10, 11] showed anti-idiotypic antibodies neutralizing the inhibitory activity of the anti-factor VIII antibodies in healthy people.

Well-known predisposing factors for inhibitor formation are genetic features of factor VIII, which include large deletions, nonsense mutations or intrachromosomal recombinations [5, 23]. Also, ethnic groups other than Caucasians (e.g. Africans) have a higher risk of developing inhibitors. Other risk factors are presumably derived from the immune system. For instance, a reduction of the inhibitor was seen with lower CD4+ T helper cell counts in HIV positive hemophilic patients [3, 4]. The development of inhibitors is very likely to be a Th-2 mediated event where cytokines and their receptors, T-cell receptors and the Major Histocompatibility Complex may also play an important role.

Theoretical Background

The substituted factor is an unknown protein for patients with a severe hemophilia.

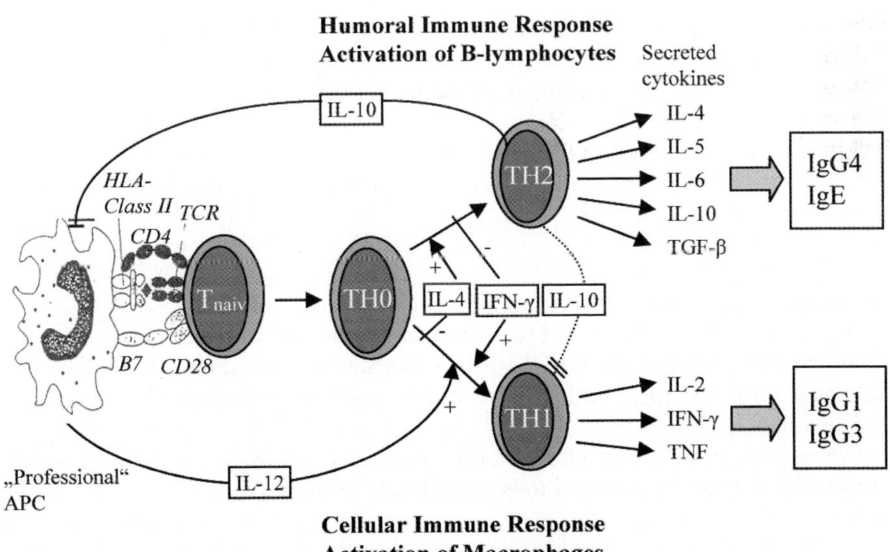

Fig. 1. The normal immunoresponse (according to BAENKLER [2])
Abbreviations: TCR – T cell-receptor; APC – antigen presenting cell

Unknown proteins are taken up in macrophages by pinocytosis, split into peptides and bound to MHC class II molecules. This complex is transported to the cell membrane and is presented to T cells on the cell surface. The peptide MHC class II complex is recognized by the T cell receptor. The T cell is activated by binding of the complex to the T cell receptor. Co-stimulatory molecules, including the B7 – CD28 interacting molecules, provide additional signals and start the differentiation into the Th-1 or Th-2 direction. Th-2 specific T cells produce IL-4, IL-5, IL-6, IL-10 and TGF-β, leading to the switch to IgG4 and IgE. Th-1 specific T cells cause the switch to IgG1 and IgG3 by production of IL-2, IFN-γ and TNF (Fig. 1).

Factor VIII and IX inhibitory antibodies are mostly IgG-type immunoglobulins, especially subclass 4, rarely subclass 1 [4]. Therefore, inhibitor development was considered to be a Th-2 mediated event. However, Reding at al. [18] could show that Th-1 specific immunoglobulins play a more important role than expected before. If the patient has a high inhibitor titer, IgG4 antibodies were more commonly found. In the case of low anti-factor VIII antibody titers, IgG1 and IgG2 immunoglobulins were dominant. This was also true when the low inhibitor titer was achieved by immune tolerance therapy. During this therapy, a switch occurred from the Th-2 to the Th-1 direction.

In previous studies, no significant association between HLA class and inhibitor development was found [1, 12, 13, 15]. Later, different studies could show a higher risk of developing inhibitors when special factor VIII mutations were combined with special HLA class II molecules. For example, higher inhibitor development was associated with HLA-DRB1*1501/ DRB1*0602/DQA1*0102 in patients with the Intron 22 inversion and with HLA-DRB1*01/DQA1*0101/ DRB1*0501 in patients without the intron 22 inversion [6, 14].

In order to have better conditions studying the development of inhibitory antibodies, mouse models were established. Partly conflicting results were reported about the dominance of either Th-2 [24] or Th-1 [20, 22] specific cytokines. All authors agree that both Th-2 and Th-1 specific T cells are involved in the development of anti-factor VIII antibodies.

Mouse models also showed that the development of anti-factor VIII antibodies was inhibited by the blockade of the co-stimulatory interactions of B7/CD28 [16, 17] and CD 40-CD40L interaction [20, 21].

The Inhibitor-Immunology-Study

The ultimate goal of this study is to find out why some children suffering from severe or moderate hemophilia develop inhibitory antibodies during replacement therapy and others do not.

Within the scope of our study we want to compare the following factors between patients with and without inhibitors and between patients and the normal population:

1. T-cell and B-cell activation by factors VIII or IX, studied by the synthesis and secretion of cytokines.
2. Genetic polymorphisms in immune-response associated genes.

Because of the small factor VIII specific T cell count the method for part I is hard to establish. So we have started with part II of this study. In the following we want to report about this part of the study.

Goal is the characterization of genetic polymorphisms of genes that are associated with the immune response and the determination of the distribution of the alleles and genotypes in comparison of patients with and without inhibitory antibodies and a normal population. Possible genes are cytokines, co-stimulatory signaling proteins and other in the immune response associated genes. Even polymorphisms in coagulation factors could play a roll. But we do not want to analyze these because other working groups will have an expertise in this.

Patients and controls are planned to be typified for the HLA class. The distributions of the alleles are analyzed by direct sequencing, ARMS, Taq-Man-PCR or restriction length polymorphism PCR.

This study is an open, longitudinal case control study. The patients are not randomized. The patients are divided into three groups. These groups are:

I. No inhibitor development
II. Low responder (< 5BE)
III. High responder (> 5BE)

The duration of the study is actually not limited. Participants can be all patients with a hemophilia needing regular factor replacement therapy.

Part 2 will start with a pilot phase in order to test how many patients would be necessary to show a significantly different distribution of genotypes between patients with or without inhibitors. This pilot phase will be the basis for the decision whether sufficient statistical power can be achieved with the available patient population to see a difference between inhibitor- and non-inhibitor patients for a specific genetic variant. If no significant differences can be expected for a variant, examination of this variant will not be pursued anymore. In addition, a control group of healthy blood donors corresponding in gender will be recruited.

There are no exclusion criteria for part two.

In the initial form is asked for dates of patients as mutation or HLA class, ethnic group, plasmatic or recombinant factor preparations. There *especially data are collected shown* to be associated in inhibitor development.

Actual Data

We have got the vote of the ethics committee of the Hanover Medical University in October 2003. We wrote to 106 hemophilic treating centers and got 15 rejections and 16 assents. 5 centers have sent probes to us. A goal is to activate more centers to an active participation. In order to minimize the expenditure of the participations we made available prepaid boxes for dispatch. If it is wished by the participant we will take over the application for the local ethics commission. We only need 1 or 2 EDTA-monovettes and the complete filled initial form.

Up to November 2005 we have collected 46 samples, 38 from patients with hemophilia A an 9 from patients with hemophilia B.

Therapy of Acquired Hemophilia – Immunoadsorption and Rituximab Treatment for Immunosuppression and Substitution of Coagulation Factors

H.-H. Wolf, A. Harba, O. Dorligschaw, and H.-J. Schmoll

Autoantibodies to coagulation factors may occur in hemophiliacs as adverse events following substitution therapy.

Especially perioperative management of hemophilia patients may be complicated by inhibitors, and in many patients bleeding complications become life threatening.

Treatment with bypassing agents of the coagulation cascade like high-dose substitution of FEIBA or rFVIIa is a useful management of acute bleeding complications, but sustained elimination of inhibitors must be the therapeutic goal in inhibitor patients.

In children with inhibitors treatment according to the Malmö protocol is the gold standard [1]. In adults, however, this protocol seems to be less effective and complete B-cell suppression might be useful to induce immunotolerance.

Therefore, we developed a new protocol combining immunomodulation by steroids, cytotoxic treatment and immunoadsorption with monoclonal anti-CD 20 antibody Rituximab. Data of the first 2 consecutive patients are discussed.

Patients` Characteristics

Patient A

A 65 year old male with mild hemophilia A was brought to admission in a local hospital for chronic obstructive pulmonary disease and fracture of the radius bone. He presented no history of severe bleeding complications.

The patient's FVIII activity was 4 %, aPTT at the day of admission was 54 sec.

There had been no hemostaseologic examination for at least 12 years.

History of substitution revealed therapy with cryoprecipitates in 1981 and with plasma derived factor VIII concentrates in 1993 for dental extraction, respectively. The patient underwent osteosynthesis of the radius on January 30th, 2005. Perioperative substitution was provided with a plasma derived factor VIII concentrate January 29th until February 5th, 2005. No bleeding complications nor prolongation of wound healing were seen.

On March 17, 2005, the patient presented in our hemophilia center with diffuse sugillations despite substitution with plasma derived coagulation factor VIII con-

I. Scharrer/W. Schramm (Ed.)
36th Hemophilia Symposium Hamburg 2005

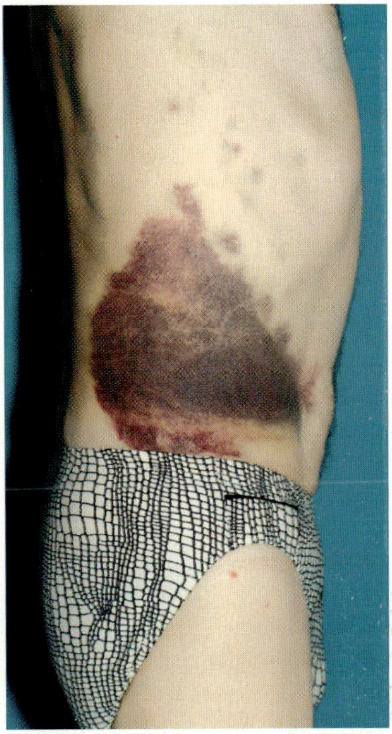

Fig. 1. 65 year old patient, FVIII inhibitor after perioperative substitution with plasma derived coagulation factor VIII concentrate

centrate. We diagnosed high-titer anti-FVIII antibody (27.6 BU) and started therapy with recombinant FVIIa (rFVII) (Fig. 1).

Patient B

A 32 year old male patient with subclinical hemophilia A presented with no history of hemorrhages but a somewhat bleeding disorder had been diagnosed in his grandfather who had expired years ago. The patient had not experienced any substitution therapy so far. August 27th, 2004, the patient faced fracture of the right humerus and underwent osteosynthesis in a local hospital. As wound healing failed the patient underwent several further surgical attempts to improve the results of osteosynthesis in two specialized traumatologic departments outside without success.

The patient's first admission to our hemophilia center was on June 9th, 2005.

We diagnosed hemophilia A (FVIII activity 18 %, aPTT 40 sec) and provided recombinant FVIII concentrate perioperatively. Surgery was done on June 14th, and substitution therapy was provided for 2 weeks. There were no perioperative bleeding complications, and the patient's dismission from the hospital took place on July 2nd, 2005.

On August 28th, 2005, the patient developed spontaneous intramuscular and joint bleedings without experience of any trauma. Despite of substitution with recom-

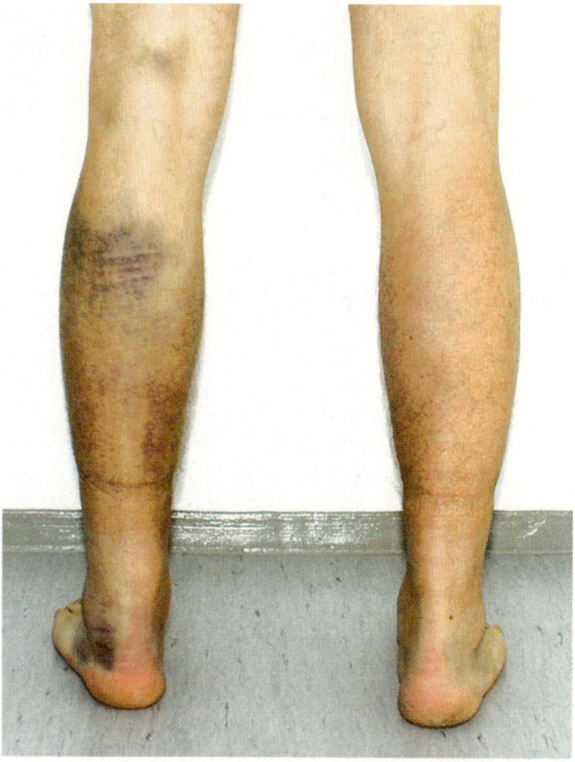

Fig. 2. 32 year old patient, FVIII inhibitor after substitution with recombinant coagulation factor VIII concentrate

binant FVIII concentrate intensity of hemorrhages increased. We diagnosed high-titer anti-FVIII inhibitor (8.4 BU) and started rFVIIa treatment (Fig. 2).

Elimination Therapy of Inhibitors with Immunoadsorption

Therapy of inhibitor patients we usually perform according to our protocol of cytotoxic and immunosuppressive therapy (steroids and Cyclophosphamide) combined with immunoadsorption, intravenous IgG substitution and substitution of rFVIIa [2].

After complete inhibitor elimination by immunoadsorption we usually started high-dose substitution with coagulation factor concentrates. The patient's admission to the hospital for immunoadsorption was necessary for about 3 weeks (see Table 1).

Table 1. Protocol of inhibitor elimination by immunosuppressive therapy with steroids and cyclophosphamide and immunoadsorption

• Prednisone	100 mg	day 1–50
• Immunoadsorption		day 4–8, 12–16, 22–24, 35–39
• IVIG	0.5 g/kg BW (body weight)	day 9–11, 17–19, 25–27, 40–42
• Cyclophosphamide	500 mg	day 3, 10, 17, 24, 45
• rFVIIa	240 kIE q 4h	day 1–7

Modified Schedule of Treatment

We modified this protocol by supplementation of anti-CD20 monoclonal antibody Rituximab. The treatment schedule of patient A is shown in Table 2, of patient B shown in Figure 3.

Patient A had to be treated in the hospital for a 15 day period due to immunoadsorption. Patient B was outpatient as inhibitor elimination proceeded fast and immunoadsorption was not necessary (Fig. 4).

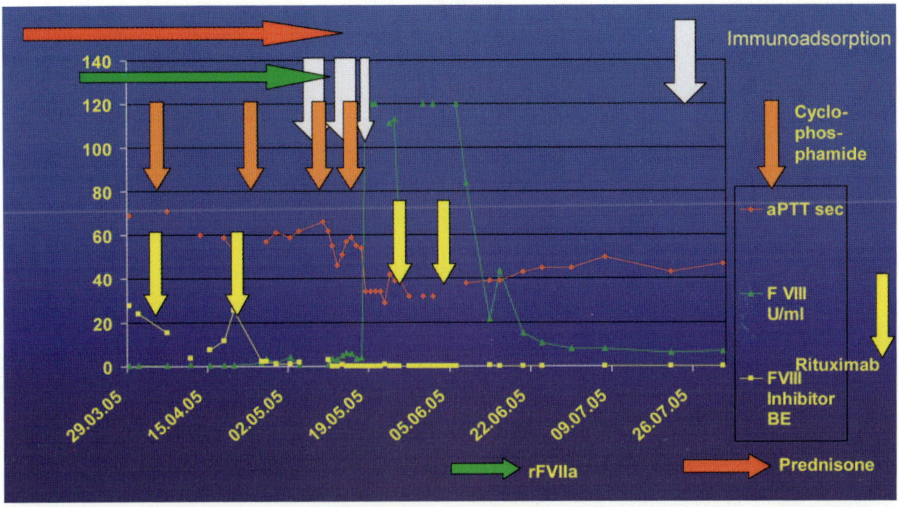

Fig. 3. Patient A, treatment schedule protocol of immunosuppressive therapy (steroids, Rituximab and Cyclophosphamide) and immunoadsorption

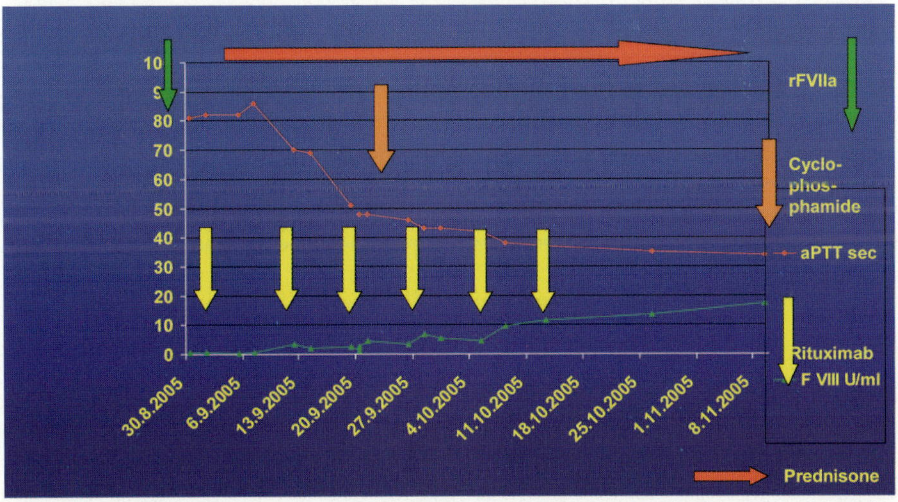

Fig. 4. Patient B, treatment schedule protocol of immunosuppressive therapy (steroids, Rituximab and Cyclophosphamide) without immunoadsorption

Table 2. Immunosuppressive treatment protocol; dosage of immunosuppressive therapy (Rituximab and Cyclophosphamide) varies in both patients

Patient A, 65a

Rituximab	1 13 50 64		Immuno- ad- sorption	34-37 41-44 47-48
Cyclo- phos- phamide	1 14 33 40			
Predni- sone	-21 bis +38		IVIG	38-40 44-46 62
Filgrastim	47- 48			

Patient B, 32a

Rituximab	1 10 17 24 32 39		Immuno- ad- sorption	none
Cyclo- phos- phamide	22			
Predni- sone	+4 bis +68		IVIG	none
Filgrastim				

Table 2 shows the complete treatment protocol of both patients.

In patient A, Cyclophosphamide therapy was administered four times resulting in granulocytopenia complicated by septicemia. Due to immunoadsorption patient A had to stay inside the hospital for several weeks.

Patient B was treated with Rituximab six times. Cyclophosphamide treatment could be reduced to one single dose as we intensified anti-CD 20 B-cell specific suppressive treatment.

Complications of Treatment

In patient A central venous access via subclavian vein led to staphylococcus epidermitis septicemia after the third application of Cyclophosphamide (May 11th, 2005). We started empirical antibiotic therapy with Teicoplanin and Piperacilin. The patient improved immediately, and CVC could remain in situ until immunoadsorption was completed. We provided IVIG substitution after immunoadsorption.

Due to cytotoxic therapy the patient experienced neutropenia grade III (leukocyte count 1.7 Gpt/l) on May 22nd, 2005, but resolved after G-CSF treatment.

In Patient B no infectious complications occurred.

Supportive Care

Following our department's guidelines for treatment of patients with hematologic malignancies we started broad antimicrobial prophylaxis at the beginning of the immunosuppressive treatment with Itraconazole 2 x 100 mg per day, Ciprofloxacine 2 x 500 mg per day, and Cotrimoxazole 2 x 960 mg twice a week, respectively.

Table 3. Prophylactic antimicrobial treatment

Ciprofloxacine	2 x 500 mg	daily dosage
Itraconazole	2 x 100 mg	daily dosage
Cotrimoxazole	2 x 800 / 160 mg	twice a week
Aciclovir	5 x 800 mg	daily dosage
Filgrastim	480 μg	in case of granulocyte count < 1,5 Gpt/l

Aciclovir was given in therapeutic dosage for the first 3 weeks only; Filgrastim treatment was started when granulocyte count was below 1,5 Gpt/l.

Lymphoid Depletion

We saw a profound and ongoing B cell depletion in both patients.

CD 20+ positive B cells were not detectable in the peripheral blood for at least 3 months.

Table 4. Leukocyte counts and lymphocyte subpopulations

Patient A, 65a 16.11. 2005, day 66

L 3.5 Gpt/l				
Lymph 30.5%	CD3+ /CD45+	70 %	CD 20	2 %
	CD16+ 56+ /CD45+	23 %	CD 19	neg
	CD19+ /CD45+	2 %		

Patient B, 32a 26.10. 2005, day 56

L 9.58 Gpt/l				
Lymph 11.9 %	CD 3+ /CD 45+	85 %	CD 20	neg
	CD16+ 56+ / CD45+	7 %	CD 19	neg
	CD19+ / CD 45+	0 %		

Substitution of Coagulation Factor Concentrates

In patient B there was a significant lower dosage of coagulation factor concentrates needed for substitution compared to patient A who underwent immunoadsorption. Patient B was treated with rFVIIa on demand before start of elimination therapy.

In patient A, however, substitution with rFVIIa had to be done prophylactically meanwhile immunoadsorption (dosage 4 x 240 kIE per day).

Follow-up

In both patients we found the combined immunosuppression regimen applicable and efficacious. After a follow up period of 14 months in patient A and 7 months in patient B FVIII inhibitor were no longer detectable despite of reexposition to coagulation factor VIII.

Table 5. Complete immunologic and hemostaseologic treatment protocol of both patients; dosage of coagulation factor concentrates administered to each patient varies significantly.

Patient A, 65 a

Rituximab	1 13 50 64		Immuno-ad-sorption	34-37 41-44 47-48
Cyclo-phos-phamide	1 14 33 40		rFVIIa	33-37 41
Predni-sone	-21 bis +38		IVIG	38-40 44-46 62
Filgrastim	47- 48		FVIII	41-68

Patient B, 32 a

Rituximab	1 10 17 24 32 39		Immuno-ad-sorption	
Cyclo-phos-phamide	22		rFVIIa	-2 bis -3
Predni-sone	+4 bis +68		IVIG	
Filgrastim			FVIII	-6 bis -7

Both patients underwent further surgeries after successful elimination therapy: In patient A inguinal herniotomy was performed 8 months after start of elimination therapy. The patient was treated with plasma derived FVIII perioperatively after two further Rituximab courses 3 weeks before undergoing surgery.

In patient B successful osteosynthesis was performed 3 months after start of elimination regimen. No reoccurrence of inhibitor production was observed. Plasma concentrations of FVIII rose up to the patients normal concentrations.

Discussion

Development of antibodies directed to coagulation factors is a serious and some times life threatening complication in hemophilia patients [3].

Genetic mutations seem to influence predisposition for development of FVIII allo-antibodies. It is not yet clear whether the type of coagulation factor concentrates – either plasma derived or recombinant products – determines the incidence of inhibitor production. Differences in immunogenicity are subject of ongoing pediatric studies in primarily untreated patients (PUP).

Usually diagnosis of hemophilia is made in early childhood, and most of the hemophilic patients receive prophylactic treatment during childhood. Therefore, adult PU patients are rare.

Immunologic response, however, seems to be different in children than in adults. Therefore, it might be necessary to modify treatment of inhibitor elimination in adult patients compared to children [4].

For primarily untreated newborns and younger children the Malmö protocol was found to be efficacious inducing long-term remissions. High-dose substitution of coagulation factor concentrates seem to bind circulating anti-coagulation factor antibodies without further stimulation of immune response.

According to this protocol the patients are treated with high-dose Prednisone and cytostatic drugs in low dosage. High-dose coagulation factor concentrate combined with mild immunosuppressive therapy may be able to overwhelm antibody production in newborns and younger children. In adult patients, however, immunologic response is different to infants, and exposure to high-dose coagulation factor concentrate is not an adequate treatment by itself [5].

In order to induce B-cell suppression we intensified treatment with steroids and cyclophosphamide by monoclonal anti-CD20 antibody Rituximab. We saw complete defect in peripheral B-Cells even 2 months after Rituximab treatment in both patients.

Combining cytotoxic drugs and Rituximab, we were aware of immunodeficiency due to hypogammaglobulinemia, granulocytopenia and even T-Cell depletion.

Therefore, supportive care is a major issue in those patients. We administered antibiotics, antimycotic and virustatic drugs prophylactically for a period of several months. In case of granulocytopenia grade IV we administered G-CSF subcutaneously. Every 3 weeks we provided complete hematologic examinations to both patients like we perform in patients with hematologic malignancies under cytotoxic therapy.

On the other hand, immunoadsorption could be avoided because of rapid decrease in inhibitor production. In both patients plasma concentrations of FVIII-antibodies diminished rapidly, and the dosage of coagulation factor concentrates administered to the patients was minimalized compared to the Malmö protocol. Immunoadsorption itself is an expensive method which induces depletion of circulating immunoglobulins, and the patient's admission to the hospital is required.

We found the protocol to be efficacious and safe. No prospective studies are available so far. Further studies in combined immunosuppression therapy of inhibitor patients are ongoing.

References

1. Zeitler H, Ulrich-Merzenich G, Hess L, Konsek E, Unkrig C, Walger P, Vetter H, Brackmann H-H. Treatment of acquired hemophilia by the Bonn-Malmö Protocol: documentation of an in vivo immunomodulating concept. Blood. 2005;105:2287–2293
2. Wolf H-H, Winkler M, Dorligschaw O, Markau S, Voigt W, Schmoll H-J. Immunomodulatory management of acquired haemophilia: Immunoadsorption, immunosuppressive treatment and factor VIIa substitution. Haemophilia. 2000;6:303
3. Wolf H-H, Harba A, Frühauf A, Schmoll H-J. Immunosuppressive Treatment in Acquired von-Willebrand`s Syndrome. In: Scharrer I, Schramm W, eds. 35th Hemophilia Symposium Hamburg 2004. Berlin Heidelberg: Springer; 2006:165–167
4. Delgado J, Jimenez-Yuste V, Hernandez-Navarro F, Villar A. Acquired Haemophilia: Review and Meta-Analysis Focused on Therapy and Prognostic Factors. Br J Hematol. 2003; 121:21–35
5. Boggio LN, Green D. Acquired Hemophilia. Rev Clin Exp Hematol. 2001;5:389–404

III. Orthopedic Treatment in Hemophiliacs

Chairmen:

I. Scharrer (Mainz)
A. Kurth (Frankfurt/Main)

Osteoporosis and Hemophilia – Is there a Correlation and Is there a Problem?

A. Kurth

As per WHO definition, osteoporosis is a metabolic bone disease characterized by a reduction in bone mass as well as destruction of the osseous microarchitecture and is thus associated with an increased risk of incident fractures. In Germany, approximately 6–7 million patients suffer from osteoporosis. However, the bone changes are only diagnosed and treated in about 20 %. Patients with manifest osteoporosis are at a high risk of experiencing further osteoporotic fractures within the year after their first fracture. One in five postmenopausal women with osteoporosis will experience another fracture within only one year after a vertebral fracture. Therefore, osteoporosis – once wrongly known as a slowly progressing disease – in fact progresses very rapidly once the first fracture has occurred. Osteoporotic fractures are associated with pain and substantial restrictions in almost all dimensions of quality of life. Therefore, both causal and symptomatic therapy is indicated in the treatment of manifest osteoporosis.

Secondary Osteoporosis

Secondary forms of osteoporosis have a clear etiology which has to be confirmed by differential diagnosis and treated causally as far as possible. The existing data reveal only very little about the incidence of secondary osteoporosis. Approximately 20 % of the women affected are likely to have osteoporosis a result of secondary causes. In men, secondary causes can be assumed to amount to as much as 60 %. Diseases that may cause secondary osteoporosis include endocrine disorders (e. g. Cushing's syndrome, hypogonadism, hyperthyroididsm, rickets, hyperparathyroidism), gastrointestinal disorders (e. g. inflammatory bowel disease, celiac disease), hematologic diseases and malignancy (e. g. mastocytosis, plasmacytoma, paraneoplastic syndrome), organ transplants, chronic inflammatory diseases (e. g. rheumatism) and genetic changes (e. g. osteogenesis imperfecta). However, drug therapies are also responsible for the development of secondary osteoporosis. Most patients receiving cumulative glucocorticoid doses develop osteoporosis. Many of the drugs used in routine clinical practice have negative effects on the bone. These drugs include anticoagulants (heparins, coumarin), immunosuppressive agents (e. g. cyclosporine), antihormone therapy, antiepileptics, and antineoplastic substances. Particularly in men, alcohol is a substance responsible for many secondary osteoporoses.

I. Scharrer/W. Schramm (Ed.)
36th Hemophilia Symposium Hamburg 2005

Hemophilia is frequently mentioned in the context of secondary osteoporosis. It is, for instance, one of the diseases associated with a loss of bone mass as mentioned by the National Osteoporosis Foundation (NOF) of the USA. Therefore, bone mineral density measurement is recommended in patients with hemophilia. In the literature, there is only little evidence of a relationship between secondary osteoporosis and hemophilia. There is no explanation whatsoever for the development of osteoporosis in hemophiliacs.

NOF recommendations, USA

Medical Conditions That May Lead to Bone Loss and Osteoporosis	
AIDS/HIV	Inflammatory Bowel Disease
Amyloidosis	Insulin-dependent diabetes mellitus
Chronic obstructive pulmonary disease	Lymphoma and leukemia
Congenital porphyria	Malabsorption syndromes
Cushing's syndrome	Mastocytosis
Eating disorders (e.g., anorexia nervosa)	Multiple myeloma
Female athlete triad	Multiple sclerosis
Gastrectomy	Pernicious anemia
Gaucher's Disease	Rheumatoid arthritis
Hemochromatosis	Severe liver disease, especially primary biliary cirrhosis
Hemophilia	Spinal cord transsection
Hyperparathyroidism	Sprue
Hypogonadism, primary and secondary (ex., amenorrhea)	Stroke
Hypophosphatasia	Thalassemia
Idiopathic scoliosis	Thyrotoxicosis
Inadequate diet	Tumor secretion of parathyroid hormone-related peptide
	Weight loss

National Osteoporosis Foundation

Diagnosis of Osteoporosis

Apart from the medical history and the assessment of risk factors (e. g. age, prevalent fracture, height loss) bone mineral density plays a decisive role in the development of osteoporosis.

In this context, the measurable bone mineral content is taken as a basis. The mean value of what is referred to as peak bone mass (the detectable bone mineral density built up during the first third of life) is the reference point for assessing the measured value.

Measured values scattered around this mean value by plus or minus one standard deviation are interpreted as normal.

Measured values deviating from the mean value of the peak bone mass by more than −2.5 standard deviations are consistent with the suspicion of osteoporosis. If no fracture has occurred when the diagnosis is confirmed, the clinical picture established will be interpreted as preclinical osteoporosis. If a first bone fracture has occurred when the diagnosis is confirmed, the presence of a clinically manifest (advanced) osteoporosis is suspected.

Measured values deviating by more than −1 and less than −2.5 standard deviations from the mean peak bone mass are assigned to osteopenia (gray area between normality and osteoporosis).

Assuming that osteoporosis is always progressive and that the risk of bone fractures is expected to increase continuously after the disease has been diagnosed it is generally agreed upon that therapy is absolutely indicated after the diagnosis has been confirmed.

At the hemophilia center of Frankfurt on the Main, a total of 52 hemophiliacs (19–72 years) have been examined osteodensitometrically regarding the presence of osteoporosis. 45 patients had hemophilia A and 7 hemophilia B. 21 patients (19 hemophilia A, 2 B) had severe hemophilia with residual factor levels below 1 %; 11 patients (10 A, 1 B) had moderate hemophilia with residual factor levels of 1–5 %; 16 patients (12 A, 4 B) had mild hemophilia with residual factor levels of > 5 %; 4 patients (A) had subhemophilia.

Apart from severity and type of hemophilia, risk factors for osteoporosis, fractures and frequency of bleeds were included in the medical record.

The bone mineral density measurements were performed in accordance with the guidelines of the German osteology umbrella organization, DVO, for the diagnosis and management of osteoporosis using a DEXA device (Hologic, QDR 4500 plus). Standard measurements of the lumbar spine and the proximal femur were performed and the usual criteria and standard values were applied for assessment of the presence of osteoporosis. At a T-Score below −2.5 osteoporosis was diagnosed and values between −1.5 and −2.5 were classified as osteopenia. Bone mineral density values corresponding to osteopenia or osteoporosis were measured in a total of 26 patients. There were 2 cases of femural osteoporosis, and 14 cases of femural osteopenia; moreover, there were 9 cases of lumbar spine osteoporosis and 13 cases of lumbar spine osteopenia. 8 of 26 positive patients had already experienced fractures typical of osteoporosis, as opposed to only 3 patients with normal bone mineral density. 13 of the 26 male hemophilacs affected were less than 50 years old.

In patients with existing osteoporosis therapy is absolutely indicated, since, if left untreated, the disease will most probably progress. So if osteoporosis is suspected in patients with hemophilia, they should be treated systematically using modern therapy on the basis of the principles of evidence-based medicine. Unfortunately, there are no recommendations on diagnostics and therapy available for patients with hemophilia.

The results of the Frankfurt investigation suggest that there is a correlation between hemophilia and the development of osteoporosis. Therefore, the experience made should be verified by a national multicenter trial. Based on the results of this trial, the procedures and therapy recommendations for patients with hemophilia should be defined by an interdisciplinary committee.

Orthopedic Evaluation of the Lower Extremity in 249 Children: A Multicenter Trial

A. Seuser, and E. Kusch

Introduction

The aim of this study was to explore typical orthopedic abnormalities of the lower extremity in children with hemophilia and to use this as a basis for developing a systematic and effective sequence of evaluations.

Material and Methods

Motion analysis has been performed to date in 318 children involved in a multicenter motion analysis trial. Datasets including orthopedic examination have been evaluated in 249 of these children, including 195 with hemophilia A, 40 with hemophilia B and 9 with von-Willebrand-Jürgens syndrome. Datasets are missing from 5 children.

Of the 195 children with hemophilia A, 137 had residual activity below 1%, 35 from 1–3% and 24 had residual activity in excess of 3%. 136 children were receiving prophylaxis and 57 received treatment on demand. Orthopedic examination in the above patient population was conducted in all cases by the same orthopedic surgeon.

The parameters studied were posture, axis deviation of the lower extremity, gait inspection, ranges of motion of the hip joint, knee joint, ankle joint and subtalar joint, periarticular tenderness for the hip joint, knee joint, ankle joint and subtalar joint, and function tests for the knee joint, ankle joint and subtalar joint. Other parameters investigated included muscle evaluations, in particular extension of the back of the leg. The pelvis and lumbar spine were examined for pelvic verticalization and spinal deformities.

Results

The joints with the greatest number of abnormalities were the ankle joint (31.3%), the knee joint (31.8%), followed by the hip joint (25.1%). The most common symptoms identified were muscular abnormalities (44.6%), axis deviation (36.7%), periarticular tenderness (33.2%), restricted mobility (28.6%) and poor posture (27.2%).

I. Scharrer/W. Schramm (Ed.)
36th Hemophilia Symposium Hamburg 2005

Hip

68.6% of the hip abnormalities concerned hypo- or hyperflexibility, 80.2% of which were due to increased internal and external rotation. This may point toward hip verticalization. Tenderness accounted for 26.3% of the hip abnormalities, with capsular tenderness in 67.7% and trochanter tenderness in 25.9%. Capsular tenderness is evidence of a joint problem and trochanter tenderness is a manifestation of a muscular problem.

Knee

The most common symptom identified in knee evaluations was tenderness. Tenderness involved the medial collateral ligament in 26.9%, lateral collateral ligament in 25% and apex of the patella in 30.8%. The second most common symptom was axis deviation, which was seen in 25.7% of cases. 82.9% of axis deviations were bow legs. The third most common symptom was synovitis (6.8%), with clinical synovitis in 50%, hyperthermia in 20% and effusion in 30%.

Ankle

The main ankle abnormalities were tenderness (59.6%), including 80.4% capsular tenderness. Anterolateral capsular tenderness was present in 46.1%, anteromedial capsule tenderness in 30.4%. Tendon tenderness was present in 17.2%, involving the Achilles tendon in 27.8% and the posterior tibial tendon in 50%. Synovitis was present in 26.9% and hypo- or hyperflexibility in 11.9%. Of the latter, hyperflexibility of the ankle joint was present in 31.8% and hypoflexibility of the subtalar joint was present in 54.5%.

Muscular

The most common symptom was shortening of the hamstring muscle group, which was present in almost 90% of the child population. Atrophy was evident in only 6.6%.

Discussion

Of the many abnormalities identified, a number of relevant manifestations can be identified as pathonomonic for effective and systematic evaluation of the lower extremity. Internal and external rotation are the primary parameters in examining the hip. This method enables the early identification and treatment of deformities. Most hip joint and muscle problems can be identified simply by pressing on the capsule and trochanter. Suitable physical therapy can be initiated on the basis of the results.

Examination of the knee joint should focus on establishing whether tenderness is present in the medial collateral ligament, lateral collateral ligament and apex of the patella. Palpitation of the kneecap is also important. These areas may be painful to palpitation although the patient may seem to have no restrictions of movement. Preventive physical measures may be initiated in such cases.

With regard to the ankle joint, tenderness in the anterolateral and anteromedial capsule is of the greatest relevance. Tenderness in these areas often reflects imperceptible chronic or acute processes in the ankle joint.

With regard to muscle tissue, shortening of the hamstrings is typically associated with disruption of the hip, pelvis and knee. Raising the extended leg is enough to show whether there is a need for prevention action.

Summary

This large-scale study of 249 children, including 195 with hemophilia A, produced an efficient and systematic examination process for the lower extremity that is easy to learn for hematologists and pediatricians, takes just about 5 minutes, and is highly likely to identify any clinically silent involvement of the joints in question.

An appropriate preventive physical therapy and training program can be instituted before the patient sustains impairment of quality of life caused by the disorders identified by the examination process.

Simultaneous Bilateral Total Knee Arthroplasty in Hemophilic Arthopathy

H. H. Eickhoff, F. W. Koch, G. Goldmann, H.-H. Brackmann, and J. Oldenburg

Introduction

Total knee replacement in advanced hemophilic arthropathy is long established. According to the literature an improvement in joint function and reduction in pain occurs in nearly all cases [1]. In contrast to the normal population there is a higher rate of postoperative complications.

The simultaneous bilateral total knee replacement is discussed controversialy. Compared to staged surgery there is a significant reduction in the amount of costs and overall hospital stay. After simultaneous surgery the patient profits directly for both joints. The disadvantages for simultaneous surgery are a longer surgery time, an increased blood loss, a more difficult postop mobilisation and especially a higher rate of complications. According to Lane et al. [2] cardiopulmonary complications are approximately three times higher, and most commonly involve arrhytmias. In the same study there was an approximately 17 times greater need for banked blood and a 4 times higher rate for postoperative confusion in the simultaneous bilateral total knee arthroplasty group. Ritter et al. [3] noted a higher percentage of patients who had thrombophlebitis in the simultaneous bilateral group (0.9%) than in the unilateral group (0.3%). On the other hand there are several studies which documented no significant difference in the rate of complications in both groups [4–8].

Case Report

The patient was a 42 year old man with severe haemophilia A. He had bilateral advanced knee arthropathy grade V according to Arnold u. Hilgartner (Fig. 1 and 2). The HSS-Score was 29 for the right and 36 for the left knee. The range of motion was markedly reduced in both knees (extension/flexion: right 0/10/50; left 0/20/30).

3$^{1}/_{2}$ years ago we implanted a cementless metal-on-metal total hip on the right side. At the same time there was performed an arthroscopy of the right knee with debridement and late synovectomy.

As concomitant disease there was a hepatitis B and C. The HIV-status was negativ.

In the case of severe knee arthropathy there was done a simultaneous bilateral knee replacement by one of the authors (H.H.E.). On both sides there was used a cemented modular knee replacement system (NexGen Version LCCK, Zimmer)

I. Scharrer/W. Schramm (Ed.)
36th Hemophilia Symposium Hamburg 2005

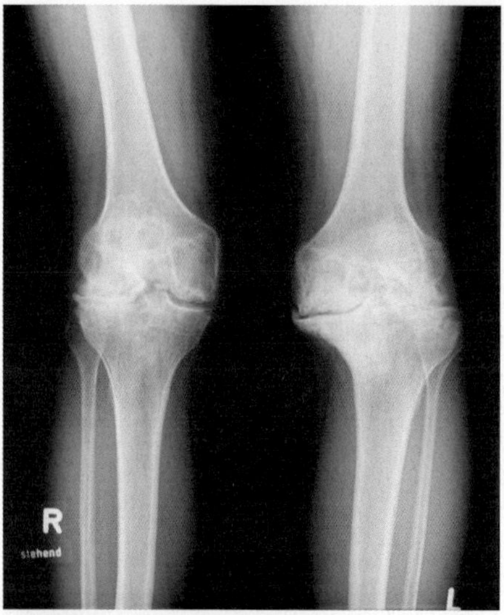

Fig. 1. Preop X-ray: both knees (a.p. view)

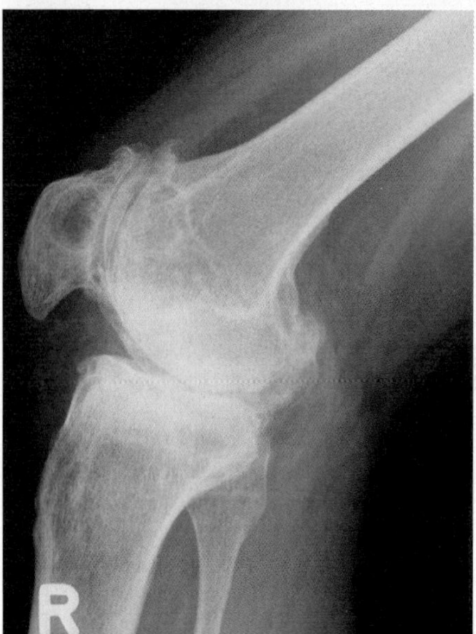

Fig. 2a. Preop X-ray: right knee (lateral view)

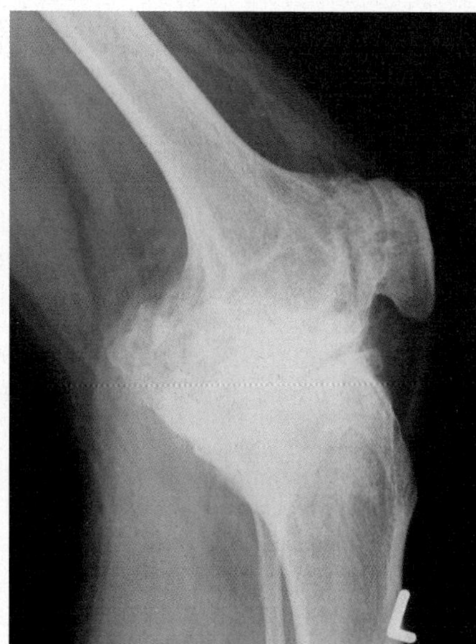

Fig. 2b. Preop X-ray: left knee (lateral view)

(Fig. 3 and 4). Because of severe joint contracture on both sides there was an extensive arthrolysis necessary, including quadriceps release, gastrocnemius release, cruciate ligament release, hamstring release and osteotomy of the tibiale tubercule. The time of surgery was 125 minutes for the right knee and 140 minutes for the left knee.

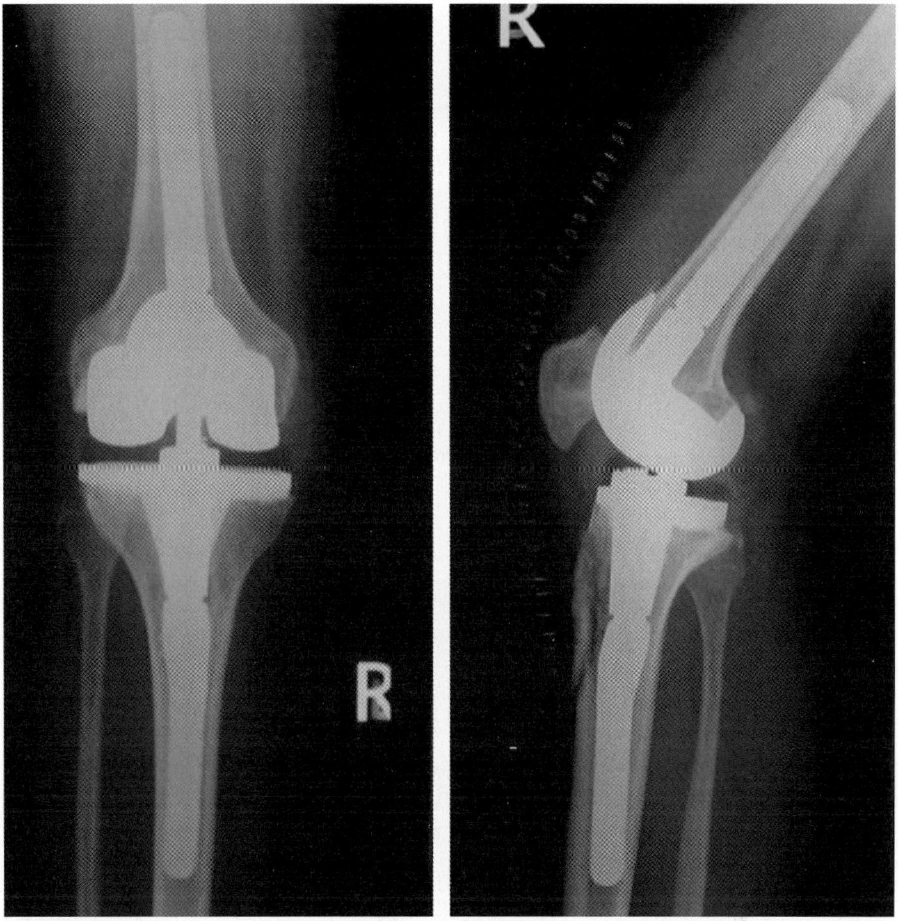

Fig. 3. Postop X-ray: LCCK total knee prosthesis, right knee

Postop the patient could be transferred from the recovery room directly to the normal ward. Mobilisation started the following day. In addition continuous passive motion machines were used. A postoperative prophylaxis with antibiotics (Cephazolin, 3 x 2 g) for three days was done. Overall five blood transfusions were needed. During the whole hospital stay the amount of 95,000 IE FVIII was given (Fig. 5). There was no complication. The hospital stay lasted 13 days.

Result

At follow-up 6 month postoperatively the patient was very satisfied. The HSS-score as well as the range of motion had improved markedly (Fig. 6 and 7).

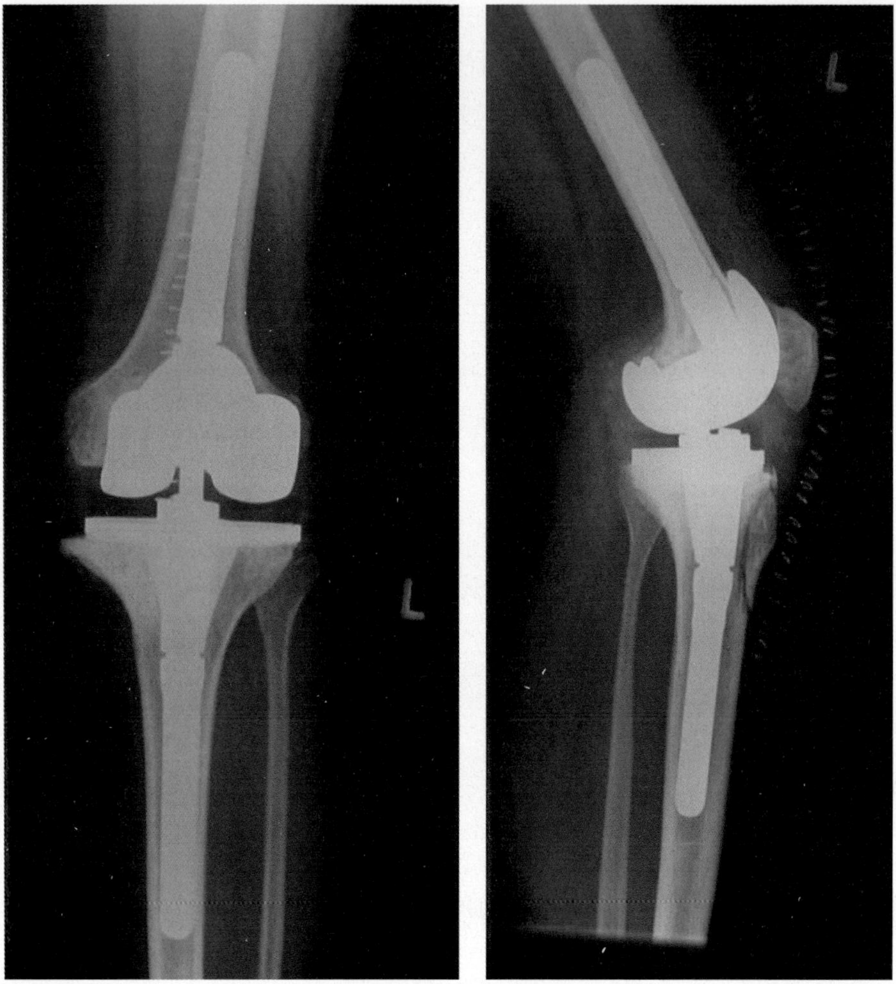

Fig. 4. Postop X-ray: LCCK total knee prosthesis, left side

Summary

This case report demonstrates that, in selected hemophilic patients, simultaneous bilateral knee replacement surgery can be performed with a good outcome without a significant increase in perioperative risk. The overall costs, especially for the FVIII replacement, are significantly lower in the simultaneous bilateral surgery than in the unilateral staged surgery. The authors continue to offer hemophilic patients the option of simultaneous bilateral total knee arthroplasties.

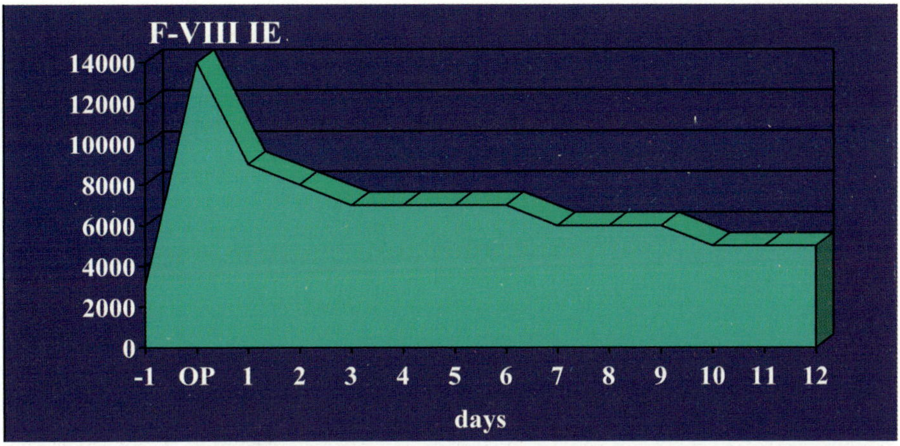

Fig. 5. Factor VIII substitution during the hospital stay. In summary 95,000 IE were given

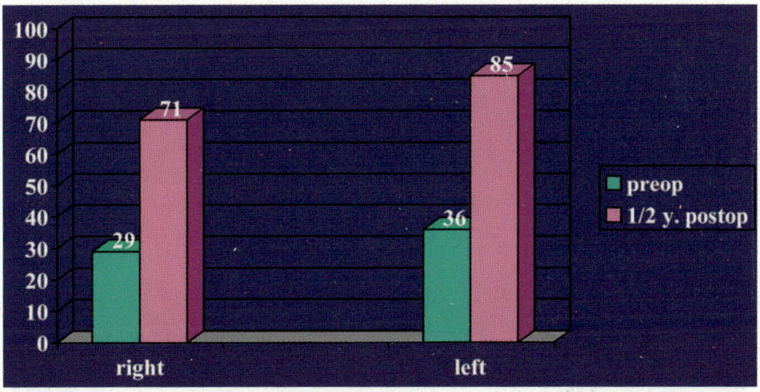

Fig. 6. Comparison of the HSS-score (preop versus ½ year postop)

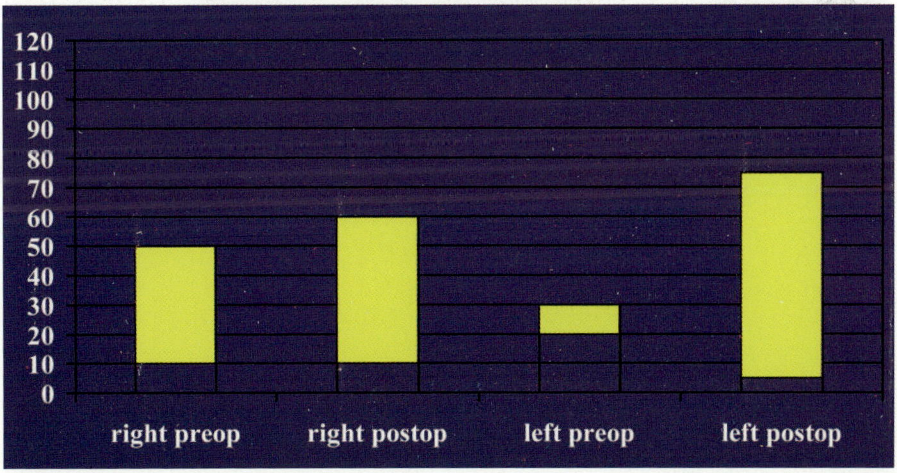

Fig. 7. Preop/postop comparison of the range of motion (acc. Neutral-Null-Method)

References

1. Rodriguez-Merchan EC, Wiedel JD. Total Knee Arthroplasty. in: Rodriguez-Merchan EC, Goddard NJ, Lee CA (eds.) Musculoskeletal Aspects of Haemophila. Blackwell Science 2000, 78–84
2. Lane GJ, Hozack WJ, Shah S, Rothman RH, Booth RE Jr., Eng K, Smith P. Simultaneous bilateral versus unilateral total knee arthroplasty. Outcomes analysis. Clin Orthop Relat Res. 1997 Dec; (345):106–12
3. Ritter MA, Harty LD, Davis KE, Meding JB, Berend M. Simultaneous bilateral, staged bilateral, and unilateral total knee arthroplasty. A survival analysis. J Bone Joint Surg Am. 2003 Aug; 85-A(8): 1532–7
4. Horne G, Devane P, Adams K. Complications and outcomes of single-stage bilateral total knee arthroplasty. ANZ J Surg. 2005 Sep;75(9):734–8
5. Stubbs G, Pryke SE, Tewari S, Rogers J, Crowe B, Bridgfoot L, Smith N. Safty and cost benefits of bilateral total knee replacement in an acute hospital. ANZ J Surg. 2005 Sep;75(9):379–46
6. Alemparte J, Johnson GV, Worland RL, Jessup DE, Keenan J. Results of simultaneous bilateral total knee replacement: a study of 1208 knees in 604 patients. J South Orthop Assoc. 2002 Fall;11(2):153–6
7. Kovacik MW, Singri P, Khanna S, Gradisar IA. Medical and financial aspects of same-day bilateral total knee arthroplasties. Biomed Sci Instrum. 1997;33:429–34
8. Ivory JP, Simpson AH, Toogood GJ, McLardy-Smith PD, Goodfellow JW. Bilateral knee replacements: simultaneous or staged? J R Coll Surg Edinb. 1993 Apr;38(2):105–7

Alternative Therapy such as the Acupuncture of the Skull for Hemophilic Arthropathy

T. A. Wallny, H.-H. Brackmann, G. Gunia, P. Wilbertz, J. Oldenburg, and Cn. Kraft

Older hemophilic patients with multiple arthropathies are often defined as chronic pain patients. E.g. due to a HIV-infection they are often forced to take multiple oral medication. In addition they may regularly need to take painkillers which have side effects in the abdominal area of stomach and bowel as well as in other internal organs.

The skull acupuncture is one of the so called microsystems of the acupuncture. These systems form a projection field, similar to the »Homunculus«, on a certain section of the body e.g. cranium, ear, oral cavity, or the metacarpal bones.

With regard to the single possible effects of the various acupuncture systems the following standard literature is named [1, 2]. Traditionally in China special point lines on the scull are assumed. These relate almost solely to the sagittal line of the skull from the back of the head to the forehead. In Chinese terminology this area is called Du Mai, translated this means governing vessel.

For the acupuncture, a needle, 25 mm long and 0.25 mm thick, is injected on this line in an easily felt groove at the back of the head. This area corresponds to rear fontanelle. The needle is injected in an angle of 45 degrees to this line from upper right or left diagonally to lower left or right. With the thumb and forefinger of the

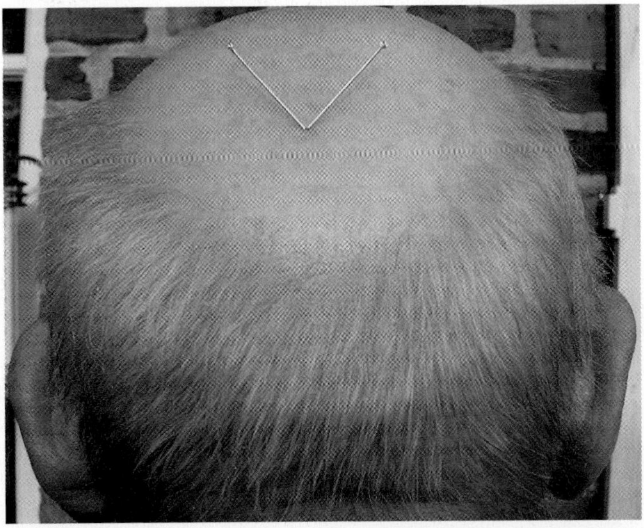

Fig. 1. Needles set for the treatment of both lower extremities

I. Scharrer/W. Schramm (Ed.)
36th Hemophilia Symposium Hamburg 2005

right hand the needle is fixed and with the thumb of the left hand the scalp is massaged in direction of the needle. After each massage the grip on the needle is let go so that prick by prick the needle is eased millimeter by millimeter under the skin. In this way the needle is lowered subcutaneously as far as the grip (see Fig. 1).

The skull remains untouched. Usually the injection of the needle itself is painless. As soon as the needle has been properly placed the grip between thumb and forefinger is fixed and the skin of the scalp is massaged once again with the thumb.

Patients and Methods

Included in the study were 12 patients with a factor VIII activity less than 1% and at least one painful arthropathy on both legs.

The patients filled in a questionnaire prior to completion of therapy and three months after. By means of a visual analogue scale (VAS) they were asked to evaluate the pain in the large joints of the upper and lower extremities before and after the therapy. Furthermore a clinical orthopedic examination was performed assessing range of motion, swelling and warmth of the target joints. Treatment was given in 15 therapy cycles per week.

After the setting of the needle and leaving the needle in place in the leg the patients are asked to move the leg for at least 30 minutes. At the same time the patient can chose to walk or move the leg while lying down. The joints of one extremity are treated with just one needle. If injected from upper right to lower left the left leg is treated and vice versa.

The location for the injection is called »DU 18«.

Based on a single blind study the patients were unaware of which side was being treated. No additional factor VIII was given. The study was approved by the ethics commission of the University of Bonn.

Criteria excluded
Painless walking distance over 1000 meters
Patients under 18 and over 65 years of age
Clinical symptoms of a HIV-infection
Sufficient pain ease by means of NSAD/opiods

Results

10 out of 12 patients showed an improvement of their subjective pain perception. The average VAS could be reduced from 6.8 to 5.0. The side not receiving treatment showed a reduction from 4.1 to 4.0.

The joints indicated as being most painful were 3 times the hip 4 times the knee and 5 times the ankle were mentioned as being most painful. 8 joints showed improvement and 4 were considered as not having changed (see Fig. 2). Whereby an improvement was only considered when at least 2 points difference in the VAS could be demonstrated.

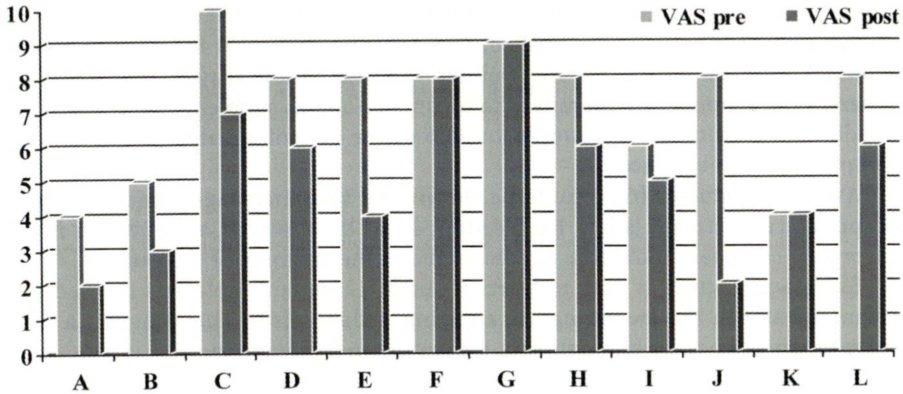

Fig. 2. VAS difference in most painful joints

6 out of 12 patients indicated that they needed less painkillers. No major differences could be detected considering range of motion and synovitis symptoms.

With special view to the knee and ankle joint it can be emphasized that 6 out of 11 painful knee joints showed improvement, and 5 remained unchanged after the therapy.

Out of the 11 ankle joints 4 showed improvement and 7 remained unchanged.

Out of the 4 as painful mentioned hips 3 showed improvement after therapy.

With regard to the upper extremities not being treated, 1 out of 24 elbow joints showed an improvement by 4 VAS points. All other joints showed similar results on the VAS or showed just a difference of just one point.

No bleeding worth mentioning could be observed where the needle was injected. There was no mention of pain or swelling in the area of the galea.

There were no infections around the injection area itself or side effects at the inner organs.

Discussion

Patients with chronic pain due to degenerative arthritis are increasingly undergoing acupuncture treatment. However the evidence is limited due to the small number of patients as well as the short follow-up [3, 4].

For hemophilic patients it also makes sense to consider an alternative therapy free from side effects which would not require any additional factor replacement.

The current study is of a pilot nature: Even if the prognosis is limited due to subjective recording of pain intensity on a visual analogue scale the unchanged pain intensity reported on the non-treated side and on the joints of the upper extremities allow the assumption that a certain achieved effectiveness cannot be ignored.

As a result of a single blind study the patients were unable to identify the side being treated. The question is how long the effects lasted!

chromogenic assays use optimized reagents for the first step, are easily automated and several commercial kits are available.

In selecting an assay, major criteria are on one-hand technical quality (i.e. accuracy, precision, ease of use) and on the other hand the ability of the assay to reflect the »true« patient situation. Technical quality is theoretically improved by reducing sample volume of patient's plasma as it is done in chromogenic assays with only about 1% patient's plasma in the whole mixture. The opposite situation is present in whole blood assays as in thrombelastography or the original method of thrombin generation test [3] with over 80% patient's blood in the mixture. It is believed, that these assays do better reflect patient's situation and that especially the thrombin generation assays are a promising tool for several indications as monitoring post-infusion plasma or in differentiation of patients with very low FVIII levels [4]. However, the available data are scientific and routine use isn't established today.

A major advantage of chromogenic assays compared to the one-stage clotting assays is the robustness against several interferences. Falsely low FVIII activities are observed in one-stage clotting assays if the analyzed plasma contains more than 0.7 IU/ml unfractionated or fractionated (measured as anti-Xa activity) heparin or a strong lupus anticoagulants activity up to a dilution of 1:80. Direct thrombin inhibitors disturb the assay result even in very low concentrations [5]. Chromogenic assays are not influenced and therefore adequate for these situations. However, one important advantage of one-stage assays is the ability to adapt the assays for measuring of low FVIII activities down to 0.1% by reducing sample dilution and a separate calibration. For these samples a better precision is observed (CV about 18% for samples of 5% FVIII activity) compared to chromogenic assays (CV ~27%) or immunoassays (CV ~30%) [5].

Calibration of assays should be based on WHO International Biological Reference Preparations. For human plasma the 5th International Standard (2003) based on a human plasma preparation containing FVIII and von Willebrand factor is available, while for measurement of FVIII concentrates the 7th International Standard (2003) based on recombinant FVIII protein is distributed by the WHO. The currently available preparations are listed online at: http://who.int/bloodproducts/ref_materials/.

Indications for FVIII Measurement

The main indications for FVIII measurement are:
1. diagnosis and classification of severity of hemophilia,
2. monitoring of therapy with (plasma-based or recombinant/recombinant B-domain deleted) FVIII concentrates,
3. labeling of FVIII concentrates by manufacturers and
4. assessment of elevated FVIII activity (>150%) in thrombophilia screening.

According to ISTH-SCC recommendation hemophilia is classified in: severe (<1% FVIII activity), moderate (1–5% FVIII activity) and mild (>5% FVIII activity) [6]. Therefore, FVIII assays must be able to differentiate FVIII levels above and below 1%. The measuring range of the regular one-stage FVIII assays is usually between

10% and up to > 200%. As mentioned above, FVIII levels as low as 0.1% can be achieved with by a separate, so-called low calibration (range: 0.1% to 10/15%). For chromogenic assays three separate calibrations are necessary to cover a measuring range of 0.5% to 400% (low: 0.5% to 5%, normal: 5% to 150%, and elevated: 100% to 400%).

A new opportunity to differentiate patients with severe hemophilia (<1%) might be the use of modified thrombin generation test. McIntosh and colleagues could show that ample amount of FIXa (14 nmol/l) in the reagent mixture (0.2 nmol/l in the original test system) gives a clear difference in thrombin generation within different patients with severe hemophilia (e.g. time to peak thrombin generation 400 sec in one patient and about 550 sec in another patient compared to about 200 sec in normals) [4]. Clinical relevance of these observations still has to be clarified.

For measurement of FVIII activity in high-purity or recombinant FVIII concentrates the following ISTH-SCC recommendations should be followed [7]:

- FVIII deficient plasma for assays should be true hemophilic plasma or immunodepleted plasma with normal content of vWF
- the assay buffer should contain 1% of albumin
- pre-dilution of patient samples should be done with true hemophilic plasma or immunodepleted plasma with normal content of vWF

However, several differences of measured FVIII levels are observed, if different assay principles are used for different types of concentrates [8]:

- high-purity plasma-based (immunopurified) concentrates showed up to 33% higher levels with one-stage clotting assays than with chromogenic assays
- B-domain depleted recombinant concentrates showed up to 28% higher levels with chromogenic assays than with one-stage clotting assays
- full-length recombinant concentrates showed no relevant discrepancy between one-stage clotting and chromogenic assays

The basic causes of the observed differences are still unknown. One theoretical approach assumes that the concentrates behave after infusion like »in vitro« (=dilution in hemophilic plasma) [9]. Based on this approach the current recommendation is to measure post-infusion samples using a FVII concentrate standard for assay calibration which is as similar as possible to the infused concentrate (»like vs like«) [10]. Using this approach most assay differences are eliminated [11]. However, for labeling of B-domain-deleted recombinant concentrates the use chromogenic assays might be necessary.

A permanently elevated FVIII level >150% is shown to be a relevant thrombophilic risk factor [12]. Therefore, FVIII assays should be able to differentiate between levels above and below 150%. This is easily done with one-stage clotting assays as described above. With chromogenic assays a separate calibration is necessary.

Summary

For daily laboratory routine work the one-stage clotting assay can be adapted to most indications. For diagnosis of severe hemophilia FVIII levels below 1% can be assessed by a separate calibration. For therapy monitoring and measurement of concentrates ISTH-SCC recommendations should be followed. Measuring »like vs. like« (optimal: assay calibration with concentrate standard the same as the infused concentrate) eliminates the major differences between assay methods. In diagnosis of thrombophilia FVIII levels above and below 150% can be easily differentiated.

Chromogenic assays might be of special use in labeling of B-domain-deleted recombinant concentrates. However, basic causes of the observed assay differences remain (partly) unknown.

References

1. Langdell RD, Wagner RH, Brinkhous KM. Effect of antihemophilic factor on one-stage clotting tests. J Lab Clin Med 1953; 41: 637–647
2. Biggs R, Eveling J, Richards G. The assay of antihaemophilic globulin. Br J Haematol 1955; 1: 20–34
3. Macfarlane RG, Biggs RA. Thrombin Generation Test: The Application in Haemophilia and Thrombocytopenia. J Clin Pathol. 1953; 6:3–8
4. Mcintosh JH, Owens D, Lee CA, Raut S, Barrowcliffe TW. A modified thrombin generation test for the measurement of factor VIII concentrates. J Thromb Haemost 2003; 1:1005–1011
5. Chandler WL, Ferrell C, Lee J, Tun T, Kha H. Comparison of three methods for measuring factor VIII levels in plasma. Am J Clin Pathol. 2003; 120: 34–39
6. White GC 2nd, Rosendaal F, Aledort LM, Lusher JM, Rothschild C, Ingerslev J; Factor VIII and Factor IX Subcommittee. Definitions in hemophilia. Recommendation of the scientific subcommittee on factor VIII and factor IX of the scientific and standardization committee of the International Society on Thrombosis and Haemostasis. Thromb Haemost. 2001; 85:560
7. Barrowcliffe TW. Factor VIII and factor IX Sub-Committee. Recommendations for the assay of high-purity factor VIII concentrates. Thromb Haemost. 1993; 70: 876–877
8. Hubbard AR, Weller LJ, Bevan SA. A survey of one-stage and chromogenic potencies in therapeutic factor VIII concentrates. British Journal of Haematology 2002; 117: 247–248
9. Barrowcliffe TW, Mertens K, Preston FE, Ingerslev J. Laboratory aspects of haemophilia therapy. Haemophilia. 2002; 8: 244–249
10. Report of a Joint WHO/WFH/ISTH Meeting: Delivery of Treatment for Hemophilia. London, United Kingdom, 11–13 February 2002. Geneva: WHO, 2002 (http://whqlibdoc.who.int/hq/2002/WHO_WFH_ISTH_WG_02.6.pdf)
11. Lee CA, Owens D, Bray G, Giangrande P, Collins P, Hay C, Gomperts E, Schroth P, Barrowcliffe T. Pharmacokinetics of recombinant factor VIII (recombinate) using one-stage clotting and chromogenic factor VIII assay. Thromb Haemost. 1999; 82: 1644–1647
12. Bertina RM. Elevated clotting factor levels and venous thrombosis. Pathophysiol Haemost Thromb. 2003–2004;33:395–400

Global ECAT Survey on Factor VIII Inhibitor Testing: Results of an Inter-Laboratory Pilot Study

P. Meijer, H. Verbruggen, J. Arnout, and M. Spannagl

Introduction

A major complication in the treatment of hemophilia patients is the development of inhibitors. This renders standard treatment ineffective. Therefore reliable measurement of inhibitors is necessary. Up to now only limited data are available on inter-laboratory comparison of factor VIII inhibitor testing. Therefore, the ECAT Foundation (an international organization for external quality assessment in thrombosis and hemostasis) conducted an inter-laboratory pilot study on factor VIII inhibitor testing. This study was meant to provide on an international scale insight in the current status of inhibitor testing in the clinical laboratory.

Study Design

A set of 3 lyophilized test samples was sent to 175 laboratories in Europe, United States and Australia. Sample A was a high titer sample (~15 BU/ml), sample B was a low titer sample (~1.5 BU/ml) and sample C was a negative sample. Sample A and B were prepared by diluting a high titer patient sample in congenital factor VIII deficient plasma. Each participant in this study received a standard report form, including questions on assay principle, reagents used, incubation time, sample dilution etc.

Results

Results were returned by 135 laboratories (~77%). The classical Bethesda assay was used by 93 laboratories (69%), the Nijmegen modified assay was used by 30 participants (22%), and 12 participants had used another method (9%). For sample A 131 numerical test results could be included in the evaluation and for sample B 124 numerical test results. Table 1 shows the overall data evaluation for sample A and B.

There are important fundamental differences between the assay design of the classical Bethesda assay and the Nijmegen modified assay. The Nijmegen modified assay uses buffered normal plasma as a source for factor VIII and factor VIII deficient plasma in the control mixture. Therefore both assay types were evaluated

I. Scharrer/W. Schramm (Ed.)
36th Hemophilia Symposium Hamburg 2005

Table 1

Factor VIII inhibitor (BU/ml)	Number	Mean	Median	Inter-laboratory variation (%)	Range
Sample A	131	14.9	13.8	56	2 – 67
Sample B	124	1.86	1.40	202	0 – 42

Table 2

Sample A Factor VIII inhibitor (BU/ml)	Number	Mean	Inter-laboratory variation (%)	Range	Number of outliers
Bethesda assay	86	14.3	41.3	4 – 29	3
Nijmegen assay	29	14.3	28.0	7 - 23	1

Table 3

Sample B Factor VIII inhibitor (BU/ml)	Number	Mean	Inter-laboratory variation (%)	Range	Number of outliers
Bethesda assay	79	1.4	47.9	0.0 – 3.0	7
Nijmegen assay	28	1.3	31.5	1.0 – 2.0	1

separately (Table 2 and 3). The results identified as outliers, i.e. > 3 times the standard deviation, were excluded from the statistical analyses.

It was further observed that 16 laboratories have reported a result below their detection limit for sample B. Thirteen of these laboratories have used the Bethesda assay. In totally we had 131 test results for sample B (including also the non-numerical results indicated as a result below detection limit). This means a sensitivity of factor VIII inhibitor testing of 92%.

For sample C (negative control) 128 laboratories returned a result. Thirty-five laboratories indicated a result below the detection limit, while 93 laboratories reported a numerical test result. Four of those numerical results were above the indicated detection limit and as such indicated as a positive sample. This means a specificity of factor VIII inhibitor testing of 97%.

It was further observed that some laboratories who indicated to perform the classical Bethesda assay also have indicated the use of buffered normal plasma and to a minor extend laboratories who indicated to use the Nijmegen modified assay who have indicated the use of non-buffered plasma. This had occurred also for the use of imidazole buffer or factor VIII deficient plasma in the control sample.

Discussion

To our knowledge this was the first large-scale inter-laboratory comparison of factor VIII inhibitor testing. Although the Nijmegen modified assay was selected by the ISTH as the reference method for factor VIII inhibitor testing still 69% of the laboratories indicated the use of the classical Bethesda assay. Because the number of laboratories who indicated the use of the classical Bethesda assay was conflicting with the number of laboratories who indicated the use of non-buffered plasma as a source for factor VIII or the use of imidazole buffer in the control sample it is questionable if laboratories exactly know the type of assay they are using. This needs to be further investigated.

The results of this study showed on general a huge variability between laboratories. When differentiated between the Bethesda assay and the Nijmegen modified assay it is clear that for both the high titer and the low titer sample the Nijmegen modified assay showed the lowest between-laboratory variation. In spite of this observation, the between-laboratory variation for the Nijmegen modified assay is still high. An important source for this between-laboratory variation may be the variation in the measurement of the residual factor VIII in the test sample (data not shown). A comprehensive evaluation of possible causes for the between-laboratory variation still needs to be explored.

It is further remarkable that the Nijmegen modified assay showed more sensitivity than the classical Bethesda assay. This, at least, should be an indication for laboratories to follow the guidelines of the ISTH to use the Nijmegen modified assay.

Conclusions

It can be concluded that in general factor VIII inhibitor testing showed a large between-laboratory variability. The results of the users of the Nijmegen modified assay are more comparable than those of the users of the classical Bethesda assay. Furthermore, testing of factor VIII inhibitors needs further standardization and improvement of the sensitivity and specificity.

A Practical Concept for Pre-Operative Identification and Improved Management of Patients at Risk for Bleeding

J. Koscielny, S. Ziemer, H. Radtke, P. Sinha, A. Salama, and H. Kiesewetter

Summary

Total of 5649 unselected adult patients were enrolled to identify impaired hemostasis prior to surgical interventions. Each patient was asked to answer a standardized questionnaire of bleeding history. Activated partial thromboplastin time (aPTT), prothrombin time (PT) and platelet counts (PC) including PFA-100 (platelet function analyzer): collagen-epinephrine (C/E) and collagen-ADP (C/ADP) were routinely done in all patients. Additional tests, bleeding time (BT) and von Willebrand factor (vWF: Ag) were performed only in patients with a positive bleeding history and/or evidence of impaired hemostasis, e.g. drug ingestion.

The bleeding history was negative in 5021 patients (88.8%) but positive in the remaining 628 (11.2%). Impaired hemostasis could be verified only in 256 (40.8%) of these patients. The vast majority were identified by PFA-100: C/E (n = 250; 97.7%). The only abnormality found among patients with a negative bleeding history was a prolonged aPTT due to lupus anticoagulant in 9 patients (0.2%). The sensitivity of the PFA-100: collagen-epinephrine was the highest (90.8%) in comparison to the other screening tests (BT, aPTT, PT, vWF: Ag). The positive predictive value of the PFA-100: collagen-epinephrine was high (81.8%), but the negative predictive value was higher (93.4%). We identified 254 out of 5649 unselected patients scheduled for surgery at our hospital as having either acquired (n = 182) or inherited (n = 72) impaired primary hemostasis (platelet dysfunction including von Willebrand disease). All patients were initially pretreated with desmopressin (DDAVP) and further anti-bleeding drugs in case of DDAVP-non-response. Response to DDAVP or subsequent treatment(s) was defined as correction of any one of the abnormal PFA-100 platelet function tests. The non-responders were additionally treated with tranexamic acid or aprotinin; those with von Willebrand disease (vWD) received factor VIII concentrates with von Willebrand factor (vWF). Those still unresponsive to therapy received conjugated estrogens and, as a last attempt, a platelet transfusion.

The administration of DDAVP led to a correction of platelet dysfunction in 229 of the 254 patients treated (90.2%). Tranexamic acid was effective in 12 of 16, aprotinin in 3 of 5 and factor VIII concentrates with vWF in all 4 patients with unresponsive to DDAVP. The remaining 6 patients were pretreated with conjugated estrogens, and 2 of these patients were additionally treated with platelet transfusion. The frequency of blood transfusion was lower, but not statistically significant (9.4%

I. Scharrer/W. Schramm (Ed.)
36th Hemophilia Symposium Hamburg 2005

vs. 12.2%: $p = 0.202$) in preoperatively treated patients with impaired hemostasis than in patients without impaired hemostasis. In a retrospective group, the frequency of blood transfusion was statistically significant higher (89.3% vs. 11.3%: $p < 0.001$) in patients without preoperative correction of impaired than in patients without impaired hemostasis.

Preoperative identification and correction of impaired primary hemostasis is possible in nearly all patients affected, and results in a reduction of homologous blood transfusions.

Introduction

Currently, pre-surgical assessment of a bleeding risk in patients scheduled for elective surgery often consists of a non-standardized bleeding questionnaire and a few standard laboratory tests, i.e. PT, aPTT and a platelet count. Several investigators have questioned the need for routine preoperative hemostatic screening of parameters such as the platelet count (PC), activated partial thromboplastin time (aPTT), prothrombin time (PT), and bleeding time (BT) [1–8]. In view of the fact that primary hemostasis defects, such as von Willebrand Disease and drug-induced platelet deficiencies, are much more frequent than coagulation defects, it is surprising that essentially no screening for primary hemostasis deficiencies is performed. Consequently, many have challenged the current routine [7, 8]. In addition, there still is a scarcity of information on the management of patients with acquired platelet dysfunction.

A few years ago, we decided in the Charité to test the clinical robustness of an improved pre-surgical concept based on a standardized questionnaire to capture patients bleeding risk and history, and addition of a platelet function screening test, as performed with the PFA-100 test system, to the standard laboratory test panel. We aimed to demonstrate that improved pre-surgical identification of patients with a deficiency in hemostasis, in combination with pre-surgical corrective therapy, would enable a practical, as well as improved, as well as cost effective pre-surgical therapeutic patient management.

Methods

A total of 5.649 (2.631 females and 3.018 males, ranging in age between 17 and 87 years) patients scheduled for elective general with vascular, thoracic, orthopedic, gynecology, urology, rhino-laryngology with head-neck or cranio-maxillofacial surgery were recruited in the study from 2nd January 2000 to 2nd January 2001.

Emergency surgeries and patients with pre-existing hemostatic disorders and anticoagulation therapies were excluded. The study was approved by the local ethics committee. Informed consent was obtained from each participant.

On entry, hemostatic screening including PC, aPTT, PT and PFA-100: collagen-epinephrine and collagen-ADP (Dade-Behring, Liederbach, Germany) was done as a part of the preoperative tests ordered by the surgeons and/or anesthesiologists.

Additionally, each patient had a complete history and physical examination by the anesthesiologist who also reviewed the reply of the patient to the bleeding history questionnaire (Fig. 1) given to him on admission. Based on previous studies [9–12] and our experiences the questionnaire was designed to cover the most common symptoms of impaired hemostasis, and to supplement the history and physical examination. The need for further hemostatic testing was determined by the anesthesiologist and hemostatic experts. Patients who seemed (on the basis of history, clinical examination or any question of the questionnaire) to have a impaired hemostasis were classified as having a positive bleeding history and/or evidence of impaired hemostasis, e.g. drug ingestion. If there was no evidence for the presence of a bleeding tendency, patients were classified as having a negative bleeding history.

Standard Bleeding Assessment – Questionnaire

1. Have you ever experienced strong nose bleeds without prior reason?
2. Did you ever have – without trauma – »blue spots« (hematoma) or »small bleedings« (at the torso or other unusual regions of the body)?
3. Did you ever have bleeding of the gums without apparent reason?
4. How often do you have bleedings or »blue spots« (hematoma): more than 1 or 2 times a week or less than1 or 2 times a week?
5. Do you have the impression that you have prolonged bleedings after minor wounds (e.g., razor cuts)?
6. Did you have prolonged or grave bleedings after or during operations (e.g., tonsillectomy, appendectomy, or during labor)?
7. Did you ever have prolonged or grave bleedings after tooth extraction?
8. Did you ever receive blood packs or blood products during an operation? If so, please describe the operation(s):
   ....
   ....
9. Is there a history of bleeding disorders in your family?
10. Do you take analgesic drugs or drugs against rheumatic disease? If so, please specify:
    ....
11. Do you take other drugs? If so, please specify:
    ....
12. Do you have the impression that you have prolonged menstruation (> 7 days) and/or a high frequency of tampon change (only for women)?

Fig. 1. Questionnaire for the detection of an increased risk for bleeding

The following parameters were additionally assessed in all patients with a positive bleeding history and/or evidence of impaired hemostasis, e.g. drug ingestion: bleeding time (Surgicutt, New Jersey, USA) and vWF:Ag (STA LIATEST vWF, Boehringer Mannheim, Germany).

The PFA-100 device simulates primary hemostasis by aspirating citrate-anticoagulated whole blood (3.2%–106mM) and high shear (5000–6000/s) through a 150 µm aperture membrane coated with collagen and either ADP or epinephrine [13]. The reference range of PFA-100: collagen-epinephrine was 72 to 150 sec. The collagen-ADP test had a reference range between 62–100 sec. The blood samples for the PFA-100 were processed within 1 hour after sample collection. The variation coefficient for collagen-epinephrine was 5.9% from day to day (same proband) compared to 5.7%, respectively, for collagen-ADP.

Von Willebrand factor (vWF):Ag was measured using the particle immunoassay (STA LIATEST vWF, Boehringer Mannheim, Germany). The cut-off used to define abnormal and suspected vWF values were $< 50\%$ and 50%–70%, respectively. The vWF multimeric analyses were performed in the follow-up period according to a luminographic procedure [14). The classification followed the guidelines laid down by the »Subcommittee on von Willebrand Factor of the Scientific and Standardization Committee of the International Society on Thrombosis and Haemostasis« [15].

If vWD and drug ingestion were excluded, the following tests were done to confirm the diagnosis of hereditary thrombopathies: platelet morphology, mean platelet volume (distribution of platelets), platelet aggregation using Born`s turbidometric method (Ristocetin, ADP, collagen, arachidon acid), flow cytometry using glycoprotein specific monoclonal antibodies CD 41a, CD 42b, CD 61, CD 62, CD 63 (PLATELET Gp kit; Biocytex, Marseille), before and after TRAP 6-stimulation (thrombocyte-receptor activating peptid 6, Bechem, Heidelberg).

The Mann-Whitney test was used to compare abnormal spot checks. The difference was considered to be significant at a level of $p<0.05$ (»Statistical View 4.5« software). Specifity, sensitivity and predictive values [16, 17, 18] are used accordingly. The effect of changes in the cut-off on the test performances i.e. sensitivity and specifity was determined by using a receiver operating characteristic (ROC) curve. The level of significance was defined as $p < 0.05$ (StatView Program 4.5). A Fisher exact test was used to compare the frequency of transfusion and costs of treatment in the different groups of patients [16, 17]. When all the single values are known, the Bayes theorem can be used to calculate the positive predictive value for »blood transfusions« out of a combination of the different variables. This study fulfills the conditions for the Bayes theorem, namely, independence of the individual tests and application of the tests in parallel [16].

Results

Pre-Surgical Identification of Patients with a Deficiency in Hemostasis [19]

Prospectively, in the course of one year, 5649 patients were included in the program, all scheduled for elective surgery, and all submitted to a **standard bleeding risk**

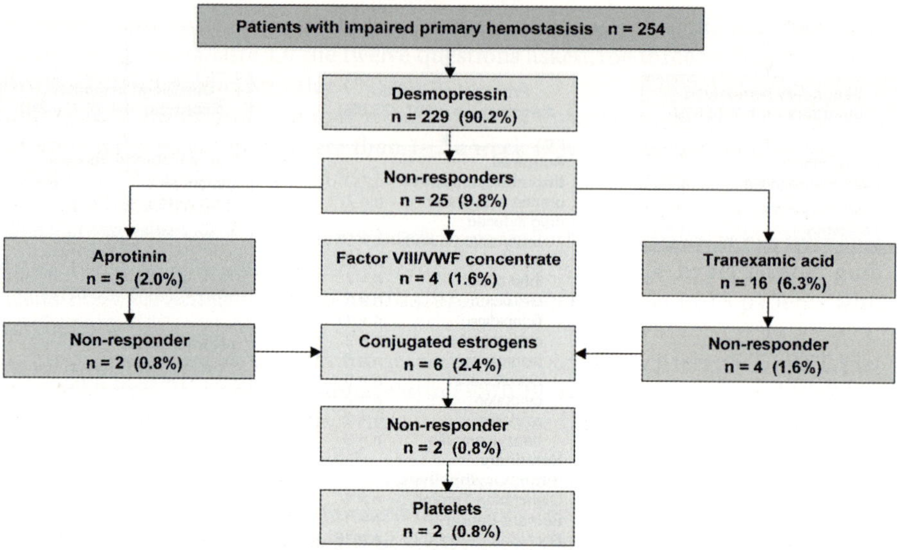

Fig. 4. Results of treatment in patients identified to have acquired and inherited platelet dysfunction including vWD (prospective group)

concentrate (Haemate HS). Any other DDAVP non-responsive patients received appropriate therapy with either Tranexamic Acid, Aprotinin, conjugated estrogens or platelet concentrates (Fig. 4).

During a retrospective study [20] with similar results on identification of patients with confirmed risk for bleeding, based on the SBA and the laboratory test panel including PFA-100 Col/Epi test, we showed a post-operative blood transfusion need in 89.3% when such patients did not receive pre-surgical prophylactic therapy (Fig. 5). In a retrospective similar group at the same hospital in 1999 we preoperatively identified 317 out of 5102 unselected patients scheduled for surgery at our hospital as having either acquired (n = 299) or inherited (n = 18) impaired primary hemostasis (platelet dysfunction including von Willebrand disease). A total of 311 patients with impaired hemostasis (n = 317) exhibited abnormal PFA-100: collagen-epinephrine, and the majority of these patients (n = 283; 89.3%) received blood transfusions. Both PFA-100 tests showed normal platelet function in the remaining patients (n = 4785).

During the follow-up of the patients receiving pre-surgical therapy in the above study cohort, the number of patients requiring post-operative blood transfusion was 9,4%; much lower than the 89.3% in the non treated retrospective group, and a bit lower, although not significant, than the 12,2% of the patients with negative SBA and negative laboratory tests. Also the patients with a positive SBA and negative laboratory tests did not show higher blood loss and transfusion need compared to the all-negative controls, illustrating the safety of the proposed clinical algorithm.

Discussion

In agreement with the results of previous studies, our study clearly shows that primary hemostatic disorders are much more common than secondary disorders. The vast majority of patients at increased risk for bleeding complications could not be identified by routine screening for platelet count (PC), prothrombin time (PT), and activated partial thromboplastin time (aPTT). These tests did not identify a single patient without prior suspicion of impaired hemostasis (positive bleeding history and/or evidence of impaired hemostasis, e.g. drug ingestion). PC and PT were normal in all patients with a negative bleeding history, and all recognizable aPTT abnormalities in these patients were related to lupus inhibitors, that reflected in our patients an increased risk of thrombosis and not of bleeding complications. Moreover, only two patients with a positive bleeding history and/or evidence of impaired hemostasis, e.g. drug ingestion, (0.3%) had plasma disorders that were detectable only by PT (one patient with dysfibrinogenemia, and one with hereditary factor VII deficiency). Similarly, the aPTT and PC did not provide any additional information. The former test was abnormal in 24 of 39 patients with vWD who also showed platelet dysfunction in 37 cases. Only two patients with vWD were undetectable by both types of PFA-100. The PC was significantly decreased in two patients with liver cirrhosis, both of whom also had detectable platelet dysfunction. Even if the bleeding time was added to the routine preoperative screening tests, about 20–30% of the patients with an increased risk of bleeding complications would escape detection by all these testing procedures. Thus, as has previously been suggested by others [1–9], these tests should only be used in cases where indicated. In contrast, the bleeding history assessment using a standardized questionnaire and tests of platelet function were highly predictive. Both methods seem to supplement each other. All patients with positive bleeding histories related to primary or combined hemostatic disorders could be identified using PFA-100: collagen-epinephrine and/or PFA-100: collagen-ADP. It is also worth mentioning that the platelet function tests detected abnormalities in 14 patients who initially failed to report antiplatelet drug use. On the other hand, many patients reported a history of bleeding, but did not appear to have a hemostatic disorder (n = 372). None of the laboratory tests revealed any abnormalities, and none of these patients developed bleeding that could be attributed to a hemostatic disorder.

In agreement with the findings of other groups [22–27], the PFA-100 is clearly superior to the bleeding time (BT). In addition, both PFA-100 tests showed high positive predictive values, and high negative predictive values (81.8% and 93.4% for the PFA-100: collagen-epinephrine, and 77.3% and 79.4% for the PFA-100: collagen-ADP). The sensitivity of the epinephrine technique was slightly superior to that of collagen-ADP. A similar discordance was recently reported by other investigators [26–28]. This discrepancy was related either to aspirin ingestion (n = 87 versus 46) or vWD (n = 52 versus 42).

The objective of the present study was to design a concept for prophylactic correction of acquired and congenital platelet dysfunctions capable of causing significant bleeding during surgical interventions. We succeeded in normalizing the hemostatic defect in nearly all patients studied. Conditions associated with plasmatic defects were corrected by administration of fibrinogen and factor VII; the two patients affected had congenital dysfibrinogenemia and factor VII deficiency. The remaining patients had acquired (more common) or inherited (less common) platelet dysfunctions that could be corrected by DDAVP in almost all cases (90.2%). In agreement with the findings in the literature [21, 29–34], 84 to 100 % of our patients responded to DDAVP (Fig. 4).

The small number of cases studied may be the reason for the low response observed in certain cases (e.g., uremic patients or those receiving benzylpenicillin). It is still unclear whether DDAVP may also help in the management of patients with thrombasthenia or Bernard-Soulier syndrome; the two such patients in our group were unresponsive. Interestingly, the majority of non-responders to DDAVP did respond to aprotinin, tranexamic acid or conjugated estrogens. Only two patients required platelet transfusions; both of these patients had liver cirrhosis.

The reason for our preferential use of DDAVP over aprotinin or tranexamic acid is the high cost of aprotinin and the relatively high frequency of severe side effects of both drugs. Adverse reactions to DDAVP are usually mild, whereas those related to the other two drugs can be dangerous [30, 35]. In the present study, a relatively large number of patients treated with DDAVP developed facial flushing, one developed hyponatremia, and one with a history of epilepsy had an epileptic seizure. In comparison, none of the 16 patients treated with tranexamic acid developed side

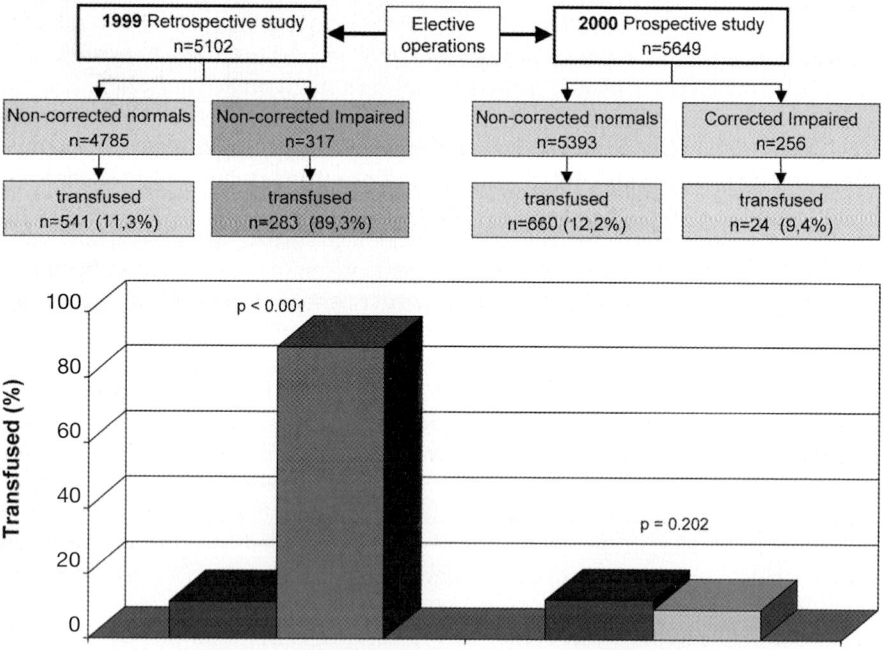

Fig. 5. Frequency of blood transfusions in patients who underwent selective operation without (retrospective data) and with pretreatment of impaired hemostasis (prospective study)

effects, whereas two of the five patients treated with aprotinin developed significant adverse reactions. Since the effect of tranexamic acid and aprotinin on platelet dysfunction seems to be comparable to that of DDAVP, these drugs can all be used at the discretion of the attending physician based on his or her own experience.

The effects of DDAVP, aprotinin, and tranexamic acid could be detected within 30 minutes of administration, whereas conjugated estrogens required 15 to 30 minutes to take effect. DDAVP may lead to improvement of hemostasis by increasing the levels of coagulation factor VIII, vWF and tissue plasminogen activator [8]. However, the mechanism by which aprotinin, tranexamic acid and conjugated estrogens influence platelet function remains somewhat unclear. There is evidence showing that aprotinin and tranexamic acid may increase the expression of GP Ib-receptor on platelets, thereby improving platelet adhesion [36, 37]. Conjugated estrogens also seem to increase platelet aggregation [38, 39]. The improvement of platelet function by these drugs was confirmed by the functional assays, particularly the collagen-epinephrine test.

Although the present study does not have data from a prospective control group for comparison, correction of the hemostatic defects was found to decrease the need for blood transfusion dramatically. The frequency of blood transfusions did not differ significantly among the groups of patients, but was lower in preoperatively treated patients with platelet dysfunctions than in their untreated counterparts (Fig. 5).

Cost Effectiveness of the New Pre-Surgical Screening and Management Concept

The SBA demonstrated high specificity in identifying patients at low risk for bleeding during surgery. These findings strongly suggest that routine laboratory testing of patients with negative SBA is not indicated. In contrast, adding PFA-100 Col/Epi testing to standard coagulation test panel for screening patients with positive SBA was clearly beneficial. A pre-surgical screening concept, represented by testing of PT, APTT, platelet count, and the PFA-100 Col/Epi closure time in case of positive SBA (11.2%), and refraining from laboratory testing in case of negative SBA (88.8%), would result in a cost reduction of around 15 million Euro/year in Germany alone (based on 5 million elective surgeries/year).

A pre-surgical correction of all identified hemostatic deficiencies, primarily by DDAVP-therapy and monitored by normalized PFA-100 test results, has been shown to improve patient management. Moreover, the proposed algorithm is again cost effective. Currently, average costs (tests, transfusion need) of patients without hemostatic deficiencies are around 190 €/case. In patients with an identified and corrected defect, these costs increase to around 340 €/case. In case no pre-surgical correction of hemostasis is applied, the initial laboratory costs remain at 190 €/case but will in many patients increase 5-fold to around 1700 €/case because of transfusion requirement and/or other post-surgical bleeding management. In this consideration patients of all operative disciplines are included. Based on a model of 3 million major surgeries/year, cost savings by ensuring adequate hemostasis prior to surgery will be around 20–25 million €/year in Germany.

Conclusion

We have shown that improved patient management is feasible by the introduction of a practical and cost effective pre-surgical concept, characterized by the usage of a standardized bleeding risk assessment (SBA) and improved pre-surgical identification and correction of hemostasis deficiencies. The concept will require testing with Col/Epi of those patients having a positive SBA, and correction of the deficiency with DDAVP, as can be confirmed with a normalized PFA-100 Col/Epi test result. Preoperative correction of impaired primary hemostasis is possible in nearly all patients affected, and results in a reduction of homologous blood transfusions. Nation wide adaptation of this practical and improved concept would annually save up to 40 million Euro in Germany.

References

1. Eika C, Havig O, Godal HC. The value of preoperative hemostatic screening. Scand J Haematol 1978; 21: 349.
2. Kaplan E, Sheiner L, Boeckmann A, Roizen M, Beal S, Cohen S, Nicoll D. The usefulness of preoperative laboratory screening. JAMA 1985; 253: 3576.
3. Barber A, Green D, Galluzzo T, Tsào C-H. The bleeding time as a preoperative screening test. Am J Med 1985; 78: 761.
4. Rohrer MJ, Michelotti MC, Nahrwold DL. A prospective evaluation of the efficacy of preoperative coagulation testing. Ann. Surg 1988; 208: 554.
5. Rodgers RP, Levin J. A critical reappraisal of the bleeding time. Sem Throm Haemost 1990; 16: 1.
6. Lind SE. The bleeding time does not predict surgical bleeding. Blood 1991; 77: 2547.
7. Velanovich V. The value of routine preoperative laboratory testing in predicting postoperative complications: A multivariate analysis. Surgery 1991; 109: 236.
8. Macpherson CR, Jacobs P, Dent DM. Abnormal perioperative hemorrhage in asymptomatic patients is not predicted by laboratory testing. S Afr Med J 1993; 83: 106.
9. Houry S, Georgeac C, Hay JM, Fingerhut A, Boudet JJ. A prospective multicenter evaluation of preoperative hemostatic screening tests. The American Journal of Surgery 1995; 170: 75.
10. Bowie EJW. Recognition of easily missed bleeding diseases. Mayo Clin Proc 1982; 57: 263.
11. Rapaport S. Preoperative hemostatic evaluation: Which tests, if any ? Blood 1983; 61: 229.
12. Borzotta AP, Keeling MM. Value of the preoperative history as an indicator of hemostatic disorders. Ann Surg 1984; 200: 648.
13. Srámek A, Eikenboom J, Briet E, Vandenbroucke J, Rosendaal F. Usefulness of patient interview in bleeding disorders. Arch Intern Med 1995; 155: 1409.
14. Böck M, de Haan J, Beck KH, Gutensohn K, Hertfelder HJ, Karger R, Heim MU, Beeser H, Weber D, Kretschmer V. Standardization of the PFA-100® platelet function test in 105 mmol/l bufffered citrate: effect of gender, smoking, and oral contraceptives. Br J Haematol 1999; 106: 898.
15. Budde U, Schneppenheim R, Plendl H, Dent J, Ruggeri ZM, Zimmermann TS. Luminographic detection of von Willebrand factor multimers in agarose gels and on nitrocellulose membranes. Thromb Haemost 1990; 63: 312.
16. Sadler J.E. A revised classification of von Willebrand disease. Thromb Haemost 1994; 71: 520.
17. Sachs L. Angewandte Statistik. Springer Verlag, Berlin – Heidelberg – New York 1984; 1.
18. Büttner J. Die Beurteilung des diagnostischen Wertes klinisch-chemischer Untersuchungen. J Clin Chem Biochem 1977; 15: 1.

19. Galen S, Gambino SR. Norm und Normabweichung klinischer Daten. Gustav Fischer Verlag, Stuttgart 1979; 4.
20. Koscielny J, Ziemer S, Radtke H, Pruss A, Schmutzler M, Sinha P, Salama A, Kiesewetter H, Latza R. A Practical Concept for Preoperative Identification in Patients with Impaired Primary Hemostasis. Clinical and Applied Thrombosis/Hemostasis 2004, 10 (3): 195–204.
21. Koscielny J, Tempelhoff GF, Ziemer S, Radtke H, Schmutzler M, Sinha P, Salama A, Kiesewetter H, Latza R. A Practical Concept for Preoperative Management in Patients with Impaired Primary Hemostasis. Clinical and Applied Thrombosis/Hemostasis 2004, 10 (2): 155–166.
22. Koscielny et al. Consensus use of desmopressin and antifibrinolytics in three university clinics. Anaesthesia 1998
23. Kundu SK, Sio R, Mitu A, Ostgaard RA. Evaluation of platelet function by PFA-100. Clin. Chem 1994; 40: 1827.
24. Despotis GJ, Levine V, Filos KS: Evaluation of a new, point-of-care test that measures PAF-mediated acceleration of coagulation in cardiac surgical patients. Anesthesiology 1996; 85: 1311.
25. Mammen E, Comp P, Gosselin R, Greenberg C, Hoots W, Kessler C, Larkin E, Liles D, Nugent D. PFA-100TM System: A new method for assessment of platelet dysfunction. Sem Thromb Haemost 1998; 24: 195.
26. Cattaneo M, Federici AB, Lecchi A, Agati B, Lombardi R, Stabile F, Bucciarelli P. Evaluation of the PFA-100 system in the diagnosis and therapeutic monitoring of patients with von Willebrand disease. Thromb Haemost 1999; 82 (1): 35.
27. Harrison P, Robinson MS, Mackie IJ, Joseph J, McDonald SJ, Liesner R, Savidge GF, Pasi J, Machin SJ. Performance of the platelet function analyser PFA-100 in testing abnormalities of primary hemostasis. Blood Coagul Fibrinolysis 1999; 10: 25.
28. Cattaneo M, Lecchi A, Agati B, Lombardi R, Zighetti ML. Evaluation of platelet function with the PFA-100 system in patients with congenital defects of platelet secretion. Thromb Res 1999; 96: 213.
29. Kundu SK, Heilmann EJ, Sio R, Garcia C, Davidson RS, Ostgaard RA. Description of an in vitro platelet function analyser – PFA-100. Sem Thromb Haemost 1995, 21 (Suppl. 2): 106.
30. Cattaneo M. Desmopressin in the treatment of patients with defects of platelet function. Haematologica 2002; 87 (11): 1122.
31. Mannucci PM. Desmopressin in the treatment of bleeding disorders: the first 20 years. Blood 1997; 90: 2515.
32. Cohen AJ, Kessler CM, Ewenstein BM. Management of von Willebrand disease: a survey on current clinical practice from the hemophilia centers of North America. Hemophilia 2001; 7: 235.
33. Ehl S, Severin T, Sutor AH. DDAVP treatment in children with hemophilia B. Br J Hematol 2000; 111: 1260.
34. Sloand EM, Alyono D, Klein HG. 1-deamino-8-D-arginine vasopressin (DDAVP) increases platelet membrane expression of glycoprotein Ib in patients with disorders of platelet function and after cardiopulmonary bypass. Am J Hematol 1994; 46: 199.
35. Despotis GJ, Levine V, Saleem R et al. Use of point-of-care test in identification of patients who can benefit from desmopressin during cardiac surgery: a randomised controlled trial. Lancet 1999; 354: 106.
36. Mannucci PM, Carlsson S, Harris AS. Desmopressin, surgery and thrombosis. Thromb Hemost 1994; 71: 154.
37. Fremes SE. Metaanalysis of prophylactic drug treatment in the prevention of postoperative bleeding. Ann Thorac Surg 1994; 58: 1580.
38. Soslau G, Horrow J, Brodsky I. The effect of tranexamic acid on platelet ADP during extracorporal circulation. Am J Hematol 1991; 38: 113.
39. Tsur H, Rasner C, Shafir R et al. The hemostatic effect of conjugated water-soluble estrogenes in rats. Ann Plast Surg 1982; 8: 387.
40. Elkeles RS, Hampton J, Mitchell J. Effect of estrogen on human platelet behaviour. Lancet 1968, 2: 315.

Intravascular Tissue Factor in Cord vs Adult Whole Blood

G. Cvirn, M. Köstenberger, J. Kutschera, U. Ferstl, W. Muntean,
P. Sedlmayr, G. Juergens, and S. Gallistl

Introduction

Recent in vitro studies using low amounts of recombinant lipidated tissue factor (TF) to initiate clot formation revealed, in accordance with the clinical observation, efficient thrombin generation and short clotting times of neonatal plasma. It has been shown that this high coagulability of cord plasma is attributable to the concomitant low anticoagulant action of the three inhibitors activated protein C, tissue factor pathway inhibitor, and antithrombin.

However, in all these experiments activation of plasma samples was performed by addition of same amounts of recombinant lipidated TF (e.g., 5 pM) to both cord and adult plasma samples. This, apparently, does not reflect in vivo conditions. Therefore, the aim of our study was to compare the capability of neonatal whole blood (WB) to form and express intravascular TF with that of adult WB by evaluating TF mRNA levels, TF exposure on the cell membrane of the monocyte, and TF procoagulant activity in the absence and presence of a stimulus (lipopolysaccharide, LPS). TF mRNA levels were determined by means of reverse transcription-polymerase chain reaction (RT-PCR), exposure of TF on the outer leaflet of monocytes was evaluated by means of flow-cytometric analysis, and the procoagulant action of the intravascular TF was studied by means of thrombelastography (TEG).

Results

GAPDH mRNA expression in cord vs adult WB GAPDH mRNA expression was utilized as internal standard. The expected single band of the RT-PCR products (265 bp) was always observed in both cord (n = 12) and adult (n = 10) WB samples. Whereby, GAPDH mRNA expression was significantly higher in unstimulated cord than in unstimulated adult WB. Quantity of RT-PCR products in cord WB was 349 ± 92 % of adult value. GAPDH mRNA expression remained unmodified whether WB samples of neonatal or adult origin were stimulated or not with LPS.

TF mRNA Expression in Cord vs Adult WB

RT-PCR products were obtained as a single band of 282 bp, the expected size of the TF cDNA fragment amplification. TF mRNA expression was significantly higher in

I. Scharrer/W. Schramm (Ed.)
36th Hemophilia Symposium Hamburg 2005

unstimulated cord than in unstimulated adult WB samples. Addition of LPS resulted in enhanced TF mRNA expression in both cord and adult WB samples. Whereby, the quantity of RT-PCR products was increased by 439 ± 112 % in cord WB samples and by 797 ± 215 % in adult WB samples. When normalized to the corresponding values from GAPDH signal, quantity of TF RT-PCR products in unstimulated cord WB was ~ 1.5 times higher than in unstimulated adult WB.

Monocyte TF Antigen Expression in Cord vs Adult WB Samples Evaluated by Means of Flow Cytometry

The monocyte population in both cord (n = 12) and adult (n = 10) WB samples was identified by gating on CD 14 positivity. The monocyte count was significantly higher in cord than in adult WB samples (661 ± 153 vs 325 ± 114 counts out of 10 000 total events, $p < 0.05$). Furthermore, significantly higher monocyte TF antigen expression was observed in cord compared to adult WB samples in the absence of LPS. After LPS-incubation (3 h, 10 μg/ml), the median of the monocyte fluorescence intensity curve was shifted to the right by 28.82 ± 3.11 units in experiments performed in cord WB and by 19.16 ± 2.54 units in experiments performed in adult WB in relation to the irrelevant, isotype-matched mouse IgG. Thus, the shift of the median of the monocyte fluorescence intensity curve due to the LPS-induced TF expression in cord WB was comparable with that in adult WB samples (19.40 ± 3.01 vs 15.11 ± 2.33 fluorescence units), indicating approximately same ability of neonatal and adult monocytes to express TF upon LPS-stimulation.

Procoagulant Activity of LPS-Induced TF Evaluated by Means of TEG

In the absence of LPS, clotting times (CTs) and clot formation times (CFTs) were significantly shorter in cord than in adult WB samples (527 ± 41 vs 592 ± 23 s, and 178 ± 23 vs 226 ± 18 s, $p < 0.05$). MCF was significantly lower in cord vs adult WB samples (50.6 ± 1.3 vs 52.9 ± 1.4 mm, $p < 0.05$). Reduction of CT due to LPS incubation (3 h, 10 μg/ml) was significantly higher in cord than in adult WB samples. CT was reduced by 29.65 ± 3.35 % in cord WB (Figure 1, panel A) and by 12.03 ± 6.23 % in adult WB (Figure 1, panel A, $p < 0.05$) compared to control (PBS, 3 h). This procoagulant activity was largely blocked by incubation with antibody against human TF (20 μg/ml, data not shown). Reduction of CFT (Figure 1, panel B) and increase of MCF (Figure 1, panel C) due to LPS incubation in cord WB was comparable with that in adult WB.

Conclusions

We found significantly higher TF (and GAPDH, internal standard) mRNA expression, TF antigen expression on the monocyte membrane, and shorter CTs examined by means of TEG in native (non-stimulated) cord vs adult WB. We speculate that the

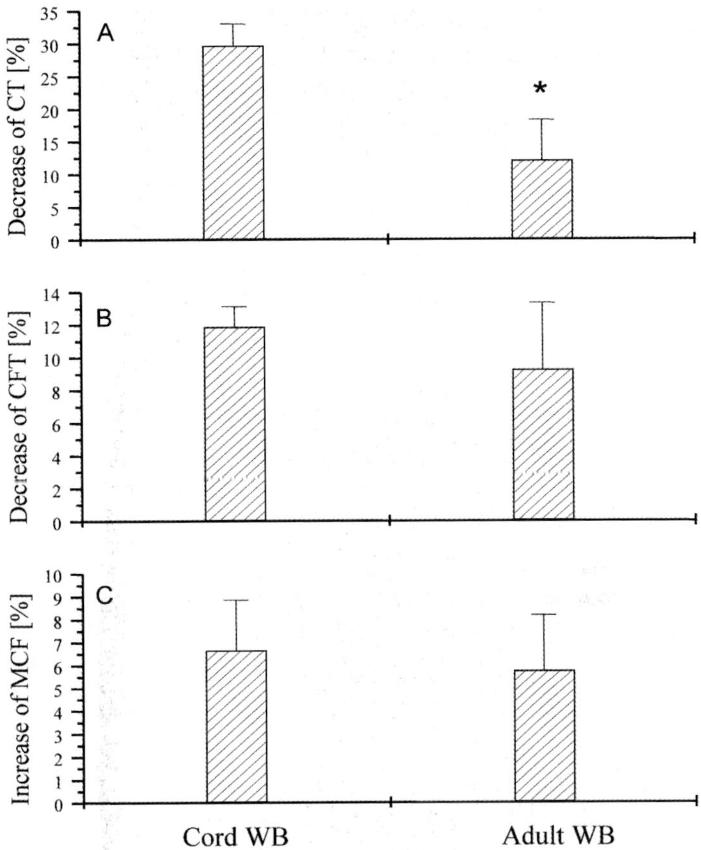

Fig. 1. Effect of LPS on TEG parameters in cord and adult WB samples. LPS incubation of cord and adult WB samples (3 h, 10 µg/ml) resulted in decreased CTs (panel A), decreased CFTs (panel B), and increased MCF (panel C). * $p < 0.05$.

high basal levels of GAPDH and TF mRNA present in human cord WB samples are attributable to the metabolic active state of neonates, e.g., increased cell proliferation in neonates compared with adults. Furthermore, we found higher TF antigen expression on the neonatal vs. adult monocyte membrane and shorter CTs of native cord vs adult WB. We demonstrate that the high TF expression and exposure levels in cord WB are paralleled by significantly shorter clotting times (CT) of native cord vs adult WB and by significantly more pronounced shortening of CTs in cord vs adult WB due to LPS-stimulation. We assume that the higher procoagulant TF activity in cord vs adult WB due to LPS-stimulation is attributable not only to the higher surface TF expression on the neonatal vs adult monocyte but also to the significantly higher number of monocytes present in cord vs adult WB.

In conclusion, we demonstrate high levels of TF mRNA expression, TF exposure on the monocyte membrane and TF activity in WB of neonatal origin prior and after LPS incubation. Together with already reported higher ability of the newborn endothelium to generate TF we assume that significantly higher amounts of active TF are available in the newborn's circulation compared with adults.

Perioperative Coagulation Screening in Children – Reasons and Results

C. Bidlingmaier, F. Sax, and K. Kurnik

Background

Laboratory assessment tests of hemostasis in children are conducted for many reasons. In most patients they are performed prior to surgery, in some because of a positive family history or patient's clinical history suspicious for an inherited or acquired bleeding disorder, in others just accidentally during routine blood drawing because of infections or during hospitalization. Because of the commonness of coagulation screening tests and the high proportion of pathological results, the workup of prolonged prothrombin time (PT) and especially activated partial thromboplastin time (aPTT) has become one of the most frequent reasons for referrals to pediatric coagulation laboratories. Our study aimed to evaluate the reasons for the initial blood drawing and the results of an extended workup of pathological coagulation profiles, especially of prolonged aPTTs prior to surgery.

Patients and Methods

We retrospectively reviewed 501 medical records of patients that were consecutively referred to our outpatient clinic during 2002 and 2005 for extended hemostatic assessments because of a preoperatively or accidentally found altered coagulation profile or a clinical or anamnestic history of bleeding. The reason for referral, patient and family history of bleeding and the history of surgery were recorded as well as the results of our standardized scheme to rule out coagulopathies, i.e. PT, aPTT, fibrinogen and platelet count, results of the platelet function analyzer (PFA 100), lupus-anticoagulant screening, cardiolipin antibodies and β2 glycoprotein antibodies and factor (F) XIII. In case of previously reported aPTT prolongation additionally FVIII, IX, XI, XII, Ristocetin-Cofactor activity and von-Willebrand-factor (vWF) antigen as well as analysis of vWF multimers were recorded and for PT prolongation FII, V, VII and X. 255 patients referred for extended coagulation workup prior to surgery were additionally contacted by phone and questioned for bleeding complications or measures taken perioperatively to prevent those. All data were recorded in a database and anonymized directly after data collection.

I. Scharrer/W. Schramm (Ed.)
36th Hemophilia Symposium Hamburg 2005

Results

Reason for Referral

Of 501 patients 291 (51%) were referred because of a prolonged aPTT, 17 (3%) because of a prolonged PT, 100 (20%) because of a personal history of bleeding without previous blood drawing and 52 (10%) because of a positive family history of bleeding. 41 (6%) were referred because of others reasons, such as medication with Valproat (Fig. 1).

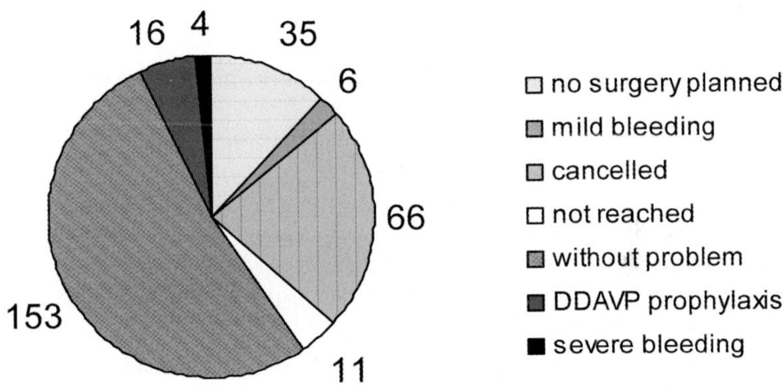

Fig. 1. Clinical Outcome of 291 patients with prolonged aPTT (determined by telephone calls)

Of the 291 patients referred after an initially prolonged aPTT the coagulation profile was assessed in 250 patients (86%) because of planned surgery (in 70% planned ear-nose and throat surgery), in 8% accidentally and in 6% because of a positive patients or family history.

Control of the aPTT

The main limitation to use global tests of coagulations as predictors for an increased bleeding risk is their sensitivity to preanalytic bias. Whereas all of the referring physicians had to send the blood to a laboratory the blood drawn in our outpatient clinic is measured in the laboratory only minutes after collection. Because of this and the exclusion of other known preanalytic sources of error by using standardized procedures to obtain and handle blood samples we found 190 of the previously 291 prolonged aPTTs to be normalized at our institution (65.3%). On the other side, normal aPTT values at our institution did not predict normal single factor concentrations. The lengths of the initial aPTT measured outside our hospital and the lengths of the aPTT measured in our outpatient clinic did not correlate.

Extended aPTT Workup

For all patients with previously reported prolonged aPTTs the laboratory examinations described in the methods section were performed. Only in 7 patients (2.4%) a relevant coagulopathy was confirmed. In 5 von-Willebrand-disease (vWD) type 2 was found, in 1 acquired vWD and in 1 subhemophilia A. There was no correlation between the length of aPTT and the presence and severity of the found coagulopathy. 2/3 of the patients showed either signs of an unspecific »lupus inhibitor«, defined by more than 2 lowered factors and positive lupus-anticoagulants screening or alterations of the coagulation system that do not lead to an increased bleeding risk (i.e. FXII deficiency). The rest of the patients showed no alterations of the plasmatic hemostasis.

Operative Course of Patients with Previously Prolonged PTT

153 of 255 children in which surgery was initially planned finally underwent surgery without problems. On the other side surgery was cancelled in 66 patients although extended hemostatic assessment did not reveal a significant coagulopathy (25.9%). Only 10 children bled during or after surgery, 6 mildly (defined as prolonged hospitalization because of mild bleeding symptoms but no reoperation or transfusion necessary) and 4 severely (defined as reoperation necessary).

Of these 10 bleeding patients 7 bled without a coagulopathy found despite extensive workup, 3 of these needed reoperation. 1 patient with vWD type I bled severely and needed reoperation, but the treating surgeon suspected rather a surgical problem than the coagulopathy to be the reason of the hemorrhage. Two patients with vWD type 2 needed prolonged monitoring because of mild bleeding symptoms despite adequate substitution with factor concentrates.

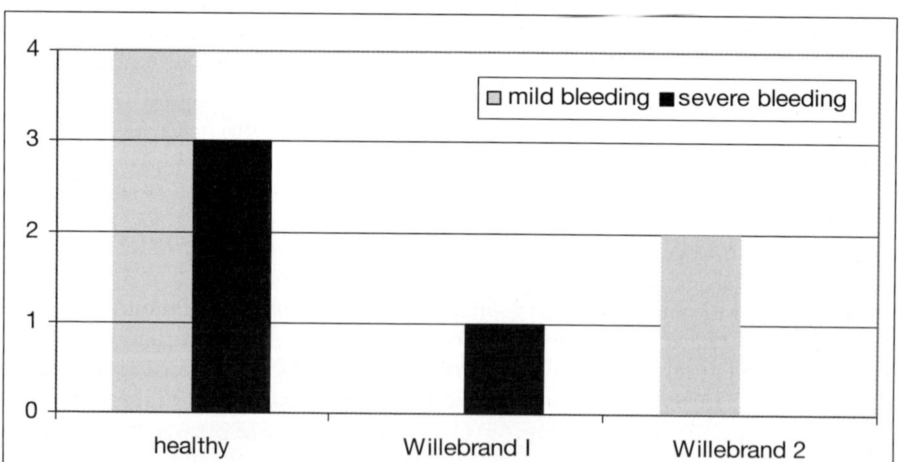

Fig. 2. Laboratory diagnosis of 10 patients bleeding after surgery with initially prolonged aPTT

Extended Coagulation Workup after Bleeding during Surgery

Of the 501 patients referred to our hospital during the study period 27 had previously suffered from severe bleeding during or after surgery despite an initially normal coagulation profile. Extended coagulation workup revealed no coagulopathy in 19 patients (70%) but vWD type I in 5 (18%) and 1 patient with thrombopathy, mild FVII deficiency or FXIII deficiency respectively. None of the 27 patients showed prolonged aPTT or PT during workup.

Discussion

Our retrospective analysis of 501 patients supports the thesis that (preoperative) clotting tests (aPTT, PT) neither do rule out the presence of a relevant coagulopathy nor predict an increased risk for bleeding complications [1]. Of 255 children with a preoperatively prolonged aPTT 10 (3.9%) bled during surgery, 7 of those without a relevant coagulopathy found during extensive workup. The bleeding frequency in our cohort was therefore comparable to the bleeding frequency in other patients undergoing surgery [2]. Otherwise we saw 27 children that had bled severely during or after surgery which did not show a prolonged aPTT or PT at any time. Of these children 8 (30%) did suffer from a relevant coagulopathy previously undetected by simple screening tests. We therefore agree with others that the routine preoperative assessment of aPTT and PT is of little value to detect coagulopathies or to predict the bleeding risk in a previously healthy child without any (family) history of bleeding [3–5]. The main reasons for aPTT prolongations are either preanalytic problems [6] or alterations of the coagulation system that are not correlated to an increased bleeding risk [7] (e.g. FXII deficiency or an unspecific inhibitor such as lupus-anticoagulants).

Moreover we stress that a normal aPTT might lead to a false illusion of safety whereas normal aPTT values do not predict a normal bleeding risk. Since most patients with vWD do not show a prolonged aPTT these patients at risk won't be identified by routine coagulation tests. To identify these patients a standardized history and the analysis of laboratory values specific for vWD remain crucial.

We also highlight that coagulation tests should only be performed if indicated. Prolonged aPTTs found accidentally after routine blood drawing because of simple infections or hospitalization do rarely mark an actual coagulopathy and lead to uncertainty for patients, parents and physicians, followed by the costly necessity for an extended workup to rule out this suspicion.

Bleeding complications are one of many risks associated with surgery. The exact incidence of bleeding complications appears to be low but is not yet fully known. It is therefore necessary to mitigate this risk by other strategies than insufficient laboratory screening tests, although clinical history alone might not fulfill this task [8]. It is also necessary to learn more about bleeding complications, their incidence and reasons and to adequately inform parents about this risk and measures to be taken if bleeding occurs.

We therefore conclude that the routine testing of aPTT/PT does not increase the safety for children undergoing surgery. In fact exactly taken clinical histories following a standardized questionnaire [6] and in selected cases – were the patient's history cannot be taken (e.g. the child is too young or there is no possibility to question the family) – an extended laboratory workup including vWF and Ristocetin-Cofactor activity seems more reasonable. Since in the end it is impossible to rule out bleeding complications the indication for surgery has to be clear and particular care has to be taken to monitor children after surgery.

Since prospective data on this issue are rare a prospective multicenter study is ongoing in Germany to increase the evidence of this thesis.

Acknowledgement. This work was supported by an unrestricted research grant from ZLB Behring (Hattersheim, Germany). The investigators analyzed and interpreted all data, analysis was not influenced by the funding source.

References

1. Chee YL, Greaves M. Role of coagulation testing in predicting bleeding risk. Hematol J 2003;4(6):373–8.
2. Windfuhr JP, Chen YS, Remmert S. Hemorrhage following tonsillectomy and adenoidectomy in 15,218 patients. Otolaryngol Head Neck Surg 2005;132(2):281–6.
3. Klinge J, Eberl W, Lischtzki G. Die präoperative aPTT-Verlängerung. pädiat prax 2004;65:57–66.
4. Derkay CS. A cost-effective approach for preoperative hemostatic assessment in children undergoing adenotonsillectomy. Arch Otolaryngol Head Neck Surg 2000;126(5):688.
5. Kang J, Brodsky L, Danziger I, et al. Coagulation profile as a predictor for post-tonsillectomy and adenoidectomy (T + A) hemorrhage. Int J Pediatr Otorhinolaryngol 1994;28(2-3):157–65.
6. Eberl W, Wendt I, Schroeder H-G. Präoperatives Screening auf Gerinnnungsstörungen vor Adenotomie und Tonsillektomie. Klin Pädiatr 2005;217:20–24.
7. Kitchens CS. To bleed or not to bleed? Is that the question for the PTT? J Thromb Haemost 2005;3(12):2607–11.
8. Gabriel P, Mazoit X, Ecoffey C. Relationship between clinical history, coagulation tests, and perioperative bleeding during tonsillectomies in pediatrics. J Clin Anesth 2000;12(4):288–91.

Thrombin Generation in Children

A. Siegemund, S. Horneff, and R. Schobess

Introduction

Newborns and children have lower concentrations of coagulation factors and inhibitors than adults. The range of thrombin concentration varies from 20 % for premature newborns and 35 % for newborns to 80 % in children [1] resulting in a lower thrombin generation (TG). But TG not only depends on age. Also patients with hemophilia A and B show a lower TG [2, 3]. The TG is very variable in patients with hemophilia, but also in healthy controls [4]. However, in hemophilia patients TG correlation between TG and FVIII concentration can be calculated only on an individual base.

There have been many attempts to correlate bleeding tendency and factor VIII consumption with TG. Assuming that the substitution of factor VIII is better documented in children compared to adults, we measured the TG in children in relation to levels of factor VIII for further investigations.

Materials and Methods

Measurement of TG was done with the original Hemker method with reagents from Thrombinoscope BV and with the Thrombinoscope software package (version 3.0.0.29, calibrated automated thrombogram). In addition an in house method and calculation procedure was used as described previously [2]. We determined the ETP (endogenous thrombin potential) and the maximum reaction velocity (V_{max}). All measurements were done in platelet poor plasma (PPP).

Plasma from children from the hemophilia center, University Hospital, Martin Luther University Halle-Wittenberg was studied. All children have documented hemophilia (hemophilia A 12 patients, hemophilia B 2 patients) or von Willebrand disease (type I/II: 8 patients, type III: 2 patients) with different severity of the underlying disease. The patients were repeatedly investigated at different time intervals. The results are expressed as standard deviation and standard error of the mean (S.E.M.).

I. Scharrer/W. Schramm (Ed.)
36th Hemophilia Symposium Hamburg 2005

Results

The corresponding FVIII levels in children younger than 6 years were comparable to those older than 6 years, whereas TG was influenced by age. Children younger than 6 years had a lower TG than older children (768 nM vs 872 nM). These differences are significant ($p < 0.001$) regarding the amount of generated thrombin and also the velocity of the reaction ($p < 0.001$). These results were expected because of the lower reference ranges especially for antithrombin, protein C and S in children. Also α_2 macroglobulin plays a different role in young children and newborns. In infants the elevated α_2 macroglobulin level compensates in part for the low levels of antithrombin.

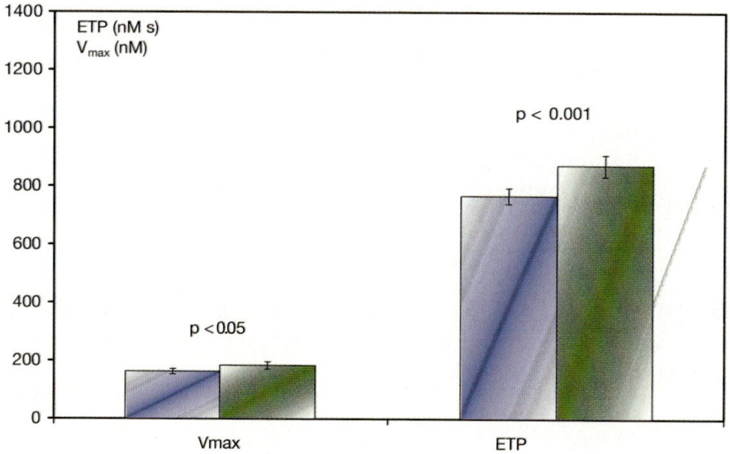

Fig. 1. Age dependent TG (expressed as V_{max} and endogenous thrombin potential, ETP)

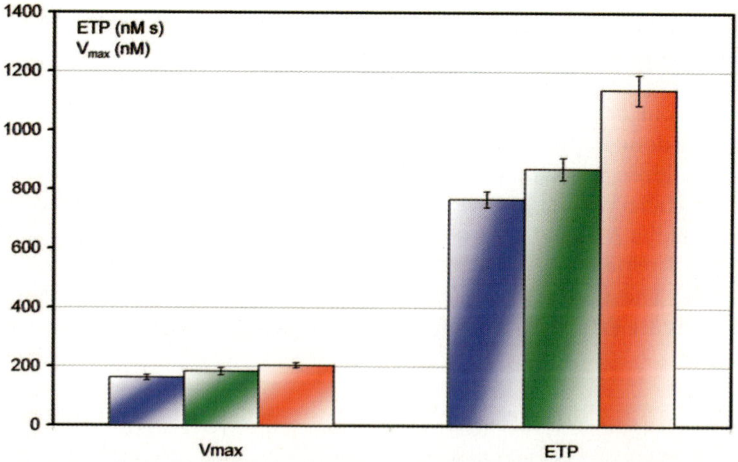

Fig. 2. ETP and V_{max} in children of different age categories compared to adults

Adults have a further increase in TG (Fig. 2). The corresponding levels of FVIII are 43.2 ± 7.3% in children with an age below 6 years, 41.6 ± 7.4% in children older than 6 years (up to 18 years) and 40.0 % ± 7.6 % in adults. The differences are significant ($p < 0.001$).

There is a relationship between TG measured as ETP or V_{max} and levels of FVIII in the patient population investigated. The correlation is poor for both methods (in house and Hemker method), whereas the correlation of the original method and the in house method is acceptable (Fig. 3 and 4). This means that FVIII influences TG, but other components also determine TG. The difference is not due to a methodical failure.

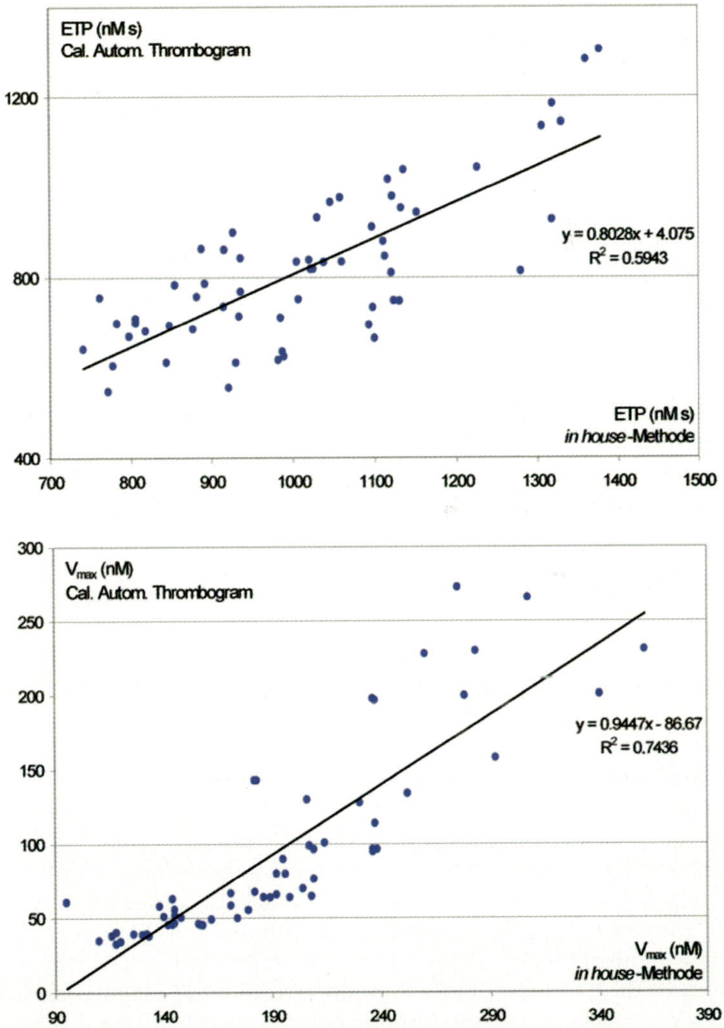

Fig. 3a, b. Correlation of two TG methods expressed as ETP and V_{max}

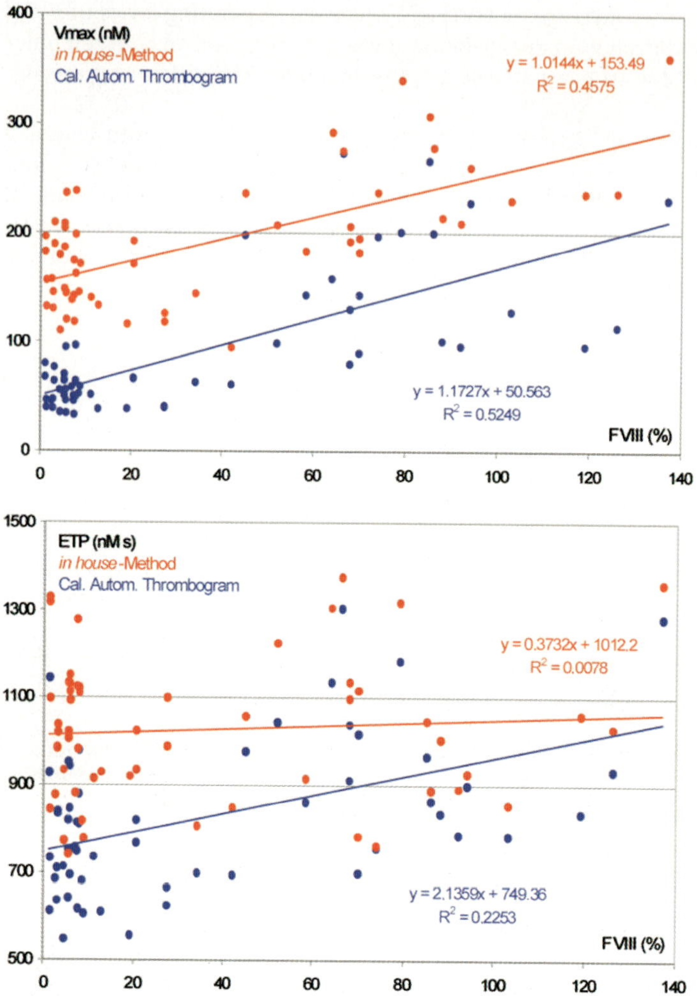

Fig. 4a, b. ETP and V_{max} depending on FVIII levels in different methods measuring TG

Differentiating between FVIII levels < 10% and FVIII levels > 10 % the following diagrams were obtained (Fig. 5). The reaction velocity was significantly influenced by the FVIII level, the influence on the ETP was neglectable and the length of the lag phase did not significantly differ in patients with lower FVIII levels. This can be explained by the cofactor function of FVIII in the coagulation system.

Despite of the great interindividual differences of TG every child with hemophilia A and B or von Willebrand disease has his own TG value which is influenced not only by the FVIII level, but also by the level of other coagulation factors, by the presence or absence of prothrombotic risk factors [5] and many other unknown parameters.

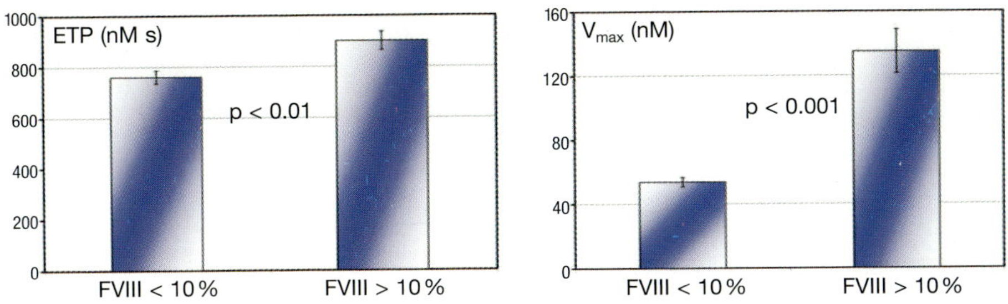

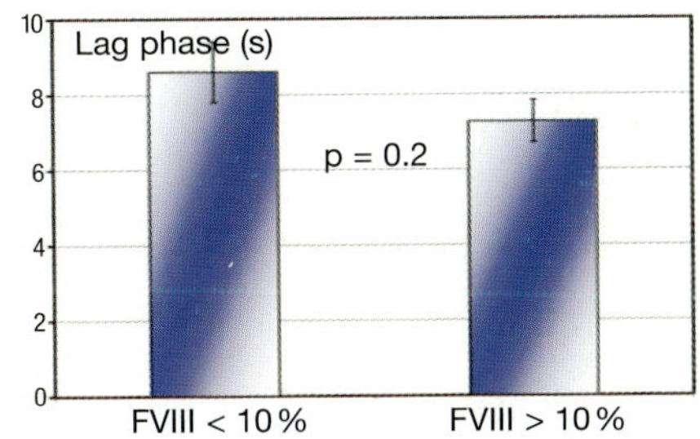

Fig. 5. TG and related parameters as function of FVIII

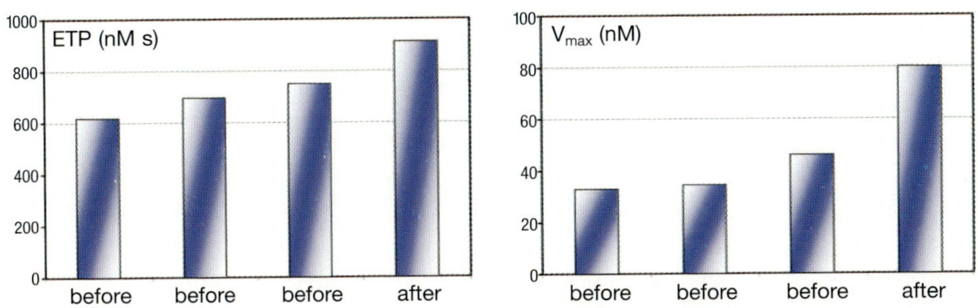

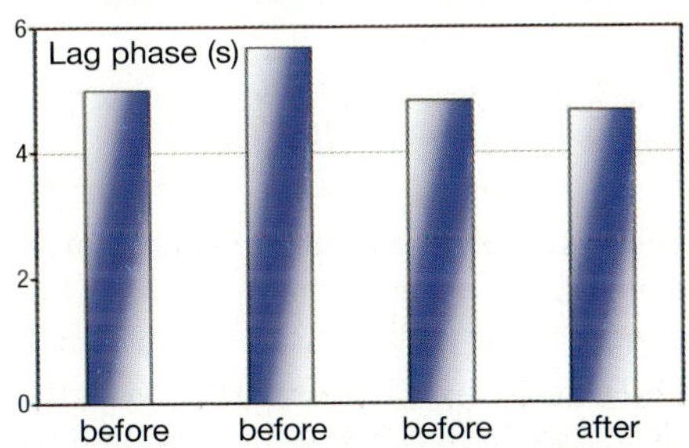

Fig. 6. TG in a patient with moderate Hemophilia A at different time intervals

Children with von Willebrand disease (vWD) have a TG within the reference range except for patients with severe vWD (type III). The TG of vWD type III patients is lower as in hemophilia A patients with the same interindividual differences caused by the massive loss of FVIII due to the lack of stabilization by the Willebrand complex.

TG can also be used to monitor children with thrombophilic risk factors. In children with prothrombotic risk factors we have the same tendency of an individual value which is influenced by therapy (Fig. 8). Figure 8 demonstrates the TG in a

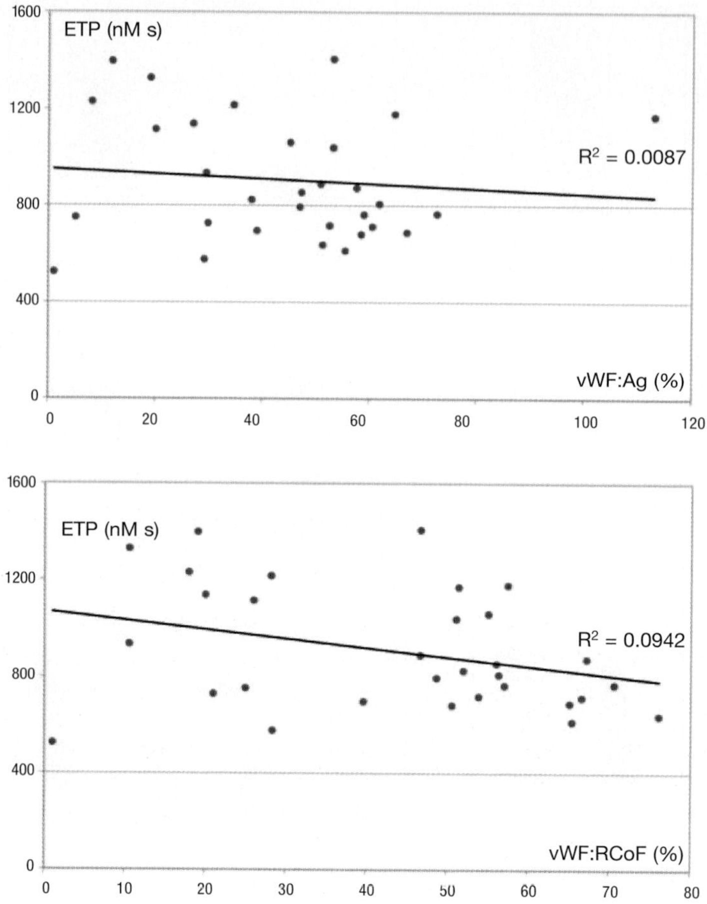

Fig. 7. TG depending on von Willebrand factor antigen (VWF:Ag) and Ristocetin cofactor activity (RCoF)

child carrying the prothrombingen mutation 20210 GA who developed a stroke after discontinuation of a therapy with UFH in a postoperative condition. Great disturbances in the coagulation system occur when one therapy is interrupted without an overlapping new therapy. The moment of stroke manifestation was the moment of the highest TG. After discontinuation of the therapy the TG arrives the initial value.

Conclusions

Similar to adults children show interindividual differences in TG, but a relatively constant individual TG.

The maximum reaction velocity, the ETP and the beginning of the thrombin generation measured as lag phase characterize TG. The maximum reaction velocity

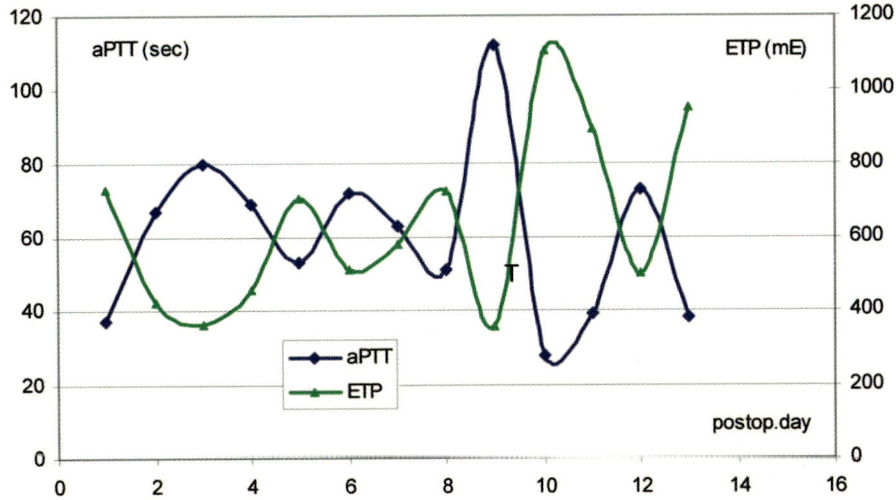

Fig. 8. Inhibitor dependent TG in a patient with stroke carrying the prothrombin mutation 20210 GA

is the parameter which best describes the situation of TG. That's why the ETP can be used as a helpful tool to monitor the substitution therapy over a long period of time.

Determining TG it is possible to monitor patients with hemophilia A and B and severe vWD (only type III) because TG reflects the overall capacity of the coagulation system to generate thrombin. The same investigations are possible in patients with thrombophilia.

Further investigations are needed to show the role of platelets, FVIII elevations because of acute-phase-reactions and factor VIII consumption in TG.

References

1. Brenner, B, Marder VJ, Conard, J. Women's Issues in Thrombosis and Haemostasis, Martin Dunitz Ltd London 2002
2. Siegemund, T, Petros, S, Siegemund, A, Scholz, U, Engelmann, L. Thrombin generation in severe haemophilia A and B: the endogenous thrombin potential in platelet-rich plasma. Thromb Haemost 2003;90:781–6.
3. Varadi, K, Turecek, PL, Schwarz, HP. Thrombin generation assay and other universal tests for monitoring haemophilia therapy. Haemophilia 2004; 10 Suppl2:17–21.
4. Brummel-Ziedins, K, Vossen, CY, Rosendaal, FR, Umezaki, K, Mann, KG. The plasma hemostatic proteome: thrombin generation in healthy individuals. J Thromb Haemost. 2005;3(7):1472–81.
5. Kurnik, K, Escuriola-Ettingshausen, S, Horneff, S, Düring, R, Schobess, R, Bidlingmaier, S, Halimeh, H, Pollmann H, Bogdanova, N, Nowak-Göttl, U. Effects of F V G1691A Mutation and the F II G20210A Variant on the Clinical Expression of Severe Hemophilia A (< 2%) in Children – Results of a Multicenter Study in 35th Hemophilia Symposium Hamburg 2004, Springer Berlin/Heidelberg 2004.

VI. Free Lectures

Chairmen:

B. Zieger (Freiburg)
R. Zimmermann (Heidelberg)

Working-Group of the German Hemophilia Assistants – History, Purpose and Goals

K. Andritschke, H. Ringkamp
for the Working Group of the German Hemophilia Assistants

Summary

The aim of this presentation is to introduce the working-group of the German hemophilia assistants to the hemophilia community. After a first initiative twenty years ago the German hemophilia assistants began to organize themselves as an working-group in 2001. Since then the group met twice a year to discuss special problems of hemophilia care, to define possible contents of a planned qualification program and to have an educational part with a coagulation specific subject. The goal is to define and to guarantee in parallel to the optimal medical treatment also an optimal care for patients with coagulation disorders.

History

A first meeting of some hemophilia assistants to discuss the experiences of disease specific care took place during the WFH congress in Bonn 1980. During the next twenty years only a few additional meetings could be arranged (Table 1). In 2001, when the assistants met in the hemophilia center of Muenster, it became very clear that an extensive exchange of experiences is necessary, because similar problems and challenges could be identified in most of the centers. Therefore it was decided to have regular meetings twice a year. Invited to take part in these meetings are examined nurses, but also other non-scientific employees of the treatment centers, which directly care for patients. For this reason the group is called 'German Hemophilia Assistants' instead of hemophilia nurses.

Table 1. Hemophilia assistant meetings between 1980 and 2001

1980	WFH Congress Bonn; first meeting of Ms. Brackmann and Ms. Beha with the International Hemophilia Nurses Group
1997	First meeting of some nurses and non-scientific employees during the Hemophilia Symposium in Hamburg
2001	Meeting of some hemophilia nurses and assistants in the hemophilia center of Muenster; since then regular meetings twice a year

I. Scharrer/W. Schramm (Ed.)
36th Hemophilia Symposium Hamburg 2005

Purposes

One of the first activities of the group was to define the tasks and responsibilities of the assistants in the German treatment centers. During the discussions it became evident that the tasks and responsibilities differ substantially between the hemophilia centers. In some centers the work of the nurses or assistants is restricted to the care of the patients only, whereas in other centers it includes also more specific responsibilities. In general the hemophilia assistant plays a central role as person of confidence for the patients, which have a lot of questions and need somebody to talk with about their personal problems. As the nurses assist the treating physicians they also play an important role as link between patients and doctor. And last but not least the assistants play an important role in the education and instruction of the patients, for example how to do self infusions, home treatment and treatment documentation. Table 2 summarizes in a detailed list the different tasks and responsibilities, which may be the duties of hemophilia assistants.

Table 2. Tasks and responsibilities of the hemophilia assistants

- Assistance of the treating physician during blood drawings and factor substitutions as well as for documentations and coordination of diagnostic or treatment measures
- Education of patients or parents in terms of special care for patients with coagulation disorders
- Handling of DDAVP and factor concentrates (ordering, reconstitution, injection or infusion, storage, etc.)
- Documentation of coagulation factor substitutions (according to the German »Transfusionsgesetz«)
- Instruction of patients for home-self-treatment
  - Aseptic working conditions
  - Re-constitution of the concentrates
  - Application of the factor as i.v.-injection or infusion via port-a-cath, perfusion pumps, injectomat, or minipump
  - Side effects
  - Documentation of bleeding events
  - Batch documentation of the substituted factor concentrate
- Explanation of the specific coagulation disorder to the patient or parents
- Informations on »living with the coagulation disease«
- Encouragement to live a normal life (school, job, sports, social activities, etc.)
- First contact person in case of problems in connection with the disease
- Informations on the patient organizations (e.g. DHG/Deutsche Hämophilie-Gesellschaft, IGH/ Interessengemeinschaft Hämophiler).
- Link between science and patient in case of clinical studies (study nurse)

Goals

The overall goal of the treatment of patients with coagulation disorders must be to guarantee optimal medical treatment, but also optimal patient care. In parallel to the medical treatment also the patient care must be further developed and optimized. The achievement of this optimization of disease-related patient care is the main goal of the hemophilia assistants working-group. Milestones on the way to the main goal are:

- Establishing of a hemophilia assistants working-group
- National and international exchange of experience
- Definition of the tasks and responsibilities
- Definition of the education contents
- Publications
- Establishing of a specialized hemophilia education
- Appreciation as qualified hemophilia assistant (long-term goal)

Some of these activities have already been started. The working-group exists since 2001 and meets regularly twice a year. In one of the annual meetings a special educational topic is always on the agenda (Table 3). In addition some publications of the group are already available (Table 4).

For the further development and to reach the mentioned goals the support of the whole hemophilia community is appreciated and necessary.

Table 3. Educational topics in the meetings since 2001

2001 in Muenster	Mobility in hemophilia
2002 in Hanover	Hepatitis C and hemophilia
2003 in Bonn	1. Psychological and social aspects in hemophilia 2. Orthopedic treatments in hemophilia
2004 in Duesseldorf	HIV and hemophilia
2005 in Frankfurt/M.	1. Handicap status of patients with hemophilia 2. Thrombophilia 3. Treatment of inhibitors
2006 in Berlin	1. Surgical interventions in hemophiliacs 2. Vessel embolization in repeated joint bleeds

Table 4. Publications of the hemophilia assistants

- »Die Hämophilieassistentin – Aufgaben und Qualifikationen«
  (Posters: Global Nurses Symposium 2003 in Miami; Hämophilie-Symposium 2003 in Hamburg; WFH Congress 2006 in Vancouver)
- »Hämophilie – eine chronische Notfallerkrankung«
  (Journal: ›Heilberufe‹)
- »Die Hämophilie – sowohl chronische als auch Notfallerkrankung«
  (Journal: ›Kinderkrankenschwester‹)
- »Hämophilie – Blutererkrankung«
  (Journal: ›Praxisnah‹)
- »Einführung in die Heimselbstbehandlung«
  (Patient brochure)
- »Handbuch: ABC der Hämophilie«
  (Patient brochure)

The Endogenous Thrombin Potential as a New Parameter for the Peri-Operative Monitoring in Conjunction with Endo-Prosthetic Supply due to Hemophilic Arthropathy

U. Scholz, A. Siegemund, T. Siegemund, and R. Scholz

Introduction

With regard to surgical procedures patients suffering from hemophilia or serious von Willebrand Jürgens syndrome (type 3) are distinguished by the increased risk of blood loss resulting from their basic illness.

For the peri-operative management substances containing factor VIII are available to aid the substitution of the plasmatic deficiency.

Through the determination of the endogenous thrombin potential (ETP) and its singular parameters conclusions regarding the development and elimination of thrombin can be drawn [1–3].

In previous studies of our research group the endogenous generation of thrombin taking place in the plasma which is rich of platelets was examined; its significance in representing the total potential of the hemostasis was studied under various clinical aspects and the results were published [4].

In the current study this method will be simultaneously observed as a way of peri-operative monitoring in cases of serious hemorrhagic diathesis and under substitution of factor VIII.

Methods

First of all the generation of thrombin was examined in a group of 9 patients (severe hemophilia A) before and after the substitution of 1000 IE factor VIII. A sample of blood was taken 30 minutes before and 30 minutes after the medication was applied.

Subsequently 4 patients (severe hemophilia A, von Willebrand Jürgens syndrome type 3, total knee arthroplasty, ankle arthroplasty) were peri-operatively treated with substitution therapy applying the medication with factor VIII. They were enclosed in the evaluation. The sample of blood was taken on a daily basis before the first substitution of the factor VIII was carried out. The determination of the endogenous thrombin potential in the plasma was realized using a Fluorescan Ascent 2.2 (Labsystems, Helsinki). The global coagulation parameters (d-dimer, prothrombin fragments, factor VIII) were obtained utilizing a BCS (Dade Behring).

The evaluation of the endogenous thrombin potential was based on the area beneath the graph of $ETP_{ges.}$ and the peak of the maximal velocity of thrombin generation V_{max}.

I. Scharrer/W. Schramm (Ed.)
36th Hemophilia Symposium Hamburg 2005

Results

The endogenous thrombin potential representing the generation of thrombin significantly increases before and after the substitution involving the substance with 1000 IE factor VIII (recovery: 30 minutes). However, the distinct raise in the generation of thrombin varies individually.

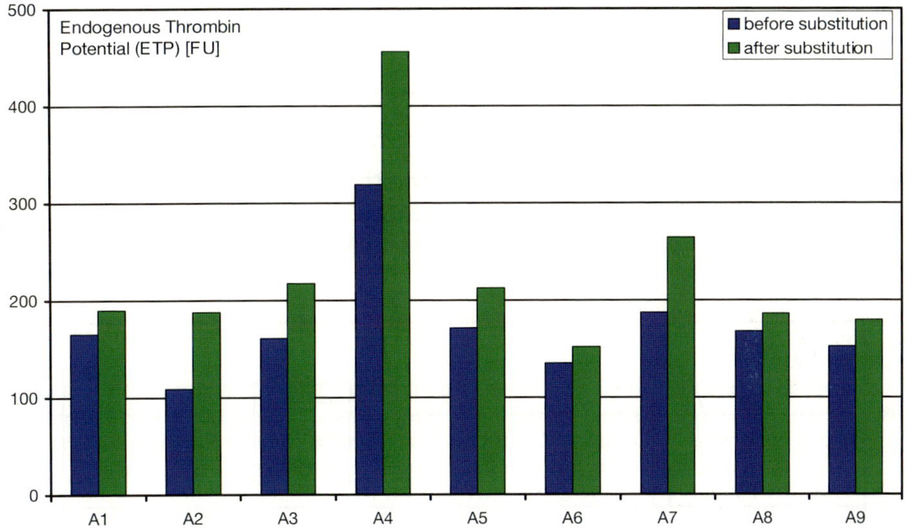

Fig. 1. Endogenous thrombin potential before/after substitution (severe hemophilia A)

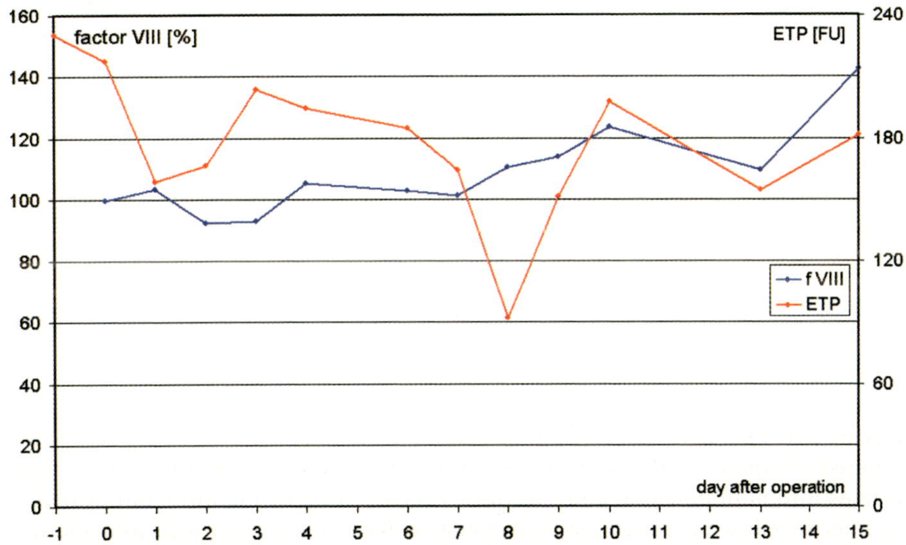

Fig. 2. Peri-operative progress of the endogenous thrombin potential and the factor VIII (severe hemophilia A)

Sequencing

The ssDNA of all positive clones was extracted and sequenced on an automated ABI sequencer. Sequencing revealed in between 48 and 71 peptide inserts for each patient. Several sequences appeared in multiple copies. Altogether for each patient 34 to 38 different sequences were identified. For patient Acq-F-01 RQPP was identified as dominant motif in most of the peptide sequences. For patients Acq-F-02 to Acq-F-04 the motifs SS-A/T-W, PxELL, YxVPxRL were repetitively identified, respectively. These motifs have been identified as »core motifs« which are flanked by other amino acids in the sequence of the peptide insert. The reactivity by ELISA reflects the presence of further amino acids in the phage sequence adjacent to the core motif.

Epitope Mapping

Using 3DEX software (see Materials and Methods), the primary sequence of the peptide inserts was compared to the primary sequence of FVIII and to the surface of a FVIII model using the structure published by Stoylova et al. [20]. For all patients epitopes have been identified in the A2 or C2 region (see Figures 4a to e): for patient Acq-F-01 and -04 epitopes have been mapped to different sites of the A2 region, whereas epitopes for patients Acq-F-02 and -03 closely overlap on the C2 domain of FVIII. For patient Acq-F-01 an additional possible epitope was identified in the A1 region of FVIII.

Discussion

Screening of phage displayed random peptide libraries is a very capable method to rapidly identify small ligands for a given molecule. In this study, small peptide ligands to FVIII inhibitors have been identified by screening phage displayed random peptide libraries with plasma from patients with acquired hemophilia A. Four patients have been analyzed so far. Small peptide sequences have been isolated for each patient that specifically bound to the patient plasma but not to control plasma. The peptides represent the epitope on FVIII for the analyzed inhibitor and are called mimotopes (mimicking epitopes). The peptide sequences were compared to the primary sequence of FVIII to identify linear epitopes as well as to the three-dimensional model of FVIII to identify conformational (or discontinuous) epitopes (see Materials and Methods). For two patients, epitopes in the A2 region have been identified and for the other two in the C2 region (see Figure 4). The epitopes identified in this study cluster around the regions that have been described before for inhibitor binding in acquired hemophilia. Also, the C2 epitopes of two patients show a great overlapping portion. The epitopes located in A2 domain are located on the opposite sites of the molecule. For patient Acq-F-01 a possible additional epitope has been located in the A1 domain. The evidence for this is weaker than for the other epitopes so that this epitope needs to be further investigated (data not shown). Synthetic peptides have been generated that correspond to the sequence of the peptide inserts identified on the phage clones isolated with plasma from patient

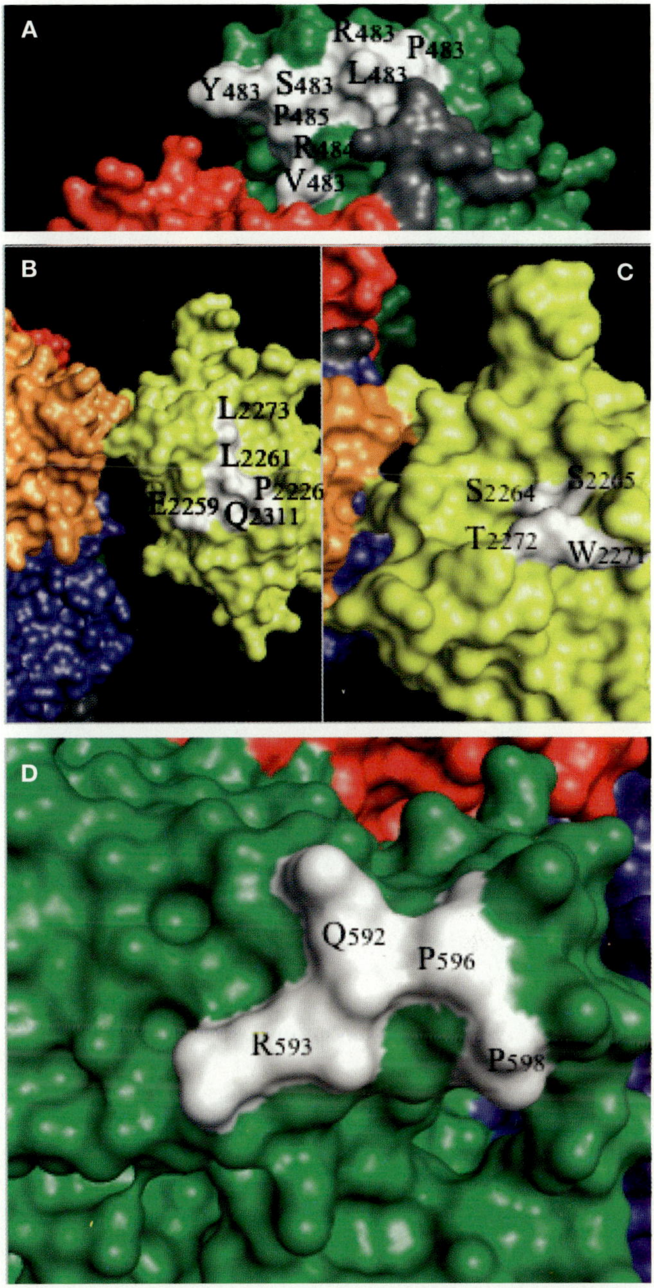

Fig. 4. Location of epitopes on FVIII. The location of identified epitopes for patients Acq-F-01 to -04 are shown on the threedimensional model of factor VIII. In a to d close ups of the epitopes of each individual patient is schown. In e all epitopes are shown as the summary. The upper and lower parts of the pictures show the molecule from different directions.

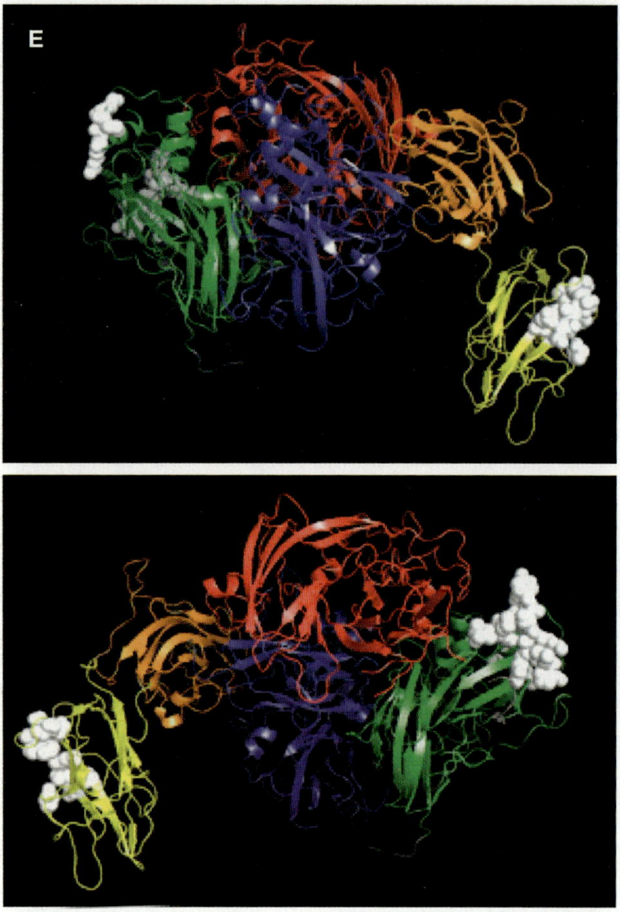

Fig. 4

Acq-F-01. Using synthetic peptides allows to determine binding to a specific sequence without the phage protein as a scaffold. Reactivity of autologous patient plasma was assessed by ELISA: the reactivity was much weaker than achieved with phage clones, but specific compared to control peptide or binding of inhibitor negative patient plasma (data not shown). The decrease in binding might be due to a different presentation of the synthetic peptides compared to the peptides displayed on the surface of the phages, due to different immobilization of a small molecule on the ELISA plate or due to amino acids of the phage coat protein being involved in inhibitor binding. This needs to be evaluated in further assays.

For phage display screenings using plasma of patients with congenital hemophilia, the percentage of positive clones isolated after the third round of screening correlated with the inhibitor titer – low BU, low frequency of positive clones, and vice versa. This reflects the amount of FVIII inhibitors present in the plasma. It is of interest to note that the BUs and percentage of positive clones do not correlate for the patient plasma examined in this study (see Table 1). The reason for this observation remains to be elucidated. This might reflect the clinical experience that BUs in acquired hemophilia do not correlate with the severity of the bleedings. It could also be an indication for different amounts of inhibitors in plasma that are not reflected by the Bethesda assay. Except for a possible second epitope for patient Acq-F-01 in the A1 domain, only one epitope has been identified for each of the other patients. Taken into consideration that a polyclonal immune response is expected in patients with aquired hemophilia, the identification of several epitopes was expected at the beginning of the study. The reason for the identification of only one epitope can only be speculated upon: »polyclonal« does not necessarily mean that several regions of FVIII are targeted by antibodies, also several clones can target the same immunodominant region and recognize different epitopes involving similar but not identical residues. This theory is supported by the fact that peptide sequences of different phagotopes have a similar core motif, which is flanked by different amino acids. Additionally, it is possible that one clone is dominating over the other anti-FVIII clones. Therefore the phage display screening might only pick up the dominant clone. Analysis of further phage clones might then reveal additional epitopes. A third explanation reflects the nature of the selection procedure: biopanning selects for structural similarities, i.e. peptide ligands are isolated that mimic the epitope without necessarily having the same sequence. Thus peptide sequences isolated for some inhibitors might very well mimic the epitope and bind to the given inhibitor without having a sequence homology. These peptides cannot lead to the identification of the location of the epitope. To address this question further analysis of additional clones and novel screening strategies are currently followed.

In this project, mimotopes of FVIII inhibitors have been isolated that are specific for plasma from patients suffering from acquired hemophilia A. The analysis of additional patients will hopefully help to closely identify immunodominant regions that are represented by mimotopes. The identified mimotopes need to be tested for cross reactivity with heterologous patient plasma to identify peptides that represent immunodominant regions that are relevant for the majority of patients with acquired hemophilia. These molecules might then lead to novel therapeutic strategies to overcome the antibody response to FVIII in acquired hemophilia A.

Acknowledgements. We thank Dr Ursula Dietrich and Margot Landersz, Georg-Speyer-Haus, Frankfurt, Germany, for sequencing support.

References

1. Barrow RT, Healey JF, Jacquemin MG, Saint-Remy JM, Lollar P. Antigenicity of putative phospholipid membrane-binding residues in factor VIII; Blood. 2001 Jan 1; 97(1): 169–74.
2. Fay, PJ & Scandella, D. Human inhibitor antibodies specific for the factor VIII A2domain disrupt the interaction between the subunit and factor IXa. J Biol Chem 1999: 274, 29826– 30.
3. Fulcher CA, de Graaf Mahoney S, Roberts JR, Kasper CK, Zimmerman TS. Localization of human factor FVIII inhibitor epitopes to two polypeptide fragments. Proc Natl Acad Sci U S A. 1985 Nov; 82 (22): 7728–32.

4. Green D, Lechner K. A survey of 215 non-hemophilic patients with inhibitors to factor VIII; Thromb Haemost. 1981 Jun 30;45(3):200–3.
5. Hay CR. Acquired haemophilia. Baillieres Clin Haematol. 1998 Jun;11(2):287–303.
6. Lenting PJ, van de Loo JW, Donath M J, van Mourik JA & Mertens K. The sequence Glu1811-Lys1818 of human blood coagulation factor VIII comprises a binding site for activated factor IX. J Biol Chem 1996: 271, 1935–40.
7. Lubin IM, Healey JF, Barrow RT, Scandella D, Lollar P. Analysis of the human factor VIII A2 inhibitor epitope by alanine scanning mutagenesis. J Biol Chem. 1997 Nov 28;272(48):30191–5.
8. Pipe SW & Kaufman RJ. Characterization of a genetically engineered inactivation-resistant coagulation factor VIIIa. Proc Natl Acad Sci U S A 1997: 94, 11851–6.
9. Healey JF, Lubin IM, Nakai H, Saenko EL, Hoyer LW, Scandella D, Lollar P. Residues 484-508 contain a major determinant of the inhibitory epitope in the A2 domain of human factor VIII. J Biol Chem. 1995 Jun 16;270(24):14505–9.
10. Kessel C, Königs C, Linde R, Escuriola-Ettinghausen C, Roland J, Stoll H, Klingebiel T, Dietrich U, Kreuz W. Epitope mapping during FVIII inhibitor elimination with rituximab reveals conformational epitopes on FVIII and identifies small molecules blocking inhibitor and targetting B cells;. in I. Scharrer und W. Schramm (Eds.), 35th Hemophilia Symposium Hamburg 2004, Springer Medizin Verlag Heidelberg 2006
11. Königs C, Rowley MJ, Thompson P, Myers M, Scealy M, Davies JM, Wu L, Dietrich U, Mackay CR, Mackay IR. Monoclonal antibody screening of a phage-displayed random peptide library reveals mimotopes of chemokine receptor CCR5: implications for the tertiary structure of the receptor and for an N-terminal binding site for HIV-1 gp120. Eur J Immunol 2000: 30, 1162–71.
12. Kopecky EM, Greinstetter S, Pabinger I, Buchacher A, Romisch J, Jungbauer A. Mapping of FVIII inhibitor epitopes using cellulose-bound synthetic peptide arrays. J Immunol Methods. 2006 Jan 20;308(1-2):90–100.
13. Mühle C et al. Epitope mapping of polyclonal clotting factor VIII-inhibitory antibodies using phage display. Thromb Haemost 2004: 91, 619–25.
14. Rowley MJ, O'Connor K, Wijeyewickrema L. Phage display for epitope determination: a paradigm for identifying receptor-ligand interactions. Biotechnol Annu Rev. 2004;10:151–88.
15. Saenko EL & Scandella D. The acidic region of the factor VIII light chain and the C2 domain together form the high affinity binding site for von Willebrand factor. J Biol Chem 1997: 272, 18007–14.
16. Sambrook J, Fritsch EF and Maniatis T (Eds.) Molecular Cloning: a Laboratory Manual, 2nd Ed., Cold Spring Habor Laboratory Press, Cold Spring Habor 1989.
17. Scandella D, de Graaf S, Mahoney S, Mattingly M, Roeder D, Timmons L, Fulcher CA. Epitope mapping of human factor VIII inhibitor antibodies by deletion analysis of factor VIII fragments expressed in Escherichia coli. Proc Natl Acad Sci U S A. 1988 Aug;85(16):6152–6.
18. Scandella D, Mattingly M, de Graaf S, Fulcher CA. Localization of epitopes for human factor VIII inhibitor antibodies by immunoblotting and antibody neutralization. Blood. 1989 Oct;74(5): 1618–26.
19. Schreiber A, Humbert M, Benz A, Dietrich U. 3D-Epitope-Explorer (3DEX): localization of conformational epitopes within three-dimensional structures of proteins. J Comput Chem. 2005 Jul 15;26(9):879–87.
20. Stoilova-McPhie S, Villoutreix BO, Mertens K, Kemball-Cook G & Holzenburg A. 3-Dimensional structure of membrane-bound coagulation factor VIII: modeling of the factor VIII heterodimer within a 3-dimensional density map derived by electron crystallography. Blood 2002: 99, 1215–23.
21. Villard S et al. Peptide decoys selected by phage display block in vitro and in vivo activity of a human anti-FVIII inhibitor. Blood 2003: 102, 949–52.
22. Zhong D, Saenko EL, Shima M, Felch M, Scandella D. Some human inhibitor antibodies interfere with factor VIII binding to factor IX. Blood. 1998 Jul 1;92(1):136–42

Spectrum of Molecular Defects and Mutation Detection Rate in Patients with Mild and Moderate Hemophilia A

N. Bogdanova, A. Markoff, U. Nowak-Göttl, R. Eisert, C. Wermes, H. Pollmann, A. Todorova, A. Eigel, B. Dworniczak, and J. Horst

Introduction

The amount of residual factor VIII (FVIII:C) determines the clinical variability of hemophilia A. About 50% of the patients have severe hemophilia A with a FVIII:C activity less than 1% of normal. Moderate (FVIII:C 2–5% of normal) and mild (FVIII:C > 5% of normal) hemophilia A occur in about 10% and 30–40% of patients, respectively. Recently we showed that the mutation detection rate in severely affected male patients is virtually 100% when testing for the common intron 22-/intron 1-inversions and big deletions, followed by genomic sequencing of the F8 gene. We also showed that protein truncating molecular defects are prevalent in those patients [1]. Here we report on the mutation detection rate and the spectrum of mutations in 136 patients with mild/moderate hemophilia A, as well as their distribution throughout the F8 protein.

Patients and Methods

Twenty four moderately and 112 mildly affected patients of German origin were included in the study. Genomic DNA was extracted from peripheral blood lymphocytes using salting procedure. The coding region of the F8 gene, the intron/exon boundaries and the F8 promoter region were subjected to sequencing analysis using primers and conditions as previously described [1]. The newly detected amino acid substitutions were scored for potential gross or local conformational changes and influence on molecular stability for every single F8 domain with available structures, using homology modeling [2–4].

Results and Discussion

Mutation Detection Rate

The performed sequencing analysis revealed a molecular defect in 121 (89%) of the patients, whereas 15 (11%) had no mutation in the coding region of the F8 gene, in the exon/intron borders or in the promoter region. All negative patients were mildly affected with exception of one patient with FVIII:C 2–3%.

Spectrum and Distribution of the Mutations

In the group of moderate hemophilia A patients 22 (91.6%) were affected by missense mutations. Four of these changes are novel: G236A, L172F (A1 domain), G236A (A2 domain) and A1779S (A3 domain). One patient (4.2%) had a small deletion of an adenine in an A-stretch in exon 14 of the F8 gene and in another one (4.2%) no mutation could be detected on genomic level.

The vast majority (83/112, 74%) of mutations detected in the group of mildly affected patients were also missense. Twenty seven of these molecular defects are described for the first time, namely in the A1 domain: G244D, V178G, T262P, I76S, I173T, D163A and V101D; in the A1/A2 boundary V357G; in the A2 domain: G563A, I548F, C630R, T657S and P526H; in the A2/B boundary C692R and T751S; in the A3 domain Y1815C, P1825H, M2010I, E2004K and V1873G; in the C1 domain R2150L, F2126S, T2154N, R2150L and S2133P and in the C2 domain G2325A and P2292H. Nine (8%) patients were shown to carry a splicing mutation and two – a deletion/insertion of an A in a poly-adenosin stretch in the B-domain. Three of the splicing errors are novel alterations, these are: D318Y/splice (A1 domain), IVS15-1 G>A (A3 domain) and IVS21 +1G>T (C1 domain).

The molecular defects are systematically presented in Figure 1. They are distributed throughout the whole sequence of the factor VIII gene, but predominantly in the A2 (mainly exon 11) and C1 (mainly exon 23) domains.

The novel amino-acid substitutions were scored for potential conformational changes and influence on the molecular stability, using homology modeling. Figure 2 illustrates the effects of the conservative mutation P1825H (A3 domain), detected in a mildly affected patient (slite change of loop conformation) as compared to P1825S previously published in a moderate affected patient (severe distortion of loop conformation).

Two molecular changes (–112G>A and –219C>T) in the promoter region of the factor VIII gene were detected in two patients with mild hemophilia A. These defects were excluded in a cohort of 100 normal males and have not been detected in more than 300 hemophilia A patients with known mutations. Both changes affect important promoter sites, thus supporting possible pathogenicity of these alterations. To our knowledge this is the first report on promoter mutations in the F8 gene.

Conclusion

Our data show that, in contrast to severe hemophilia A, the analysis on genomic level fails to detect the molecular defect in about 4% of the moderately and in 12.5% of the mildly affected patients. While the mutation detection rate in moderate hemophilia A is still high (<95%), it is significantly lower in the mildly affected cases (87.5%), thus suggesting that the reduction of the F8 activity could be due to other (probably unknown) reasons at least in a part of these patients.

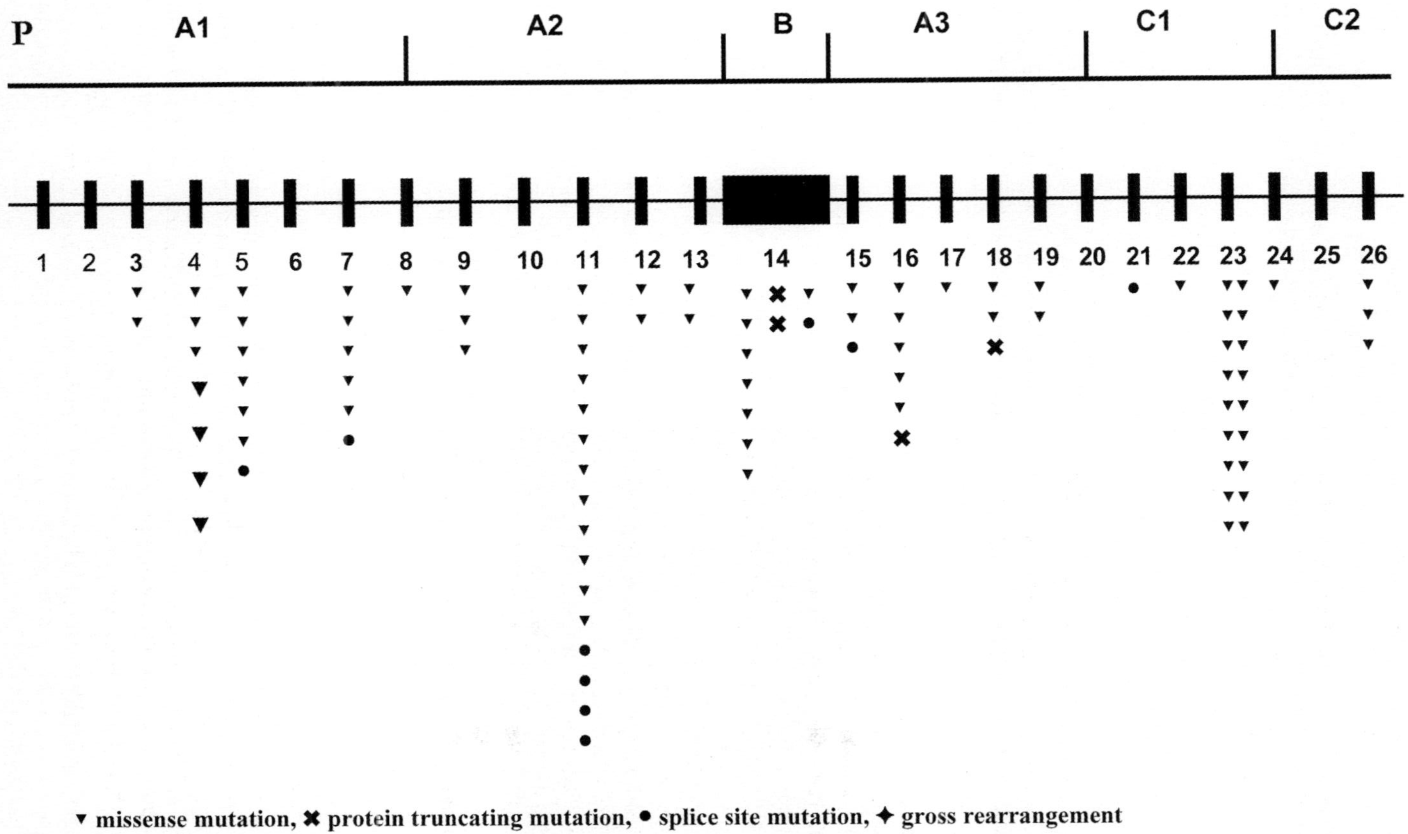

Fig. 1. Spectrum and distribution of the mutations in the F8 gene, identified in 24 moderately and 112 mildly affected hemophilia A male patients.

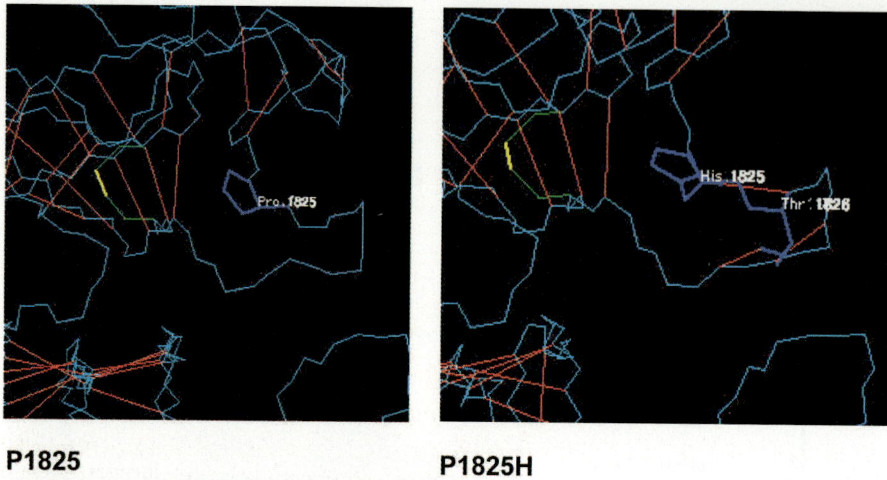

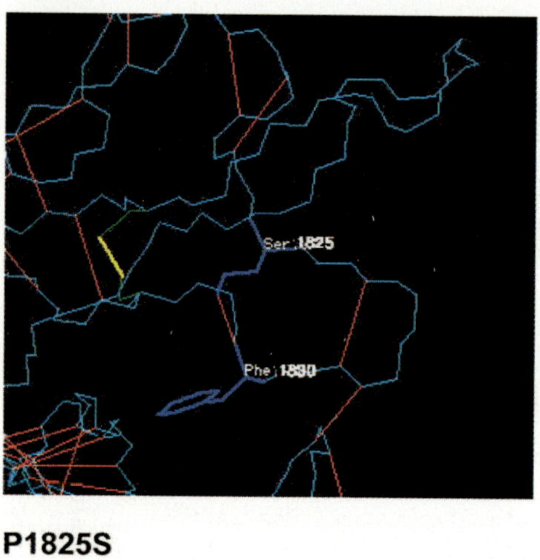

Fig. 2. Dreiding model images of a part of the F8 A3 domain around P1825 (left panel) with the mutation P1825H (middle panel) and with the mutation P1825S (right panel). Protein chains are colored in light blue, selected amino acids are dark blue. Disulfide bonds are presented in yellow, hydrogen bonds in red and ionic bonds in magenta. Residues participating in ionic bonds are highlighted in green (where not selected in dark blue).

References

1. Bogdanova N, Markoff A, Pollmann H, Nowak-Göttl U, Eisert R, Dworniczak B, Eigel A, Horst J. Prevalence of small rearrangements in the factor VIII gene F8C among patients with severe hemophilia A. Hum Mutat. 2002; 20(3):236–7
2. Lund O, Frimand K, Gorodkin J, Bohr H, Bohr J, Hansen J, Brunak S. Protein distance constraints predicted by neural networks and probability density functions. Protein Eng. 1997; 10: 1241–1248
3. Pemberton S, Lindley P, Zaitsev V, Card G, Tuddenham EG, Kemball-Cook GA molecular model for the triplicated A domains of human factor VIII based on the crystal structure of human ceruloplasmin. Blood. 1997; 89(7):2413–21.
4. Stoilova-McPhie S, Villoutreix BO, Mertens K, Kemball-Cook G, Holzenburg A. 3-Dimensional structure of membrane-bound coagulation factor VIII: modeling of the factor VIII heterodimer within a 3-dimensional density map derived by electron crystallography. Blood. 2002; 99(4):1215–23

Recombinant Factor VIIa for Major Surgery in Severe Factor XI Deficiency: Pharmacodynamic Monitoring Using Thromboelastometry

H. Dehmel, J. Priesack, R. Eisert, and A. Tiede

Introduction

Factor XI (FXI) deficiency is a rare autosomal recessive disorder characterized by abnormal bleeding after trauma or surgery. FXI replacement therapy using fresh frozen plasma (FFP) or FXI concentrate has been associated with important side effects including inhibitor formation, arterial and venous thromboembolism and volume overload [1].

The type of FXI gene mutation strongly influences the risk of inhibitor formation. In an Israeli cohort study of 64 unrelated subjects with severe deficiency (FXI < 15 IU/dL), two mutations accounted for > 90% of cases, a nonsense mutation Glu117Stop (known as type II mutation) and a missense mutation Phe283Leu (type III). Homozygotes for type II and III have a residual FXI activity of 1 and 10 IU/dL, respectively, whereas compound heterozygotes (II/III) have a mean residual activity of 3 IU/dl. Inhibitors against FXI were observed only in patients homozygous for the type II mutation, who were exposed to plasma-derived FXI. The cumulative incidence was 7 out of 21 (33 %) [2]. Thus, patients with a FXI residual activity < 1 % seem to be at high risk for inhibitor formation.

The successful use of recombinant activated factor VII (rFVIIa) for surgical prophylaxis has been reported in two cases with severe deficiency and inhibitor [3, 4]. Moreover, in a pilot study 14 consecutive patients (5 severely deficient, one with inhibitor) underwent 15 procedures (5 major, 4 minor, 6 dental) [5]. For the major procedures, patients received 90 µg/kg 2-hourly for 13 doses followed by 90 µg/kg 4-hourly for 6 doses. All procedures were successfully performed without any evidence of bleeding. The use of rFVIIa is potentially advantageous in FXI deficient patient by avoiding the risk of inhibitor formation and volume overload.

In the above mentioned cases, dosing of rFVIIa was similar to the treatment of patients with inhibitors against factor VIII (FVIII). It is unclear whether this dose is actually required in FXI deficient patients who seem to have a milder bleeding phenotype compared to patients with hemophilia and FVIII inhibitors. Adequate monitoring assays to support dosing decisions in these patients are currently not available. Here, a severely FXI deficient patient was treated using rFVIIa and pharmacodynamic monitoring was performed using rotation thromboelastometry.

I. Scharrer/W. Schramm (Ed.)
36th Hemophilia Symposium Hamburg 2005

Subject and Method

Subject

The patient reported here is a 65 year-old male who was diagnosed with FXI deficiency after a prolonged aPTT had been observed. FXI activity measured at several occasions was < 1 % (< 1 IU/dl) without detectable inhibitor. There was no history of trauma or surgery. However, he noticed markedly prolonged bleeding following tooth extractions. Concurrent diagnoses included obesity (120 kg body weight), grade III heart failure and osteoarthritis of the hip. He was scheduled for elective total hip replacement surgery (HRS).

Rationale for Treatment and Prospective Treatment Schedule

For surgical procedures in FXI deficient patients, FFP infusion therapy targeting a FXI activity of 15 to 20 IU/dl is recommended [6]. FFP infusions of at least 20 ml/kg was not considered an appropriate option because of obesity and heart failure in this patient. A FXI concentrate is not licensed in Germany. Furthermore, FXI concentrate would be considered high risk for inhibitor development in this patient because he had a residual FXI activity of < 1 %. Therefore, recombinant factor VIIa (rFVIIa) was used for replacement therapy.

A dosing schedule was derived from the preliminary reported of the above mentioned pilot study: 90 μg/kg 2hourly for 13 doses followed 90 μg/kg for at least 6 doses. Using this schedule, five major surgical procedures were performed without increased bleeding, although the type and extent of the procedures was not stated in the report [5].

Pharmacodynamic Monitoring

Citrated blood samples were collected at the indicated time points. aPTT and PT were determined in platelet-poor plasma using standard reagents and equipment (Roche, Mannheim, Germany). Factor XI activity was determined using aPTT-based one-stage assay (Dade Behring, Marburg, Germany). Thromboelastometry was performed in duplicate in citrated whole blood using standard equipment (Pentapharm, Munich, Germany) with a minute amount of tissue factor (tif-TEM A) and calcium (star-TEM) as activating and starting reagents, respectively. Reference values were determined using citrated whole blood from 12 healthy donors activated with tif-TEM A and star-TEM. The 2 s interval was used to define lower and upper limits for the reference range.

Results

Thromboelastometry

At baseline, the clotting time (CT, 888 +/–43 s, reference range 386–744 s) and the clot formation time (CFT, 495 s, reference range 166–321 s) were prolonged. Following the first dose of rFVIIa (90 µg/kg), a correction of the CT (after 10 min: 484 +/–35 s; after 120 min: 593 +/–74 s) and CFT (after 10 min: 128 +/–3 s; after 120 min: 173 +/-76 s) was observed. Continued dosing with 90 µg/kg in 2-hour intervals according to O'Connell, resulting in a further shortening of the CT (329 +/– 8s) and CFT (113 +/–16 s) after 24 hours. Following a dose reduction to 40 µg/kg given in 6-hour intervals, the CT (523 to 561 s) was within the normal range, whereas the CFT (100 to 126 s) remained shortened.

Routine laboratory assays

The PT (Quick), given in per cent, was > 200 % at all times during treatment with rFVIIa (not shown). The aPTT was prolonged at baseline (97 s, reference range 25 to 35 s). During treatment, the aPTT was shortened, but remained above the upper normal limit. Likewise, FXI activity measured by aPTT-based one-stage assay was also increased from < 1 U/dl to up to 44 U/dl during treatment with 90 µg/kg, and to up to 5 to 14 U/dl during treatment with 40 µg/kg.

Clinical Effectiveness and Safety

Hemostasis was normal as judged by the surgeon during the operation. Estimated blood loss (500 ml) was within the expected range for unilateral HRS. There were no clinical signs of excessive bleeding or thromboembolism during the entire postoperative course. The patient fully recovered without delay.

Discussion

There is little experience in the use of rFVIIa during surgery in FXI deficient patients. Most of the published experience was made during minor surgery in patients with severe FXI deficiency and inhibitor secondary to plasma replacement. Lawler et al. reported on the management of cataract extraction using a starting dose of 90 µg/kg immediately before surgery followed by continuous infusion of 20 µg/kg per hour for 18 hours. This regimen resulted in an uncomplicated clinical course [4]. Bern et al. reported on a patient undergoing uneventful knee arthroscopy, who received 90 µg/kg in 2-hour intervals for 8 hours, after which intervals were prolonged to 3-hourly for 6 hours and 4-hourly for 16 hours. A preliminary report on a prospective open-label study indicated that five major procedures were successfully managed using a dose of 90 µg/kg in 2-hour intervals for 24 hours, followed by 90 μg/kg in 4-hour intervals for another 24 hours. However, the severity of FXI deficiency in the patients undergoing the major procedures was not stated.

Dose finding studies for the optimal use of rFVIIa in FXI deficiency are not available. Salomon et al. demonstrated restoration of thrombin generation in FXI-deficient plasma spiked ex vivo with rFVIIa [8]. Correction of the endogenous thrombin potential to 80% of normal was obtained in 6 out of 8 samples using a concentration [illegible]

[illegible]

[illegible] therapy was administered in a dose of 90 μg/kg every 2 hours. Further studies are needed to evaluate [illegible]

[illegible]

8. Salomon O, Steinberg DM, Zucker M, et al. Inherited factor XI deficiency confers no protection against acute myocardial infarction. J Thromb Haemost 2003;1:658–661.

Establishment of a Web-Based Documentation System for Quality Assurance of Hemophilia Treatment in Mecklenburg/Western Pomeranian: a Pilot Study

B. Steiner, P. Bruhn, B. Berthold, D. Hähling, B. Meyer, A. Grainacher, F. Herrmann, U. Kyank, B. Gombert, C. Burstein, and M. Freund

The quality of the overall management of hemophilia critically depends on the communication between patients, primary care physicians and specialized treatment centers. In addition to the management of acute bleeding events and infectious issues, diagnostic and therapeutic approaches to diseases not primarily associated with the inherited bleeding tendency require increasing awareness. The latter issue has received little attention. We selected an internet-based database approach to overcome this shortage of information. Within four years of its implementation, we have documented data obtained from patients with hemophilia (n = 131) and von Willebrand's disease (n=18) aged between 12 and 84 years. An optimized substitution regimen was introduced for 46 patients and fully documented. Additional aspects toward improved overall quality included the diagnosis and treatment of viral infections (n = 22) and documentation and completion of vaccination status (n = 26). Conservative and/or surgical treatment of the skeletal system was started in 48 patients. Cardiovascular surgery was performed in 8 patients requiring a multi-team approach to the hemostaseological management before, during, and after surgery. Two hemophilia patients started regular hemodialysis for chronic kidney failure under optimized coagulation control. Four patients received chemotherapy for malignancy. Laboratory diagnosis and monitoring data are available from 56 patients.

The continuous communication between patients, primary care providers, and specialized centers is a prerequisite for acute bleeding events as well as accompanying diseases. Based on our experience over the last four years, the web-based documentation approach represents a helpful communication tool to improve care provided for patients suffering from bleeding disorders.

I. Scharrer/W. Schramm (Ed.)
36th Hemophilia Symposium Hamburg 2005

Successful Angiographic Embolization of Recurrent Elbow Joint Bleeds in one Patient with Severe Hemophilia A

R. Klamroth, S. Gottstein, E. Essers, M. Orlovic,
and M. Wilaschek

Introduction

In patients with severe hemophilia A spontaneous joint bleeds lead to cartilage destruction and secondary arthrosis. In joints with high-grade arthropathy bleedings occur, that do not respond to substitution of factor VIII. The reason may be pathologic reactive angiogenesis in chronic synovitis. Bleeds from those vessels typically show a sudden onset of symptoms with massive soft swelling of the joint. Patients often perceive the bleeding as »atypical«.

Patient

One patient, 56 years old und 72 kg bodyweight, with severe hemophilia A experienced recurrent massive bleeds of the right elbow in absence of trauma in the beginning of 2005. He had high-grade hemophilic arthropathy of multiple joints. He was on home-treatment and had many years experience with self intravenous-

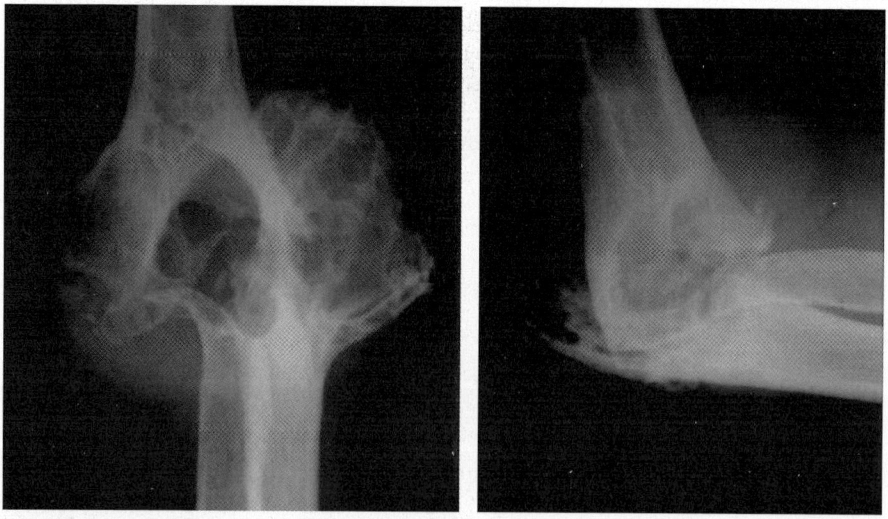

Fig. 1. X-ray right elbow

I. Scharrer/W. Schramm (Ed.)
36th Hemophilia Symposium Hamburg 2005

injection on demand. He used a recombinant factor VIII concentrate (Advate, Baxter Inc.) and had no history of factor VIII inhibitor. He was HIV-negative but had chronic hepatitis C.

On clinical examination tenderness, soft swelling and (further) reduction of range of motion were found.

Conventional X-rays show nearly complete destruction of the elbow joint (Fig. 1). After initial application of factor VIII concentrate (50 IU/kg bodyweight) there was only slow and never complete relief of symptoms. Despite intensive secondary prophylaxis with 30 IU/kg bodyweight daily holding the factor VIII level in plasma at minimum 70%, new massive bleeding at the same location occurred. Vascular bleeding was suspected. The patient had been treated 3 months earlier with particle embolization.

Method

After normalization of factor VIII-levels (2 times 2000 IU factor VIII concentrate prior puncture) angiography of the arteries of the right arm was performed via the right femoral artery by catheterization of the brachial artery. After contrast fluid application two vessels were identified as possible bleeding sources considering location and morphology. One vessel was originating from the ulnar artery, and after its embolization a second branch of the ulnar artery supplying the elbow was displayed (Fig. 2 and 3).

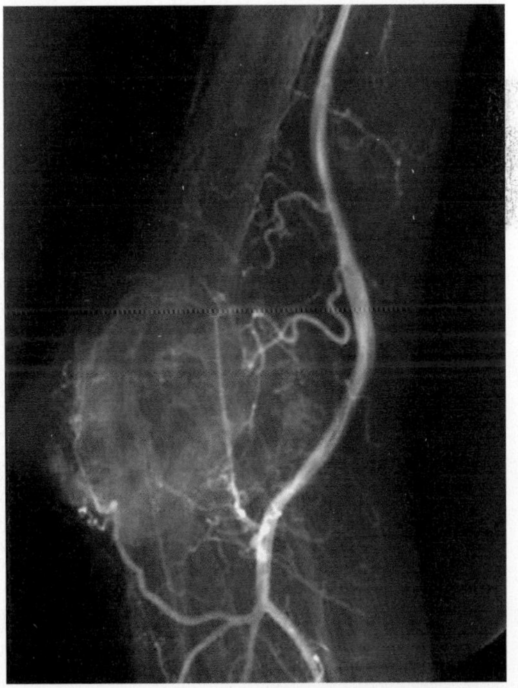

Fig. 2. Elbow arteries before embolization

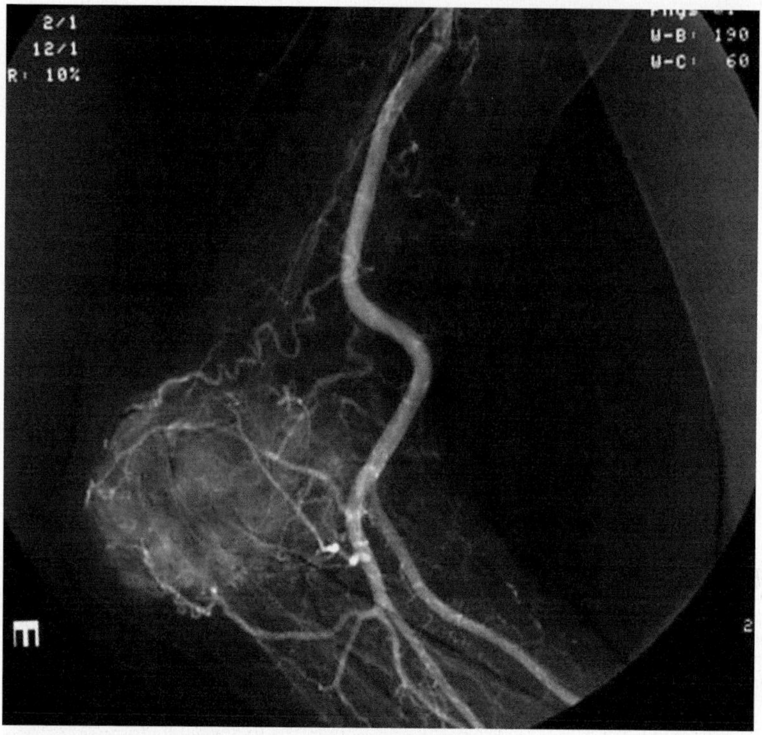

Fig. 3. Elbow arteries before embolization

The first embolization in April 2005 was performed with microparticles (Polyvenyl alcohol; 250–355 nm) per microcatheter (0,014 inch). The second embolization with embolization fluid (Ethylen vinyl alcohol copolymer, Onyx) was performed in July 2006 (Fig. 4).

Factor VIII substitution was continued after the procedure aiming at minimum factor VIII levels of 70% for 5 days and 30% for another week. Thereafter the dose was further reduced to prophylaxis.

Results

After the first embolization with microparticles the patient was free of bleeds for 8 weeks. Due to new severe bleeds in the elbow joint we decided to perform a second attempt. The angiography showed an opening of the same vessels as before embolization with microparticles.

So this time we used an embolization fluid (Ethylen vinyl alcohol copolymer, Onyx) which leads to complete irreversible occlusion of the artery.

The patient complained about severe, though quickly resolving pain during Onyx application despite prior analgesic medication (morphine derivates i.v.).

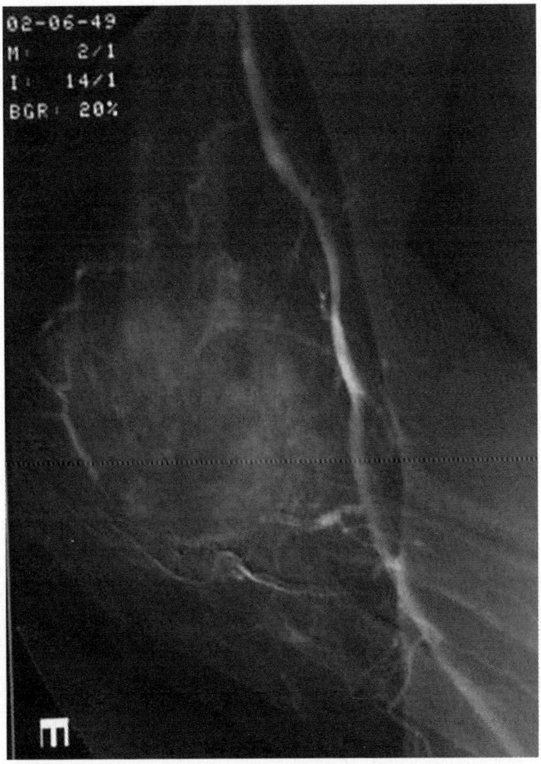

Fig. 4. Elbow arteries after embolization

Under low-dose prophylactic treatment (15 IU factor VIII/kg bodyweight 3 times/week) no recurrent bleed in the right elbow joint occurred after elective embolization of pathological arteries in the cubital region (10 months follow up). There were no complications after the procedure.

Conclusion

In joint bleeds not responding to substitution of factor VIII to normal factor VIII levels angiographic embolization might be considered as a therapeutic option, especially if surgical treatment is not possible. Embolization with embolization fluid might be more promising than use of microparticles, because microparticles are resolving after 8 weeks and there is the danger of insufficient thrombosis and reopening of the vessel in patients with severe hemophilia.

References

1. Mauser-Bundschoten EP, Zijl JAC, Mali W, von Rinsum AC, van den Berg HM, Rosendaal G. Successful treatment of severe bleeding in hemophilic target joints by selective angiographic embolization. Blood (2005) 105(7), 2654–2657

Evaluation of Thrombotic Events in Hemophiliacs Undergoing Major Orthopedic Surgery Without Thrombosis Prophylaxis

M. Krause, Ch. von Auer, A. Kurth, M. Böhm, L. Hovy, and I. Scharrer

Background

Major orthopedic procedures (hip and knee replacement) and the presence of thrombophilia are risk factors of thrombotic events. Besides the FV G1691A mutation and the FII G20210A variant, high levels of factor VIII above 150% are associated with a 5 fold risk for venous thrombosis.

In absence of any prophylaxis, the incidence of venography detected deep vein thrombosis range from 40% to 60% and that of clinically venous thromboembolism between 2% and 5%. Non-pharmacologic methods of prophylaxis, including graduated compression stockings, reduce the incidence of venous thrombosis less effective than anticoagulant based prophylaxis. The importance of thrombosis prophylaxis with heparin/LMWH in the postoperative period in patients with hemophilia undergoing hip or knee replacement is still unknown.

The aim of the retrospective study was to evaluate the occurrence of thrombotic events in hemophiliacs undergoing major surgery without thrombosis prophylaxis.

Patients

Between 1989 and 2005 a total of 32 patients with hemophilia A, median age: 47 years, undergoing 44 procedures were analyzed in our hemophilia treatment center. Patients with inhibitors were excluded. Surgical interventions were performed using recombinant (n=37) or plasma-derived (n=7) FVIII for 12 to 15 postoperative days. All patients received thrombosis prophylaxis with graduated compression stockings only. In addition to factor VIII activity, APC resistance, FV G1691A mutation and the FII G20210A variant were investigated.

CHARACTERISTICS

Patients [n=32]	median age: median BMI:	47 years 23.1	[range: 27 - 73 years] [range: 18.2 – 30.5]
Hemophilia A: orthopedic procedures [n= 44]: FVIII - replacement therapy:	severe: 27 / moderate: 4 / mild: 1 hip replacement: 9 / knee replacement: 35 recombinant: 37 / plasma-derived: 7		

I. Scharrer/W. Schramm (Ed.)
36th Hemophilia Symposium Hamburg 2005

Results

No thrombotic event in the postoperative period was documented.

The median initial dose of FVIII was 82 IU/kg^{-1}, followed by median FVIII doses of 54 IU/kg^{-1} over the first four days. The median FVIII activity was 153%, and median body mass index (BMI: kg/m^2) was 23.1. During the first four postoperative days FVIII levels > 150% were measured in 24/44 operative procedures. BMI > 25 were shown in 12/32 patients, and age > 40 years was documented in 23/32 patients. In 1/31 patient APC resistance and none of our patients FII G20210A variant were identified.

RESULTS I

BMI > 25	patients: 12/32 [38%]	
age > 40 years	patients: 23/32 [72%]	
APC resistance	patient: 1*/31 [3%]	*gene analysis not available
FV G1691A mutation	patients: 0/22	
FII G20210A variant	patients: 0/22	

RESULTS II

initial dose of FVIII:	median: 82 IU/kg^{-1}
postoperative days 1-4:	
FVIII dose	median: 54 IU/kg^{-1}
FVIII activity	median: 153% [range: 85–347%]
FVIII activity > 150%	patients: 24/44 [55%]

Discussion and Conclusion

Venous thrombotic events are rare complications in hemophilic patients. Despite the normalization of hemostasis after factor VIII replacement therapy, heparin thromboprophylaxis in the postoperative period is not currently standardized in the hemophilia centers.

In our study group elevated FVIII levels (FVIII > 150%) and additional risk factors (BMI > 25, age >40 years) seem not to relevant influence the occurrence of thrombotic events in patients with hemophilia undergoing hip or knee replacement without thrombosis prophylaxis. Further prospective studies are required to confirm whether a thrombosis prophylaxis with heparin is needed in hemophiliacs undergoing high risk surgery.

References

1. Kyrle PA. High factor VIII and the risk of venous thromboembolism. Hämostaseologie 2003; 23:41–44
2. Rosendaal FR. Risk factors for venous thrombotic disease. Thromb Haemost 1999;82, 610–619
3. Agnelli G. Prevention of venous thromboembolism in surgical patients. Circulation 2004; 110:IV 4-IV-12
4. Geerts WH, Heit JA, Clagett GP, et al. Prevention of venous thromboembolism. Chest. 2001; 119(suppl 1): 132S–175S.
5. Franchini M, et al. Absence of thromboembolic complications in patients with hereditary bleeding disorders undergoing major orthopaedic surgery without antithrombotic prophylaxis. Thromb Haemost 2003; 91: 1053–1055

Motivating Patients and Parents to Document Treatment Correctly

S. Jenkins

Background

The idea for a poster came originally from the German hemophilia nurses' meeting in Düsseldorf. We were asked to bring ideas for a collective poster. The aim was to produce a poster for the outpatient's department. After talking about this to our doctors I found that very few patients document correctly, including all the points listed in the poster. It seems that the fact that it is a legal requirement makes no difference. I became increasingly more interested in how I could motivate people to do this correctly. The most common problem seems to be: no reason given for injections just time, date and batch number. Sometimes in the stress of emergency situations parents forget that the health insurance companies also require evidence of substitutions as so many other problems need their attention. We need to alert them to deal with this quickly and carefully to prevent difficulties with insurance and to promote a clear picture for future research.

It would appear that the problem lies in awareness of what information is useful as well as forgetting or just lack of motivation.

I know from my experience in other fields that people must understand the importance of something if they are to do it well. Otherwise it is done badly or not at all.

It is also clear to me that many children are cared for not just by their parents but also by grandparents, other relatives or childminders to varying degrees. Therefore, I wanted to address all these people personally and also to include those children and teenagers who document their own treatment. So I decided to design it like a letter.

The first draft I produced in A4 form sending it to parents who had experienced problems, for example that some information was missing. This included changes like patients moving from purely »as required« substitutions to prophylactic treatments with extra substitutions due to a bleed. Many people had heard about the problems of HIV transmission without realizing the need to trace recipients of particular batches. Careful management is then required to ensure people understand that a minimal risk is always in the background, but the greater risk is that joint damage will impair their quality of life. Then I followed up by discussing whether other help was required. Then I incorporated these changes into the final version. This is now also handed out to new patients to start them off correctly.

I. Scharrer/W. Schramm (Ed.)
36th Hemophilia Symposium Hamburg 2005

Datum	Uhrzeit	Chargennummer CH-B Nr.	Menge in E	Präperat Name	Grund	Name des Arztes	
14.12.04	8⁴⁰	[redacted] 500 Ch.-B. 33665011C	500 IE	[redacted]	Prophylaxe	Dr. [redacted] Kinderärzte [redacted]	
27.12.04	11⁴⁵	[redacted] 500 Ch.-B. 33665011C	500 IE	[redacted] 500	Prophylaxe	Dr. [redacted] Kinderärzte [redacted]	
30.12.04	11¹⁵	[redacted] 500 Ch.-B. 36065011C	500 IE	[redacted] 500	Prophylaxe	Dr [redacted] Kinderärzte [redacted]	8460g. 73cm
03.01.05	11²⁰	[redacted] 500 Ch.-B. 35965011F	500 IE	[redacted] 500	Prophylaxe	Dr. [redacted] Kinderärzte [redacted]	
07.01.05	9⁰⁰	[redacted] 500 Ch.-B. 35965011F	500 IE	[redacted] 500	Prophylaxe	[redacted] Peter [illegible] Tel 08721 [illegible] 8430 [illegible]	
9.1.05	4³⁰	[redacted] 500 Ch.-B. 36065011C	500 IE	[redacted] 500	Sturz aus Bett	[redacted] Abteilung für Pädiatrie Chefarzt Prof. Dr. [redacted] Dr [redacted]	
10.1.05	19³⁰	[redacted] 500 Ch.-B. 35965011F	500 IE	[redacted] 500	Sturz aus dem Bett 2. Gabe	Abteilung für Pädiatrie Prof. Dr [redacted] 84503 Altötting · Tel 08671/509-1333	
13.1.05	11³⁰	[redacted] 500 Ch.-B. 36065011C	500 IE	[redacted] 500	Prophylaxe	Dr. [redacted] Kinderärzte [redacted]	12.01.05 8650g

Fig. 1

Documenting Hemophilia Treatment Implications and Guidelines for you!

Dear Children, Parents, and everyone who care for our children with Hemophilia!

Our aim for our patients is that they should understand why proper documentation is essential and enjoy the best quality of life:

- Legal requirement by the act governing blood products.
- Safety.
- Therapy is clearly defined.
- Which batch numbers were used?
- What product was given, when and why?
- What helped?
- Is the required amount changing?

Optimum therapy is achieved by working together!

What is important for good documentation?

Date, time and *batch number* are legally required due to safety reasons.

Reasons for substitution

- Prophylaxis or on demand therapy (due to a bleed or operation)?

- The reason for a substitution and its effectiveness (for example was one injection required or substitution for a whole week?)
- Is an inhibitor developing?

Other factors which help to obtain a clear picture

- Weight (we recommend weighing once a month as factor dosage is calculated by weight).
- The documentation of other events (for example chickenpox, etc.).
- Sensible format (our center recommends A4 as a copy is stored in the notes.)

Optimal therapy and documentation go together!

Documentation

- is a legal requirement following the problems of infection in the 1980´s.
- is important now because we can see whether the prescribed treatment is effective.
- is important in case of emergency as the paramedics can decide on effective treatment.
- is important in 10 years time because nobody knows what information will be important at that time (as medicine will have made considerable progress due to the information we receive from you today).

Fit for Life Competition: Everyone's a Winner

A. Seuser, G. Auerswald, W. Eberl, S. Gutsche, P. Böhm,
R. Klamroth, and A. Kurme

Introduction

The 5-item fitness check has now been conducted in more than 200 children with hemophilia. The results show that hemophilia is associated with specific limitations in terms of fitness. However, these skills can only improve if everybody concerned is motivated enough to perform suitable exercises several times a week. A sport recommendation program was written on the basis of an algorithm and upgraded to create an option for matching specific exercises with the individual fitness requirement. The children's motivation was further enhanced by a competition based on the 5-item fitness check.

Material and Methods

A competitive arena was fitted with the flexibility, strength, aerobic fitness, coordination and body fat equipment already known to the entrants. The procedure was designed to resemble a real-life competitive event as closely as possible. The teams registered the night before the competition took place.

Four teams were set up representing Bremen, Hamburg, Schleswig-Holstein and Lower Saxony. Each team was made up of a team leader (therapist), two hemophiliac families (a child with hemophilia, a parent and any other family member), and another three hemophiliacs from the respective center. The competition was organized so that a representative from each team completed the test course alternately. The scores achieved in each case were demonstrated to the audience in the arena on a large screen shortly after the respective performance. The last to perform were the team leaders (therapists).

Result

The individual team scores are shown in Figure 1. This figure shows the individual team results. With reference to the overall score of 2.5, only Hamburg managed to produce slightly above-average fitness scores. Hamburg was clearly superior in terms of aerobic fitness and balance. The Hamburg team was well placed with regard to coordination, flexibility, back strength and body fat. Poor aerobic fitness

I. Scharrer/W. Schramm (Ed.)
36th Hemophilia Symposium Hamburg 2005

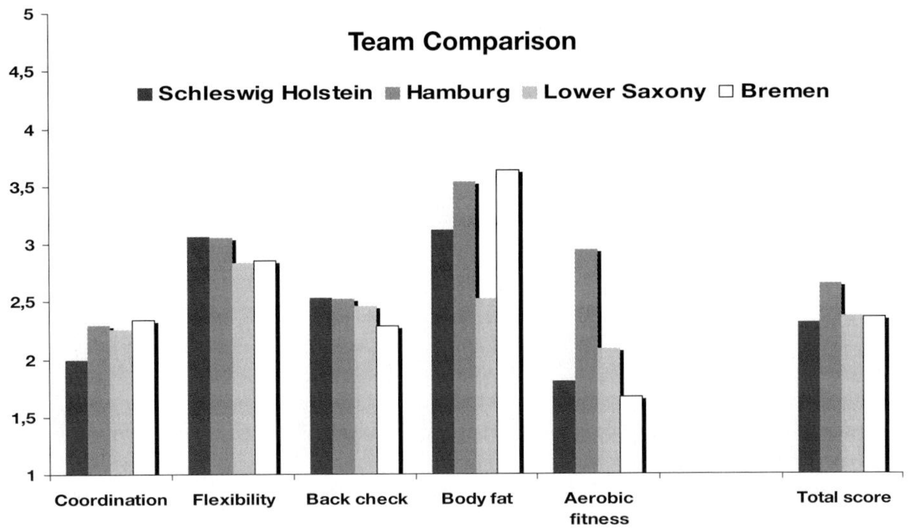

Fig. 1. In the team score, Hamburg took first place with an average of 52.92 points followed by Lower Saxony with 47.29 points, Bremen with 47.1 points and Schleswig-Holstein with 46.3 points.

lost Bremen points. All the teams scored well below average for coordination. Considerable catching-up needs to be done here. Coordination and back check results were borderline for all teams. As is often the case, a poor balance between abdominal and back muscle was the problem. Coordination is the least well-developed basic physical attribute in the whole Fit For Life study. The Lower Saxony team had the best nutritional status results.

The best individual score was achieved by T.H. from Hamburg with 60.44 points. A family score was also established. The various individual top scorers qualified for the final, following the conduct of similar events in the West, South, North and East.

The biggest winner was F.M., date of birth June 17, 1994, who was the top individual scorer in the back check category. He was the child with the best balance between abdominal and back muscle. Because of his hemophilia A and massive bleeding in the left cerebral hemisphere at the age of 10 months, F.M. has poorly controlled focal epilepsy requiring anticonvulsant therapy with 3 different antiepileptic drugs.

He also has a severe form of right-sided hemiparesis and the associated contractures. He attends a normal school where he receives the support of a personal assistant. He had not previously been able to perform sports. This young patient was no longer the same boy after the Fit For Life competition, as his delighted mother reported.

The overall results were evaluated not only on the basis of a team comparison; the participants were also analyzed in groups. We split the population into hemophiliacs, non-hemophilic family members, and therapists. Again, the competition results revealed surprising distribution patterns.

Table 1. Frequency of blood borne infections in the general population

Frequency		1986	1991-1995	1996-2000
HAV/100.000/year		135.2	131.44	73.82
HBV/100.000/year		25.2	20.86	18.64
HBsAg positivity in healthy population	children			4.7%
	adults			1.3–3.1%
Anti-HCV positivity in general population	children			1.3%
	adults			0.1–2%

Table 2. Characteristics of blood donors

Proportion of repeated donors	> 80%
Screening of AgHBs - since	1966 (immunodiffusion), 1990 (Elisa)
Screening of anti-HCV since	1993
Screening of ALAT/ASAT - since	1993

Table 3. Viro-serological profile of blood donors (repeated donors)

Antibodies	2000	2001	2002
HCV	0.16%	0.14%	0.12%
HBV	0.263%	0.203%	0.192
HIV		0.0004%	
HTLV I		0 %	
HTLV II		0.006%	

Patients and Methods

There have been 224 persons with hemophilia (PWH) A or B, with an age range of 1-35 years enrolled in the study. Their replacement therapy was performed with FFP and/or CPP supplemented with factor concentrates. (Fig. 1, 2).

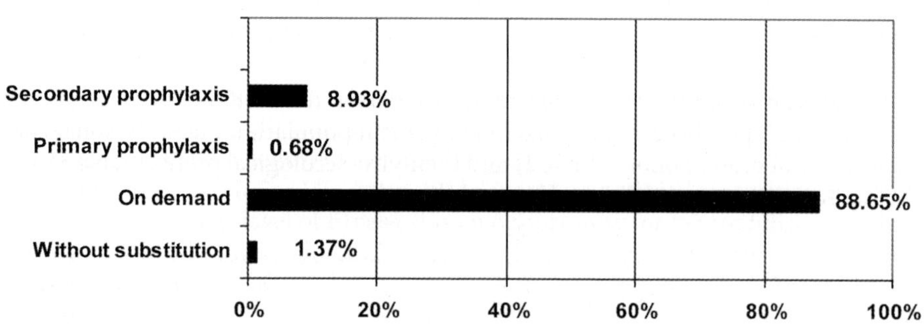

Fig. 1. Main treatment modalities and products used in hemophiliacs

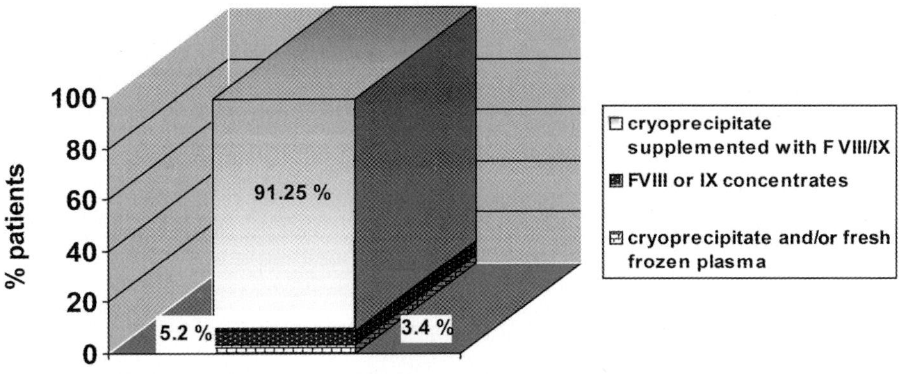

Fig. 2. Products used for substitution in hemophiliacs

Screening of IgG ± IgM-anti HAV, HbsAg, IgG anti-Hbs, IgG anti-HCV, IgG anti-CMV, IgG anti-HTLV I, IgG anti-HTLV II, Anti-HIV 1,2 by ELISA method was performed in all patients.

In HBsAg positive persons HBeAg, IgM anti-HBc, IgG-antiHBe were also controlled. In case of DNA-HBV positivity, viral load by PCR method was assessed.

In anti-HCV positive persons, RNA-HCV, and in case of its positivity genotyping were performed (RT/QRT-PCR TRUGENE VHC-NS-SB).

Results

The viro-serological profile of our patients was quite different from the one of persons with hemophilia (PWH) from other countries. It was dominated by viral hepatitis markers, with a relative low frequency of retroviral infections (HIV, HTLV) (Fig. 1, 3). PWH in our experience had not only an important risk of HCV infection,

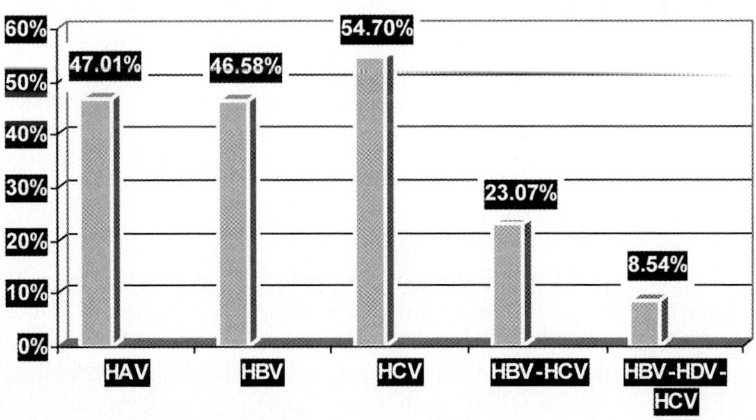

Fig. 3. Infectious status of hemophilia patients – hepatitic viruses

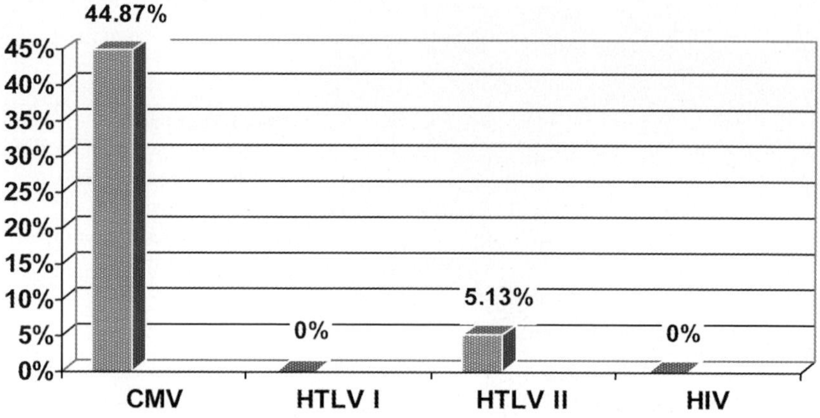

Fig. 4. Serologic profile of hemophilia patients

but according to the epidemiological peculiarities of the country (Tab. 1–3) also a great risk of HBV, HDV and HAV. This challenge is directly connected to the treatment modalities and replacement products used.

Missing the »safety tripod« procedures aiming the safety of plasma derivates (selection of blood donors, testing of donations, viral removal from the product or intermediates during manufacture), NBP maintain a high level of risk for classical transfusion transmitted infections (Fig. 3).

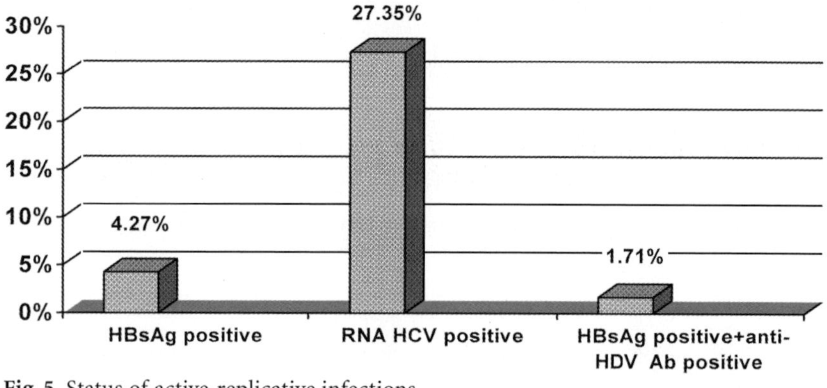

Fig. 5. Status of active-replicative infections

Our replacement therapy explains the present infections profile of PWH. The high proportion of 4.27% HBsAg and 27.35% RNA-HCV positivity (Fig. 5) represent a real threat for life quality and expectancy, cirrhosis and hepatocarcinoma alike being the main long-term complications of PWH. The high viral load and the specific viral genotype (1b HCV in all patients) represent an additional risk for an unfavorable evolution (Fig. 6, 7).

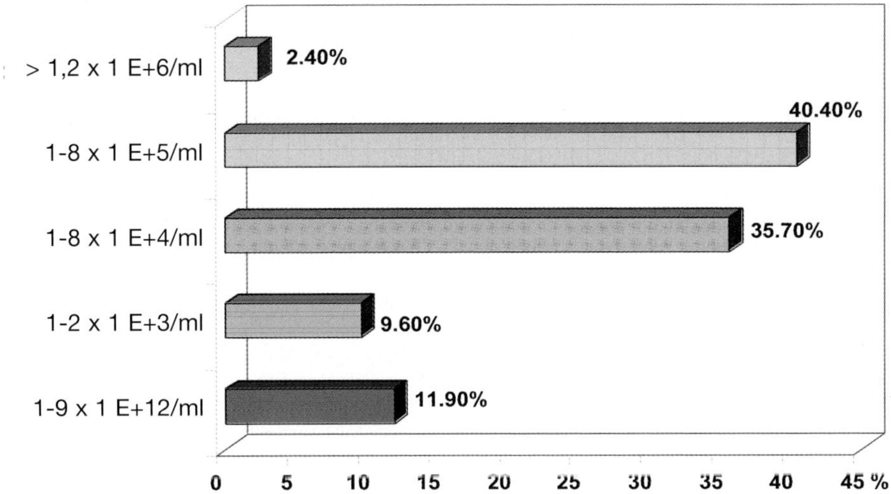

Fig. 6. Viral load in HCV positive PWH

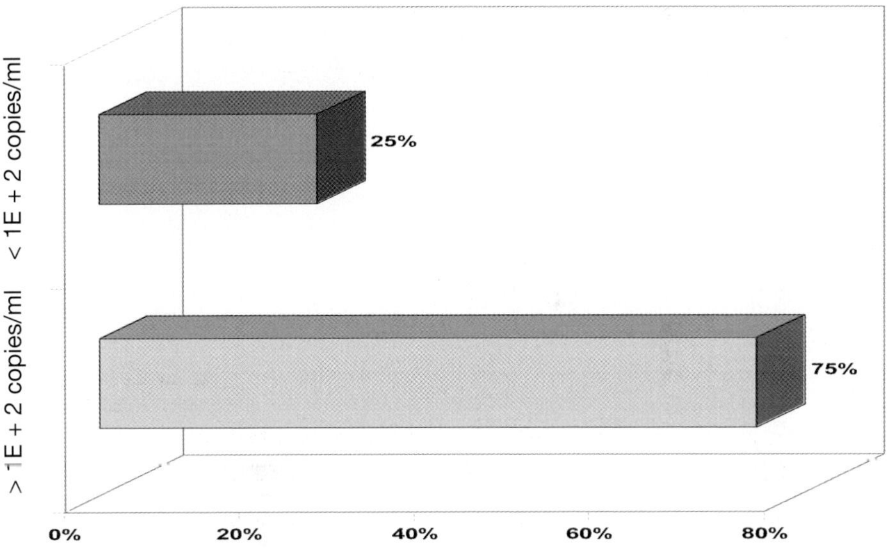

Fig. 7. Viral load in HBV positive PWH

Conclusions

NBP are still a factor of concern in patients with hemophilia despite the more efficient screening methods introduced in the last decade in our country. From this perspective, clotting factor concentrates are much more efficient and safe, but the limited access to them in our patients makes imperative to use the combination with CPP or FFP. Mandatory vaccination against HBV and the introduction of serological screening methods for donors in Romania after 1993 has led to the decrease of the risk for hepatitis transmission.

References

1. Adamowicz-Salach A, Pawelek K, Loch T, Zdzieblowska-Pawinska A, Brojer E, Walewska-Zielecka, Rokicka-Milewska R. Incidence and treatment of hepatitis C virus infection in children with haemophilia in Poland. Haemophilia, 1999, 5, 436–440
2. Giangrande P.L.F. nvCJD and Blood Products in the UK. Scharrer I, Schramm W., (Ed), 35th Haemophilia Symposium Hamburg 2004, Springer, 29–32
3. Gürtler L.G. Update on the Safety of Clotting Factors, Mainly Regarding the Risk of Transmission of vCJD (Variant Creutzfeldt Jakob Disease). Scharrer I, Schramm W. (Ed.), 35th Haemophilia Symposium Hamburg 2004, Springer, 21–29
4. Farrugia A. Evolving perspectives in product safety for haemophilia. Haemophilia, 2002, 8, 236–243
5. Ragni MV, Belle SH. Coinfection with hepatitis C virus and HIV in hemophilic men. J.Infect.Dis.,2001,183 (7), 1112–1115
6. Sabin CA, Emery V, Devereux HL, Griffioen A, Bishop J, Dusheiko G, Yee TT, Herrero-Martinez E, Lee CA. HCV-RNA levels in patients with bleeding disorders. J.Med..Virol. 2002,68 (1),68–75
7. Sousi J.M., Richardson LC. Risk factors for infection with HBV and HCV in a large cohort of hemophiliac males. Transfusion,2001,41 (3),338–343

Hemophilia Center Frankfurt – Twinning Center for Nairobi/Kenya

W. Miesbach, G. Asmelash, M. Boehm, and I. Scharrer

On the initiative of the WFH (World Federation of Hemophilia), members of the staff of the hemophilia center Frankfurt (led by Prof. Scharrer) participated in a workshop on the laboratory diagnosis of hemophilia in Nairobi, Kenya.

Throughout the world there are about 400,000 patients suffering from hemophilia. With regular medical care and treatment with factor concentrates, it is possible for hemophilia patients to lead a normal life in the long term. Without therapy however, their life expectation is greatly reduced because of the effects of recurrent bleeding and the occurrence of joint and organ damage. Unfortunately, only about 25 % of all hemophiliacs receive adequate treatment.

The goal of the WFH therefore is to improve the medical care of hemophiliacs, especially in developing countries. These countries are to be provided with centers as a »twinning« partner. To this end Professor Scharrer's hemophilia center at the University Hospital Frankfurt, was chosen as a twinning center. In 2003, the foundations for this twinning were laid in the context of a hemophilia seminar in Nairobi, Kenya.

The concept of twinning goes back to 1993, when Prof. Guglielmo Mariani demanded that medical care be strengthened in developing countries, in order to establish »comprehensive care centers« there. These should be understood as medical centers, which, despite economic weaknesses, combine their resources to give extra attention to the treatment of hemophilia. This requires a team of nurses, physiotherapists, technicians and doctors. Hemophilic patients are specially trained by the team to deal with bleeding and are also cared for at home. Since then, a world-wide network of hemophilia centers has been established, with more than 20 centers world-wide.

In June 2004, the members of the staff of the Frankfurt hemophilia center went to Nairobi to carry out a workshop on laboratory diagnosis of hemophilia in the Kenyatta National Hospital. The Kenyatta National Hospital is the largest hospital in Kenya, with over 1400 beds. However, these are occupied by over 3500 patients. Several thousand patients visit the outpatients' departments daily. The chair of the Kenyan hemophilia society is the senior consultant of the department of hematology & blood transfusion of the Kenyatta National Hospital, Dr. W. Mwanda.

Over 30 leading laboratory technicians gathered at the workshop from all over Kenya. For three days, they were given practical and theoretical training in working out the coagulation parameters as well as factor VIII and factor IX and inhibitors. Training in the avoidance of virus transfer also played a major role in view of the

I. Scharrer/W. Schramm (Ed.)
36th Hemophilia Symposium Hamburg 2005

Table 1. Type of orthopedic and surgical interventions

Hemophilia type	Intervention type	No. of interventions
A without high-titer inhibitors	Arthroscopic synovectomy	15
	Orthopedic reduction	4
	Corrective osteotomy	2
	Osteosynthesis	2
	Excision of osteoid osteoma	1
	Excision or incision of hematomas, cysts, pseudotumor and abscesses	7
	Colostomy	1
	Hydrocele excision	1
	Strabismus correction	1
A with high-titer inhibitors	Excision or incision of hematomas, cysts, pseudotumor and abscesses	6
	Shank/thigh amputation	3
	Amputation stump remodeling	1
	Wound excision	3
B	Orthopedic reduction	1
	Corrective osteotomy and open synovectomy	1
	Osteosynthesis	1
	Nephrectomy	2
	Tonsillectomy	1
	Excision of hematoma	1

We evaluated:
- *direct medical costs:* therapy and hospitalization costs of all orthopedic and surgical interventions;
- *direct non-medical costs:* home-hospital travel costs;
- *indirect costs:* morbidity costs; loss of income of family members who forfeit paid employment for hemophilia patient home care; average number of days off at school or work;
- *socio-economic consequences of the treatment:* treatment compliance.

Data regarding orthopedic and surgical interventions, replacement therapy and hospitalization duration were obtained from patients' medical charts. Because in a developing country an economic analysis is difficult to ascertain, unitary costs of clotting factor and hospitalization were expressed in €, at average exchange rate communicated by the National Romanian Bank for the last year of the study period:
- 1 hospitalization day in IIIrd Pediatric Clinic $\approx$ 99 €
- 1 hospitalization day in a Surgical Clinic $\approx$ 101 €
- 1 cryoprecipitate/FFP Unit $\approx$ 10 €
- 1 IU FVIII/FIX $\approx$ 0.5 €
- 1 IU APPC $\approx$ 1 €
- 1 kIU rFVIIa $\approx$ 12.8 €

For direct non-medical costs, indirect costs and socio-economic consequences of the treatment evaluation, a questionnaire containing questions regarding these aspects was administered to the patients who expressed their agreement to participate in our study. All patients offered complete answers to all questions.

Results

Direct medical costs

Substitution costs represented 91.14% of total direct medical costs, varying according to hemophilia type and inhibitors presence (Fig. 1).

The most costly interventions were those performed in hemophilia A with high-titer inhibitors (Table 2).

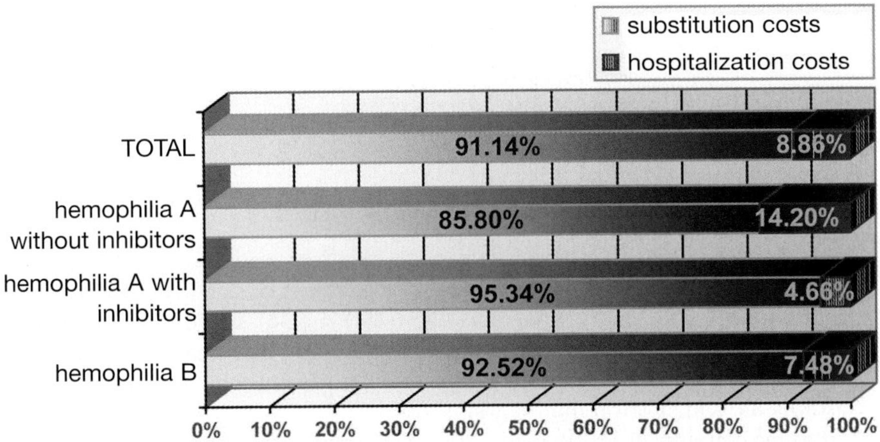

Fig. 1. Direct medical costs distribution according to hemophilia type and inhibitors presence

Table 2. Direct medical costs of orthopedic and surgical interventions

Hemophilia type	Intervention type	Substitution	Direct costs (€) hospitalization	Substitution and hospitalization
A without high-titer inhibitors	Orthopedic	15 320	3 939	19 259
	Surgical	167 565	42 319	209 884
	Synovectomy	223 700	21 008	244 708
	Total	*406 585*	*67 266*	*473 851*
A with high-titer inhibitors	Surgical	541 798	26 462	568 260
B	Orthopedic	9 250	1 414	10 664
	Surgical	86 980	6 363	93 343
	Total	*96 230*	*7 777*	*104 007*
All Patients	All Interventions	1 044 613	101 505	1 146 118

Direct non-medical costs

Means of transportation used by our patients were: car (64.9%), train (21.6%), bus (24.3%), taxi (32.4%) and ambulance (54.3%) of cases. One home-hospital travel cost represented important percents of mean family or patient income (Table 3), leading to a poor treatment compliance.

Table 3. Direct non-medical costs

Mean of transportation	Car	Train	Bus	Taxi	Ambulance
Travel cost (€)	6.34	8.57	1,84	1,16	Supported by society
% of MFI*	3.47	5.66	1.27	0,50	
% of MFI/MB**	11.25	16.01	4.28	1.63	
% of MPI***	21.61	32.30	4.78	5.09	

*-mean family income/month;
**-mean family income/no. of family members/month;
***-mean personal income/month

Indirect costs

1. Morbidity costs. Mean personal income per month in our patients was: preschool children-10.5 € (SD = 0), students-11.32 € (SD = 6.34), university students-35 € (SD = 0.86), employees-132.5 € (SD = 53.03), handicapped with social support-35 € (SD = 0). Monthly morbidity cost of hemophiliacs who underwent orthopedic and surgical interventions was 97.5 €.
2. Loss of income of family members who forfeit paid employment in order to offer home care for hemophiliacs who underwent orthopedic and surgical interventions in an important consequence of hemophilia. In our patients, in 72.98% of cases, a family member forfeited employment in order to offer home care for hemophilia patient (Fig. 2), mcan family income being lower in these families

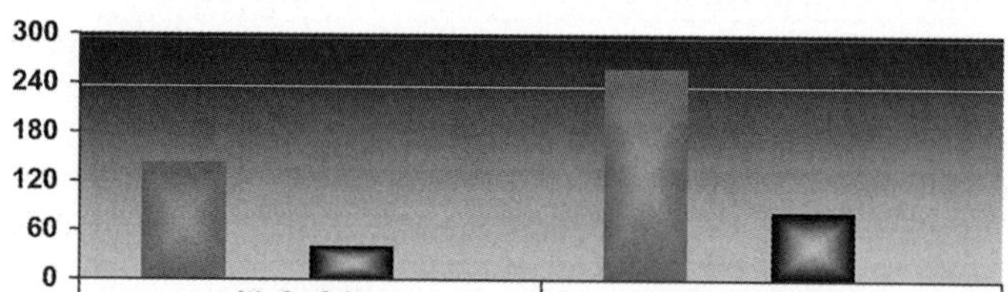

	with forfeiture	without forfeiture	
MFI*-mean (€)	142.96	258	p=0.0001
MFI*-SD	34.73	120.92	
MFI/MB**-mean (€)	40.21	84.05	p<0.0001
MFI/MB**-SD	12.89	35.79	

*-mean family income/month; **-mean family income/no. of family members/month;

Fig. 2. Comparison of mean family income/month and mean family income/no. of family members/month, according to paid employment forfeiture of a family member

(difference=115.04 € for mean family income/month and 43.84 € for mean family income/no. of family members/month).

3. Average number of days off at school or work was significantly higher in patients with orthopedic and surgical interventions than in other hemophiliacs, in all hemophilia severity forms and age groups, the differences being statistically significant (Table 4).

Table 4. Average number of days off at school or work

Category		Patients without interventions		Patients with interventions		p
		mean	SD	mean	SD	
Hemophilia severity	severe	52.27	21.16	77.50	34.71	0.0007
	moderate	27.20	16.75	50.00	13.23	0.0361
	mild	20.00	8.65	52.00	0.00	0.0024
Age group	< 18 years	39.98	23.55	65.75	19.50	0.0002
	> 18 years	39.81	22.74	90.83	54.35	0.0004
Total		39.92	23.11	72.59	33.25	< 0.0001

Socio-Economic Consequences of the Treatment

Poor social integration of the patients and loss of income of their family members lead to financial problems, which can affect treatment compliance. In our case, 81.1% of the patients who underwent orthopedic and surgical interventions missed hospitalization, for financial reasons, on an average of 12.1 times/year (SD = 8.9), and 78.4% of the patients came too late at the hospital, for financial reasons, on an average of 13.8 times/year (SD = 6.9), mean income being significantly lower in these families (Table 5, 6). In the case of hemophilia, any delay in substitution administration or absence of substitution leads to complications appearance, some of them requiring surgical interventions.

Table 5. Mean income of patients who missed hospitalization for financial reasons, compared to patients who didn't miss hospitalization

Mean income/month (€)	Patients who missed hospitalization		Patients who didn't miss hospitalization		p
	mean	SD	mean	SD	
MFI	149.83	51.06	277.85	123.08	0.0001
MFI/MB	44.38	19.36	84.95	40.12	0.0003
MPI	22.76	18.46	47.28	55.33	0.0473

Table 6. Mean income of patients who came too late at hospital, for financial reasons, compared to patients who didn't come too late

Mean income/month (€)	Patients who came too late		Patients who didn't come too late		p
	mean	SD	mean	SD	
MFI	150.17	51.94	260.63	123.94	0.0005
MFI/MB	44.31	19.70	80.17	39.54	0.0010
MPI	23.19	18.64	42.69	52.85	0.1003

Financial problems of the patients and their families were not the only reason of poor treatment compliance. All patients mentioned numerous other factors associated with this poor compliance (Fig. 3).

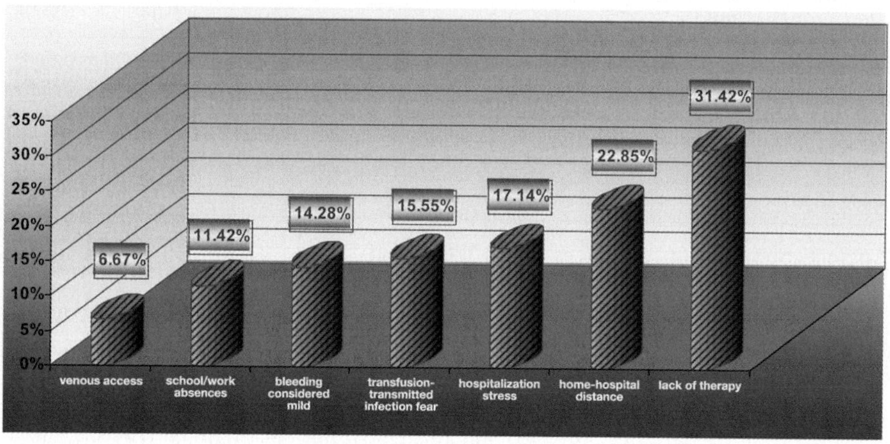

Fig. 3. Other reasons for poor treatment compliance

Discussion and Conclusions

Inadequate resource allocation leads to severe complications in hemophiliacs, which can be life-threatening, requiring costly surgical interventions. Substitution costs of orthopedic and surgical interventions represented 91.14% of direct medical costs; the higher proportion of these costs in hemophilia B patients (92.52%), compared to hemophilia A patients without inhibitors (85.8%) is explained by the use of fresh frozen plasma and cryoprecipitate (together with FVIII concentrates) in the therapy of hemophilia A, which are cheep products, while in hemophilia B, substitution was represented only by clotting factor concentrates;

In the absence of home therapy programs, patients have to travel long home-hospital distances to receive substitutive therapy. Poor social integration has a negative impact on patients' income, and, by the other hand, one home-hospital travel represents an important percentage from patient and family income, all these factors having a negative impact on patients' compliance.

In our study group, morbidity cost was 97.5 €; in many cases (72.98%), a family member had to forfeit employment in order to offer home care for hemophilia patient, mean family income being statistically significant lower.

Patient satisfaction with different aspects of medical care has been reported to influence treatment compliance. Estimating the effects of specific factors on treatment adherence is important in having a greater insight into the determinants of poor compliance. This information could be useful for developing strategies aimed at improving compliance.

Lack of substitutive products was the mean reason of poor compliance, but any delay in treatment administration or the absence of therapy led to severe complications, which can require surgical interventions, so that poor treatment compliance may lead not only to negative health outcomes for the patient but also to wasting of economic resources. Besides, treatment adherence might be related not only to the clinical severity of the disease and quality of life but also to the psychological or psychiatric well-being of the patient.

All these aspects support the need of a better financial resource allocation for hemophilia treatment, not only for increase direct medical costs, but also in order to offer a better social protection of the patients and to improve their life quality.

References

1. Evans C, Crawford B. Patient self-reports in pharmacoeconomic studies. Their use and impact on study validity. Pharmacoeconomics 1999; 15(3):241–156
2. McLoughlin V, Leatherman S. Quality or financing: what drives design of the health care system? Qual Saf Health Care 2003; 12:136–142
3. Robertson J, Lang D, Hill S. Use of pharmacoeconomics in prescribing research. Part 1: Costs-moving beyond the acquisition price for drugs. J Clin Pharm Ther 2003; 28(1):73–79
4. Schramm W, Szucs TD. State-of-the-art principles and practices of medical economics. Haemophilia 1998; 4:491-497 Szucs TD, Offner A, Schramm W. Socioeconomic impact of haemophilia care: results of a pilot study. Haemophilia 1996; 2:211–217
5. Schramm W. Towards the Best Use of Safe Clotting Factor Concentrates. Hämostaseologie 1996; 16:269–273
6. Wilkinson RG. Socioeconomic determinants of health: Health inequalities: relative or absolute material standards?. BMJ 1997; 314:591
7. Xu K, Evans DB, Kawabata K, et al. Household catastrophic health expenditure: a multi-coutry analysis. Lancet 2003; 362:111–117

VIIb. Inhibitors in Hemophilia

The Occurrence of Factor VIII Inhibitor in a Patient with Mild Hemophilia A – During Treatment with Interferon for Chronic Hepatitis C

W. Miesbach, B. Llugaliu, G. Asmelash, Ch. von Auer, and I. Scharrer

Only a few case reports describe the occurrence of factor VIII inhibitor during the treatment with Interferon [1–3]. The use of Interferon has been the treatment of choice for patients with chronic hepatitis C infection (HCV).

However, the use of interferon has also been associated with the development of autoimmune disorders.

This case report marks out the occurrence of factor VIII inhibitor in a patient with mild hemophilia A, two months after the start of the treatment with Interferon.

The patient is a 56-year-old male with mild hemophilia A (factor VIII activity: 10 %; factor VIII gene mutation: missense mutation ARG (CGA) 1941 Leu (CTA). 17 years ago, the patient presented with a transient factor VIII inhibitor (24 Bethesda units, BU) after substitution with Haemate HS after an operation. The patient has a more than 20-year history of asymptomatic HCV infection (genotype 1a) and hepatitis A and B infection.

The measurement of factor VIII activity and factor VIII inhibitor was carried out two months before and after the start of treatment with Peginterferon alfa-2b and Ribavirin for chronic HCV infection.

Two months before the initiation of this treatment, during a tooth extraction, the patient was treated with recombinant factor VIII concentrates (Kogenate Bayer) and presented with an increase of the factor VIII levels at the normal range and had no bleeding symptoms. The patient was also treated with recombinant factor VIII (Kogenate) due to a tooth extraction two years ago.

Two months after the initiation of the treatment, a factor VIII inhibitor was detected in a titer of 16 BU and the factor VIII activity was 25 %.

The discrepancy of the relatively »high« factor VIII levels of 25 % and the inhibitor titer of 16 BU does hint on an autoantibody caused by Interferon.

The Peginterferon/Ribavirin was discontinued. Up to now the patient did not show any increased bleeding symptoms and no immunosuppressive treatment was started.

Factor VIII inhibitor occurs in up to 30 % of patients with severe hemophilia A and is a major cause of morbidity in these patients [4].

The occurrence of a factor VIII inhibitor in patients with mild hemophilia, however, is less common. Several risk factors for the development of inhibitors in patients with mild hemophilia A have been proposed, such as factor VIII gene mutation, the continuous infusion of factor VIII concentrates or the use of certain drugs [5–7].

I. Scharrer/W. Schramm (Ed.)
36th Hemophilia Symposium Hamburg 2005

This case report emphasizes the necessity for regularly measurement of the factor VIII activity and the factor VIII inhibitor in patients receiving Pegintereferon/Ribavirin.

Although it cannot be excluded that the treatment with factor VIII concentrates may have resulted in production of factor VIII inhibitor, the treatment with Peginterferon/Ribavirin may be responsible for the factor VIII inhibitor production in patients even with mild hemophilia A as it is the case with patients with acquired inhibitor hemophilia [1–3].

References

1. Herman C, Boggio L, Green D. Factor VIII inhibitor associated with interferon. Haemophilia 2005;11:408–10.
2. Regina S, Colombat P, Fimbel B, et al. Acquired inhibitor to factor VIII in a patient with Hodgkin's disease following treatment with interferon-alpha. Haemophilia 2001;7:526–7.
3. Stricker RB, Barlogie B, Kiprov DD. Acquired factor VIII inhibitor associated with chronic interferon-alpha therapy. J Rheumatol 1994;21:350–2
4. Ehrenforth S, Kreuz W, Scharrer I, et al. Incidence of development of factor VIII and factor IX inhibitors in haemophiliacs. Lancet 1992;339:594–8.
5. von Auer C, Oldenburg J, von Depka M, et al. Inhibitor development in patients with hemophilia A after continuous infusion of factor VIII concentrates. Ann N Y Acad Sci 2005;1051:498–505.
6. Bril WS, MacLean PE, Kaijen PH, et al. HLA class II genotype and factor VIII inhibitors in mild haemophilia A patients with an Arg593 to Cys mutation. Haemophilia 2004;10(5):509–14.
7. d'Oiron R, Volot F, Reynaud J, et al. Impact of choice of treatment for bleeding episodes on inhibitor outcome in patients with mild/moderate hemophilia a and inhibitors. Semin Hematol 2006;43(1):S3–9.

Severe Hemophilia A Patient with High-Titer Inhibitor, use of TGA in the Monitoring of Bypassing Therapy

A. Hluší, P. Novák, V. Krčová, and L. Slavík

Introduction

Hemophilia patients with inhibitors are treated with bypassing agents: activated prothrombin complex concentrates (FEIBA) or concentrates containing FVIIa. Their mechanism of action is based on inducing of thrombin generation. Monitoring of these bypassing therapies is still problematic: The minimum rate of thrombin generation to achieve effective hemostasis in hemophiliacs is unknown.

Aim

The aim is to evaluate the potential of thrombin generation assay (TGA) for monitoring of bypassing therapy in a hemophilia A patient.

Subject and Method

We report a case of severe hemophilia A patient with a high-titer of inhibitor, who experienced large intracranial bleeding. The 49-year-old patient with long-time low-titer inhibitor was initially treated for intracranial hemorrhage by factor VIII concentrates (Immunate). After ten days of successful therapy this substitution became ineffective and high titer of FVIII inhibitor was induced and laboratory findings proved high-titer inhibitor (140 BU). The substitution therapy was stopped and immunosuppressive therapy was indicated (Prednison, IVIG, Cyclophosphamide and Rituximab). During following period recurrent hematuria occurred. For these complications FEIBA (50 IU/kg every six hours) was applied and bleeding stopped after few infusions. In our clinical monitoring we used TGA which quantitatively measures the potential of plasma to generate thrombin. The TGA parameters (Lag-phase, slope, peak-thrombin, inactivated phase) were studied before and 30 min, 3 h, 6 h after administration of FEIBA to evaluate the correction of thrombin generation capacity.

I. Scharrer/W. Schramm (Ed.)
36th Hemophilia Symposium Hamburg 2005

Result

TGA curves show the difference in amount of maximum generated thrombin or lag phase after substitution therapy with Immunate in samples before and after inhibitor increase (455 nM, 14 min, resp. 3.4 nM, 40 min in sample with inhibitor 9.4 BU). TGA curves after FEIBA administration show relatively less amount of generated thrombin (34 nM after 30 min, 12 nM after 3 hours). Though, this amount was clinically sufficient for hemostasis.

Conclusion

In our first experience with TGA we observed its high sensitivity to inhibitor development. Generation of thrombin comes slower in despite of using by-pass agent. Minimum rate of thrombin sufficient for hemostasis is unknown and probably is individual. Duration of the measurement should be prolonged over 90 minutes. The assay has a potential for bypass therapy monitoring.

EUREKA – an European Registry for Orthopedic Surgery in Hemophiliacs with Inhibitors

A. Kurth

The development of inhibitors in hemophilia patients is a serious complication that is not infrequent. Elective orthopedic procedures constitute a challenge in inhibitor patients and have only been performed at certain centers and in a small number of cases. Clear therapeutic guidelines for perioperative substitution are not available. It is only due to published data in the literature that there is a certain level of assurance, and necessary surgical procedures could be carried out. Despite this situation an increasing number of inhibitor patients will have to undergo orthopedic surgery in the future.

The literature suggests that factor rVIIa is a useful »first-line therapy« in such procedures.

Since most centers in Europe only treated a very small number of patients in the past and will continue to do so in the future, a multinational approach has been initiated. The objective of this initiative is to collect data on these patients and their clinical course, and to evaluate the data to create therapeutic recommendations.

The **EUREKA** project is a European registry for endoprostheses of the knees in inhibitor patients (**EU**ropean **RE**gistry on **K**nee **A**rthroplasty performed in hemophilia patients with recombinant factor VIIa as first line treatment). The presentation will introduce the background, experiences and approach of the EUREKA project.

I. Scharrer/W. Schramm (Ed.)
36th Hemophilia Symposium Hamburg 2005

VIIc. Casuistics

Double Balloon Enteroscopy (DBE) with Argon Plasma Laser Coagulation (APC) for a Patient with Heyde's Syndrome

A. Trummer, F. Wiedbrauck, and S. Hollerbach

Background

The striking combination of clinical significant aortic valve stenosis (AS) and considerable gastrointestinal bleeding (GIB) of unknown localization was first described by Heyde 1958 in a short letter to the editor of the New England Journal of Medicine [1]. In the following decades a debate was raised whether this was a significant correlation which could be explained pathophysiologically. Just recent work and data in larger patient populations could proof a correlation of AS and GIB [2], a more frequent occurrence of arteriovenous malformations (AVM) in patients with AS compared to a normal population [3] and finally a direct correlation between stenosis grade and severity of a von Willebrand syndrome (vWS) type 2a with loss of high molecular multimers. The incidence of skin and mucosa bleedings between patients with Heyde's syndrome ranges around 20% [4, 5]. As bleeding episodes do not account for valve replacement indications so far, patients with Heyde's syndrome often require an individual and interdisciplinary therapeutic concept and represent both a time and cost intensive problem, especially in the case of occult small bowel bleedings (OSBB) by AVM.

Until the introduction of capsule endoscopy (CE) in 2000 push and intraoperative endoscopy were the sole procedures for the investigation of OSBB but were rarely performed due to low sensitivity and high invasivity. In contrast, CE today represents the method of choice for investigation of OSBB with a sensitivity of 89% and a specificity of 95% [6]. Still biopsies or therapeutic interventions are not possible so far. Therefore double balloon enteroscopy, developed and first described by Yamamoto in 2001, for the first time allows the non-invasive treatment of AVM by APC. The technical principles are shown in Figure 1 and described in detail elsewhere [7, 8].

Case Report

We report the case of a 81-year-old male patient who was repeatedly treated on ward with blood transfusions [2 units every 2–3 weeks) due to recurrent melena and anemia. He had been both under oral anticoagulation as well as low-molecular heparin (LMH) in consequence of a mechanical aortic valve replacement at the age of 74.

I. Scharrer/W. Schramm (Ed.)
36th Hemophilia Symposium Hamburg 2005

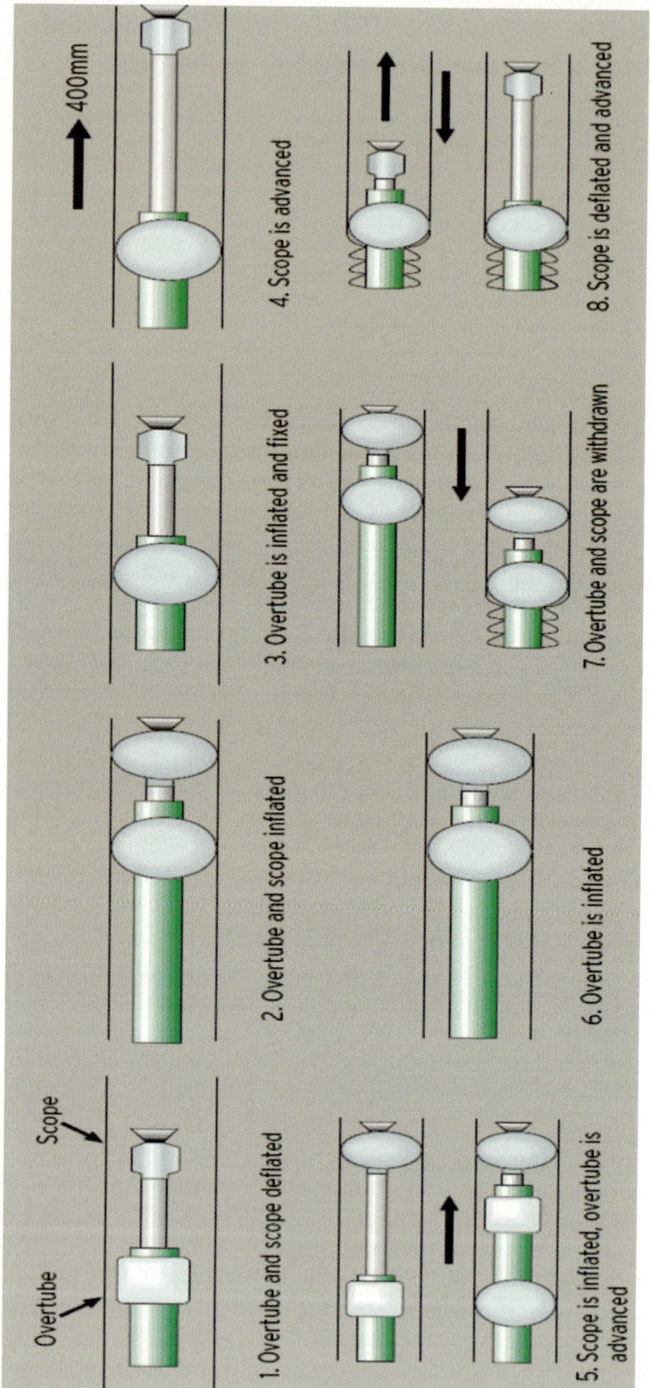

Fig. 1. Principles of double balloon enteroscopy

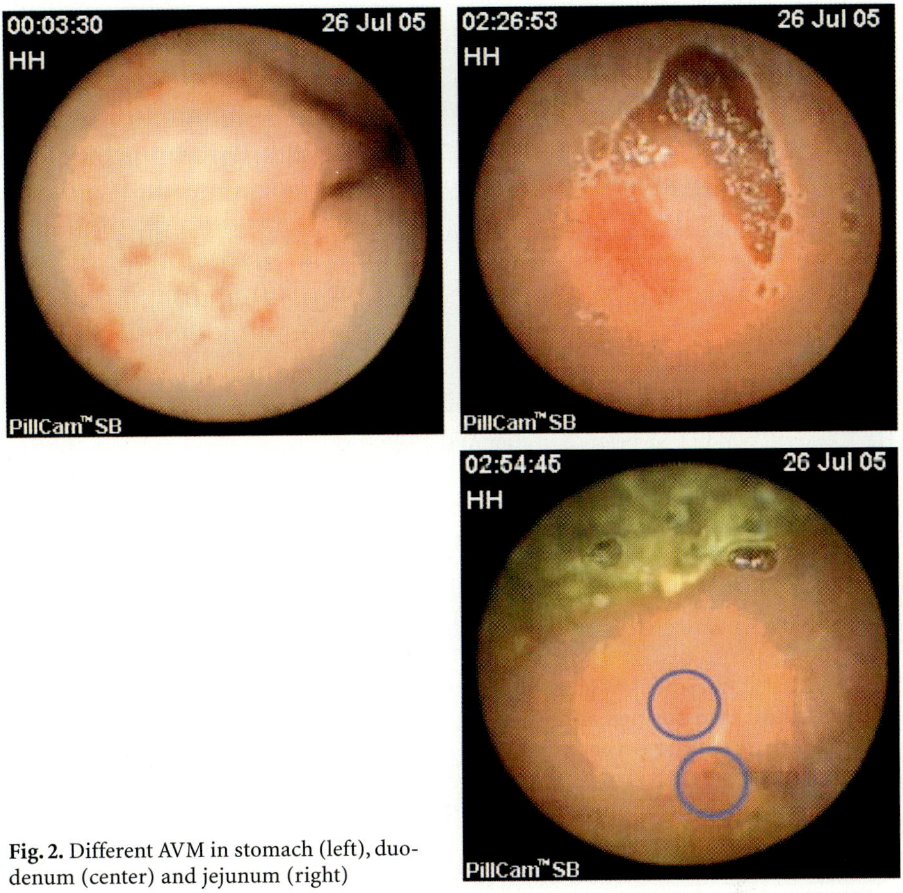

Fig. 2. Different AVM in stomach (left), duodenum (center) and jejunum (right)

Endoscopic examination (gastroscopy, coloscopy, CE) revealed multiple AVM in the entire gastrointestinal tract (see Figure 2). Despite of repeated APC of AVM reachable by standard endoscopy and reduction of LMH to prophylactic dose the frequency of the blood transfusions remained stable about several months. Thus DBE was finally performed and showed more than 30 AVM of a size up to four millimeters, mainly in the duodenal and jejunal tract, of which 17 could be treated by APC (see Figure 3). Due to the considerable cardiac restrictions of the patient the procedure was stopped after nearly 150 min. The OSBB suspended at first. But in the later course a spontaneous soft tissue bleeding occurred at the left hip which prompted us to perform a vWS diagnostic program. It showed a relative decrease of the high molecular multimers and a reduced ratio (0.72) of von Willebrand factor antigen (254%) and Collagen binding activity (182%). Therefore the diagnosis of vWS type 2a was made and a low-dose therapy of DDAVP initiated (1 puff = 10 μg/day). Subsequently no further soft tissue or skin bleedings occurred and the blood transfusion demand declined to 2 units every 8 weeks while melena had been attenuated.

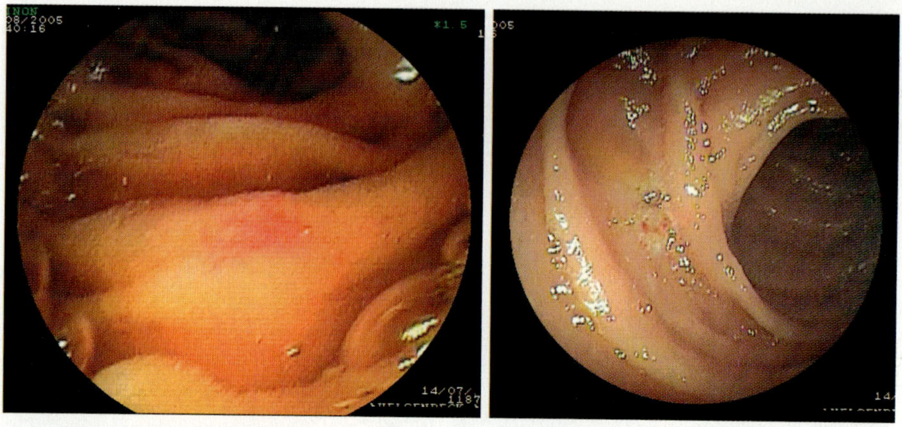

Fig. 3. Jejunal AVM in DBE before and after APC

Unfortunately the patient died 5 months after the DBE due to his progressive heart failure.

Discussion

The successful treatment of gastrointestinal AVM in patients who are in continuous need of blood transfusions abolishes the transfusion demand in nearly 80% of the cases [9]. One- and two-year probabilities for the event-free survival are around 86% and 80%, respectively [10]. The positive and negative predictive value for CE to make the correct indication for DBE are 94.7% and 98.3%, respectively. Thus CE has become both »indication filter« as well as »access path finder« for DBE (oral vs anal, also depending on the investigators skills) [11].

In summary, DBE offers a new option for the treatment of OSBB which cannot reached by conventional endoscopy, even in patients of higher age and relevant comorbidity which might not be eligible for surgery. By this way the need for blood transfusions and/or clotting factor containing products for hemorrhagic disorders can be reduced. The complications of the procedure have been quoted to be around 1% and include acute pancreatitis, paralytic ileus and perforation [12–14].

As the frequency of AVM and thus Heyde's syndrome increases with the AS grade (this correlation is independent from age and gender) [3] and as most acquired vWS cases resolve after valve replacement [4], therapy should always be preceded by an interdisciplinary decision making process including cardiologists, heart surgeons, gastroenterologists and hemostaseologists. The following parameters should be considered in detail:

a) Transfusion requirement and severity of anemic symptoms
b) Necessity and frequency of treatment with vWF containing products
c) Grade of AS or patient-prosthesis mismatch (see below)
d) Operability
e) Endoscopic treatment options

The patient-prosthesis mismatch (PPM) is present when the effective orifice area (EOA) of the inserted aortic prosthetic valve is too small relative to the patient's body surface area (BSA). This occurs in 20-71% of aortic valve replacements and leads to persistence of high transvalvular pressure gradients [15]. A vWS which has resolved after valve replacement at first can recur due to a relevant PPM within a period of 6 months [4, 5] pointing to the need of a surgical revision [15].

Patients with Heyde's syndrome therefore remain an interdisciplinary challenge and thus should primarily be treated in health-care centers with the required facilities.

References

1. Heyde EC. Gastrointestinal bleeding in aortic stenosis (letter). N Engl J Med.. 1958:259:196.
2. Pate GE, Mulligan A. An epidemiological study of Heyde's syndrome: an association between aortic stenosis and gastrointestinal bleeding. J Heart Valve Dis. 2004 Sep;13(5):713–6.
3. Batur P et al. Increased prevalence of aortic stenosis in patients with arteriovenous malformations of the gastrointestinal tract in Heyde syndrome. Arch Intern Med. 2003 Aug 11-25;163(15):1821–4.
4. Vincentelli A et al. Acquired von Willebrand syndrome in aortic stenosis. N Engl J Med. 2003 Jul 24;349(4):343–9.
5. Yoshida K et al. Acquired and reversible von Willebrand disease with high shear stress aortic valve stenosis. Ann Thorac Surg. 2006 Feb;81(2):490–4.
6. Pennazio M et al. Outcome of patients with obscure gastrointestinal bleeding after capsule endoscopy: report of 100 consecutive cases. Gastroenterology. 2004 Mar;126(3):643–53.
7. Yamamoto H et al. Total enteroscopy with a nonsurgical steerable double-balloon method. Gastrointest Endosc. 2001 Feb;53(2):216–20.
8. May A et al. Double-balloon enteroscopy: preliminary experience in patients with obscure gastrointestinal bleeding or chronic abdominal pain. Endoscopy. 2003 Dec;35(12):985–91.
9. Kwan V et al. Argon plasma coagulation in the management of symptomatic gastrointestinal vascular lesions: experience in 100 consecutive patients with long-term follow-up. Am J Gastroenterol. 2006 Jan;101(1):58–63.
10. Olmos JA et al. Argon plasma coagulation for prevention of recurrent bleeding from GI angiodysplasias. Gastrointest Endosc. 2004 Dec;60(6):881–6.
11. Gay G et al. Outcome of capsule endoscopy in determining indication and route for push-and-pull enteroscopy. Endoscopy. 2006 Jan;38(1):49–58.
12. Heine GD et al. Double-balloon enteroscopy: indications, diagnostic yield, and complications in a series of 275 patients with suspected small-bowel disease. Endoscopy. 2006 Jan;38(1):42 8.
13. Attar A et al. First case of paralytic intestinal ileus after double balloon enteroscopy. Gut. 2005 Dec;54(12):1823–4.
14. Yamamoto H, Kita H. Double-balloon endoscopy. Curr Opin Gastroenterol. 2005 Sep;21(5):573–7.
15. Blais C et al.. Impact of valve prosthesis-patient mismatch on short-term mortality after aortic valve replacement. Circulation. 2003; 108:983–988.

Successful Liver Transplantation in a Patient with Anti-Thrombocyte Antibodies and Severe Hemophilia A

W. MIESBACH, C. ZAPLETAL, G. ASMELASH, B. LLUGALIO,
W. O. BECHSTEIN, and I. SCHARRER

Hepatitis C (HCV)-related liver cirrhosis and development of hepatocellular carcinoma (HCC) is a major problem in patients with hemophilia A. Up to 30% of patients with hepatitis C infection will develop liver cirrhosis [1].

Liver transplantation has been shown to cure hemophilia and give the patients a long-term benefit in life-quality [2]. Nevertheless transplantation of a patient with coagulation disorders remains challenging especially if hemophilia is combined with any further coagulation disorder.

We report on our experience with liver transplantation in a patient with a combination of severe hemophilia A and anti-platelet antibodies.

The patient is a 53-year old man with severe hemophilia A (FVIII activity < 1%) combined with thrombocytopenia in a HCV-related liver cirrhosis Child-Pugh-Status C who was listed for liver transplantation 08/2004 and upgraded to urgency T2 in 11/2004 (69 days waiting-time). He had been regularly exposed to clotting factor concentrates but experienced several bleeding episodes due to gastrointestinal bleedings.

The patient stayed in hospital over this period due to decompensated liver function and recurrent bleeding episodes. Due to the long hospital stay he got contaminated with MRSA diagnosed in routine swabs.

In January 2005, the patient underwent liver transplantation. In the explanted liver, liver cirrhosis and incidentally, HCC pT2, G2 was diagnosed. The loading dose of factor VIII (Kogenate; Bayer) was 100 IU/kg 1 h pre operation. Boli of 50 IU/kg followed depending on intraoperative factor VIII activity. The treatment was continued until 20 hours postoperative. Laboratory tests were carried out initially every two hours and after the first day of operation every five hours. The cumulative dosage given was 36,000 IU.

The activity of factor V normalized within 24 hours. On the third postoperative day, FVIII activity reached 93% (normal range: 64–167%) corresponding to the endogenous synthesis of FV activity of 75% (normal range: 70–120%) and FVII activity of 57% (normal range: 70–130%) (Fig. 1).

The thrombocyte count before operation was 35/nl. After substitution of thrombocyte concentrates on the day of operation, the thrombocyte count increased to 70/nl but decreased to 40/nl within one day. Thrombocytopenia and allergic reaction to platelet transfusion aggravated. On the second postoperative day, no reaction to platelet transfusion could be found. The platelet count dropped to 3/nl on the second day after operation. HLA-antibodies against platelets were diagnosed. Lupus anticoagulants had been present prior to operation, but were not longer detectable

I. Scharrer/W. Schramm (Ed.)
36th Hemophilia Symposium Hamburg 2005

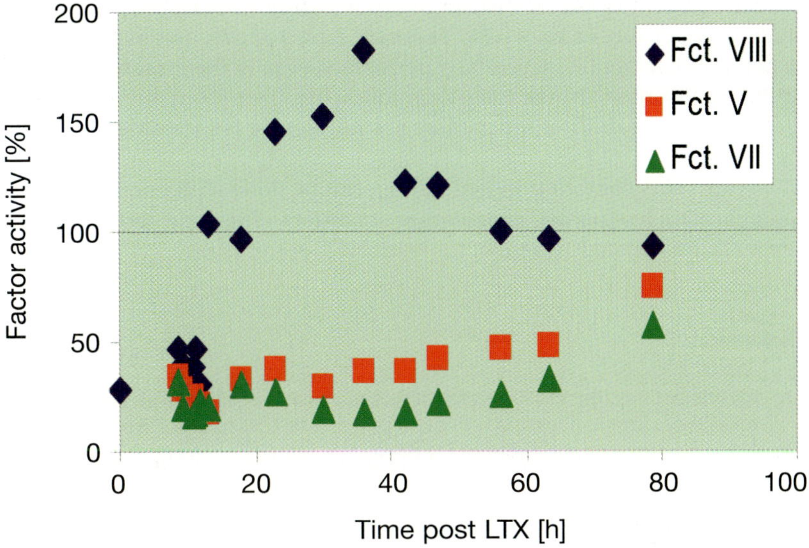

Fig. 1. Activities of factor V, VII and VIII during and post transplantation

following the transplant. The transfusion of HLA-identical platelets, however, was performed without success. We initiated treatment with human immunoglobulins (Pentaglobin; Biotest) in a dosage of 5ml/kg over 3 days. On the seventh day post operation, the platelets increased to 40/nl under substitution with thrombocyte concentrates. The platelet count increased to over 80/nl ten days after operation and no further treatment was needed (Fig. 2).

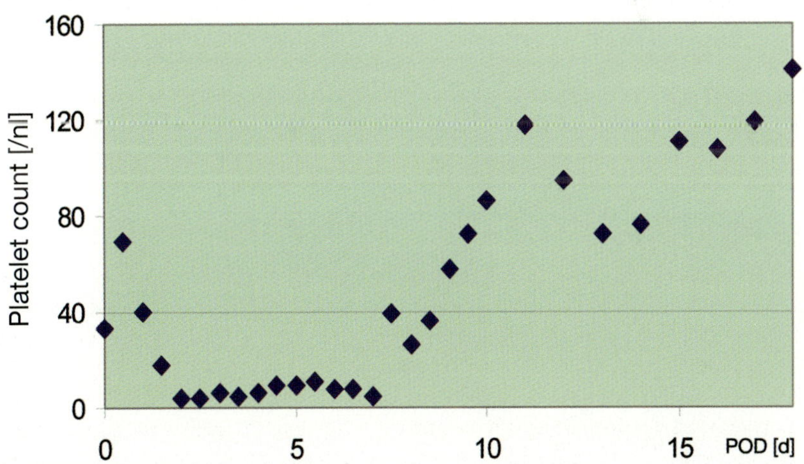

Fig. 2. Treatment of thrombocytopenia

The patient could be discharged in a significantly improved condition after a total hospital stay of six weeks. This case report shows that liver transplantation in a hemophiliac can be successfully performed even in the presence of additional coagulation disorders. In the long-term follow-up, liver function and coagulation tests remained normal. Until today there are no signs of HCV reinfection or HCC recurrence.

Liver transplantation in hemophilia can be done with good success even if it is complicated by further coagulation disorders. The long-term success, however, depends on hepatitis C reinfection and HCC recurrence.

References

1. Makris M, Preston FE, Rosendaal FR, Underwood JC, Rice KM, Triger DR. The natural history of chronic hepatitis C in hemophiliacs. Br J Haematol 1996;94:746–52.
2. Lewis JH, Bontempo FH, Spero JA, Ragni MV, Starzl TE. Liver transplantation in a hemophiliac. N Engl J Med 1985;312: 1189–90.
3. Scharrer I, Encke A, Hottenrott C. Clinical Cure Of Haemophilia A By Liver Transplantation. The Lancet, October 1, 1988;800–801.

Peri- and Postoperative Course of 95 Patients with von-Willebrand's Disease

CH. VON AUER, K. LOTTER, S. HEINSDORF, and I. SCHARRER

Objectives

Von Willebrand's disease (vWD) is the most common inherited bleeding disorder in humans, exhibiting quantitative and qualitative defects in the von Willebrand factor. To find out about the peri- and postoperative course of patients with vWD, we conducted a retrospective data analysis in our center. vWD is divided into several types and severity grades which show different bleeding patterns and require different treatment options. Thus the exact definition of type and severity is mandatory for the correct therapy in case of bleeding or surgery.

Methods

We retrospectively looked at data of 95 patients with vWD who went for surgery in our university hospital between 1981 and 2003. In detail we looked at peri- and postoperative courses of these patients regarding bleeding complications. Our own patient data were checked but also data from each involved surgery department (Abdominal surgery, neurosurgery, gynecology, otolaryngological surgery, thoracic surgery and orthopedic surgery).

vWD types were defined by the following diagnostic criteria:

Type 1: Ratio vWF:RCoF/ vWF:Ag >0.7
Severity: vWF:RCoF >30% = mild, 10–30% = moderate, <10% = severe;

Type 2A: Ratio vWF:RCoF/ vWF:Ag <0.7 and/or multimers and/or gene analysis

Type 2B: Ratio vWF:RCoF/ vWF:Ag <0.7 and/or pathologic
RIPA and/or gene analysis

Type 2N: low FVIII-binding test and gene analysis

Type 3: vWF:RCoF and vWF:Ag not detectable, no multimers in platelets.

Additionally we looked at the patient's bleeding history and present bleeding symptoms.

I. Scharrer/W. Schramm (Ed.)
36th Hemophilia Symposium Hamburg 2005

Results

From 1983 to 2003 we counted 173 surgical interventions in 95 patients with vWD. 59 Patients had type 1 vWD (two severe, three moderate, 54 mild). 16 patients had type 2 vWD (14 2A, one 2B, one 2N) and 11 patients type 3 vWD. Nine patients with type 1 vWD had an additional factor deficiency (five FXII-, two FVII- and two FV-deficiencies).

We counted 54 orthopedic surgeries, 41 abdominal surgeries, 15 angiographies, 12 endoscopic surgeries, 10 otolaryngological surgeries, 11 mamma surgeries, 10 neurological surgeries, 8 soft tissue surgeries, 7 thoracic surgeries, 3 thyroid gland surgeries and 2 biopsies.

vWD-Treatment

Most patients (108/173) were treated with Haemate HS during the pre-, peri- and postoperative phase. 33 patients were treated with Minirin (33/173), 9 patients received both products. Three patients received other plasmatic FVIII-concentrates, 20 patients had no therapy for their coagulation disorder.

Complications

16 patients had peri- or postoperative bleeding complications (10 type 1, three type 2, three type 3 vWD). Nine patients with bleeding complications had been treated with Haemate HS (9/108 = 8.3%), four with Minirin (4/33 = 12.1%), three patients had no therapy. Most bleeding complications were reported in thoracic surgery (2/7 = 28%), gynecological (3/11 = 27%) and otolaryngological surgery (2/10 = 20%). Retrospectively 15 bleeding complications could be explained by surgical technique, thrombosis prophylaxis, inefficient substitution therapy and additional thrombocytopenia.

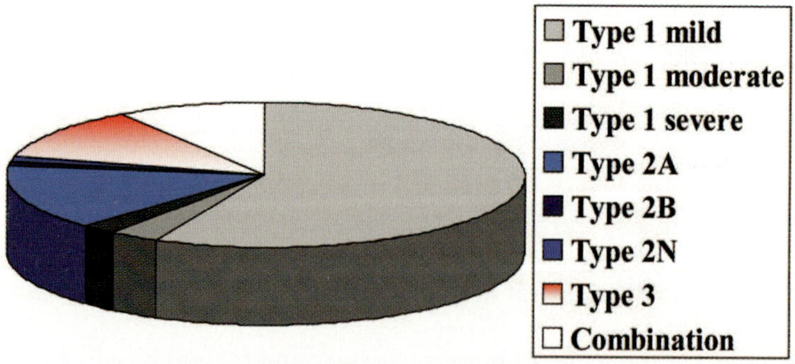

Fig. 1. vWD-Types (all patients)

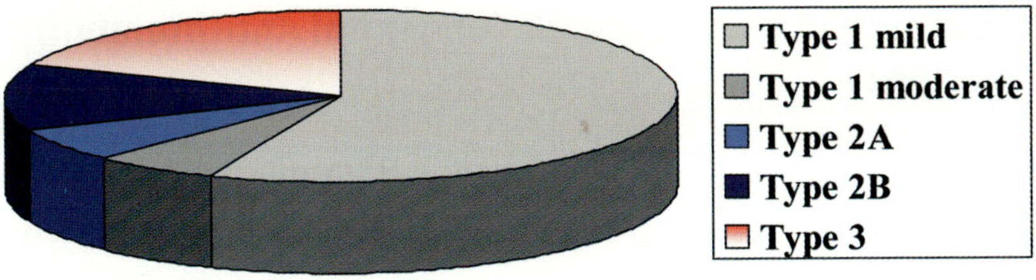

Fig. 2. vWD-Type distribution in bleeding complications

Conclusion

The finding of 16 bleeding complications in 173 surgical interventions is low (9.2%). Most bleeding complications were seen in patients with vWD type 2B and 3. Patients who underwent major surgery and who received only Minirin had more often bleeding complications.

Our evaluation of bleeding incidents in the context of surgery in vWD patients reveals the necessity of special hemostaseologic care for these patients. Substitution therapy should depend on vWD-type and type of surgical intervention. We recommend a therapy with vWF containing FVIII-products for major surgery in vWD-patients.

Especially during thoracic surgery, gynecological and otolaryngological surgery a careful peri- and postoperative hemostaseologic management as well as careful coagulation techniques of the surgeon are required.

Pregnancy in a Patient with Congenital Antithrombin Deficiency

B. Maak, L. Kochhan, Ch. Estel, and P. Heuchel

Among the hereditary thrombophilic states antithrombin deficiency is one of the most powerful factors. The disorder was first described in 1965 by Egeberg [6]. The pattern of inheritance of familiar antithrombin deficiency is autosomal-dominant, meaning men and women are equally affected.

The prevalence of this disorder has been found at between 0.2/1000 and more recently, 11/1000 [1]. The manifestation of antithrombin deficiency occurs often before the age of twenty, in the majority of the patients the first thrombotic events are localized within the deep veins of the lower extremities (more than 90%) and in many cases (more than 40%) pulmonary embolisms are typical complications [10, 13]. In antithrombin deficient women the use of estrogen-containing pills as an oral contraceptive drug is a well known risk factor for the development of venous thrombosis.

Pregnancy and puerperal period are also associated with a markedly increased risk of thrombotic complications [4]. In nearly 70% of antithrombin deficient women severe thromboembolic events occur especially during the first months of pregnancy [7]. Moreover, it had been suggested that antithrombin deficiency may be associated with placental insufficiency and fetal losses [9]. Therefore, antithrombin deficient women should be carefully observed during pregnancy and, in the case of a thromboembolic event, therapeutic intervention must be immediately performed. Unfortunately, there is only a small number of studies concerning therapeutic strategies in such situations. The use of antithrombin concentrates alone or in combination with heparin has been reported but also the use of heparin alone [2, 3, 5, 7, 8, 12].

Therefore, we present here the history of a pregnant young woman with congenital antithrombin deficiency and describe the combined use of subcutaneous administered low molecular weight heparin (LMWH) and antithrombin concentrate to treat a thrombotic occlusion and to prevent against further thrombotic complications.

Case Report

The patient was born in 1969. She suffered from her first thrombotic event in her left leg shortly after beginning an oral contraceptive treatment with an estrogen-containing pill in 1987. A second thrombosis occurred twelve years later and in 2000

I. Scharrer/W. Schramm (Ed.)
36th Hemophilia Symposium Hamburg 2005

a thrombosis of the V. tibialis posterior and V. poplitea of her right leg was diagnosed. At another clinic the following results of laboratory investigations were obtained: factor V Leiden absent, mutation G 20210 A within the prothrombin gene undetectable, antithrombin activity 65%, antiphospholipid antibodies negative. In this hospital it was not believed that the low antithrombin activity may be responsible for the recurrent thrombotic events.

The woman became pregnant in 2004. Because of the patient's history a prophylactic treatment with a LMWH was instituted immediately after the diagnosis of pregnancy. During weeks 10–11 a painful swelling of her right leg occurred and thrombotic occlusions of the popliteal vein and the superficial femoral vein were detected sonografically and the patient was admitted to our hospital.

Shortly after admission the following results of laboratory investigations were obtained:

antithrombin activity 51%, D-dimer concentration 2183 μg/l.

As cause of the reduced antithrombin activity we identified a Cys 21 (TGC) > Ser (TCC) exchange within the exon 2 of the antithrombin gene in the heterozygous state. Also in the heterozygous state the HR 2-haplotype (A 4070 G) within the factor V gene could be found. Within the factor XIII the Val 34 allele was homozygous present.

First, we increased the dosage of the LMWH, however the thrombotic occlusions showed no change. As the next step we decided to add antithrombin and ten days later the thrombus had almost completely disappeared. After discharge from the hospital the LMWH (enoxaparin, 60 mg per day) was given once per day and also an antithrombin concentrate (Atenativ).

The dosage of the antithrombin concentrate was adjusted to result in antithrombin activities between 75 and 94% twenty four hours after the application. During this treatment the D-dimer concentrations have been found in a range typical for pregnant women (185–549 μg/l) and no clinical symptoms of any thrombosis were observed.

The patient was readmitted to our hospital after 36 completed weeks of gestation. After the beginning of labour (February, 3rd) we doubled the anti-thrombin dosage and reduced the LMWH dosage from 60 mg per day to 40 mg per day. On the same day a healthy girl (3000 g, 50 cm) was born spontaneously after 37 weeks of gestation.

Three days after childbirth the D-dimer concentration in the woman rose to 1509 μg/l (see Figure 1) and no clinical signs of thrombosis were observed. However, a small thrombus in the left popliteal vein was detected by ultrasound. After raising the antithrombin- and LMWH-doses a reduction of the D-dimer concentration was observed and after ten days the thrombus was no longer present.

Conclusions and Recommendations

The patient described here suffers from antithrombin deficiency. Both of her parents showed normal antithrombin activities (mother: 88 per cent, father 101 per cent), in her mother the base exchange in the antithrombin gene was absent and the

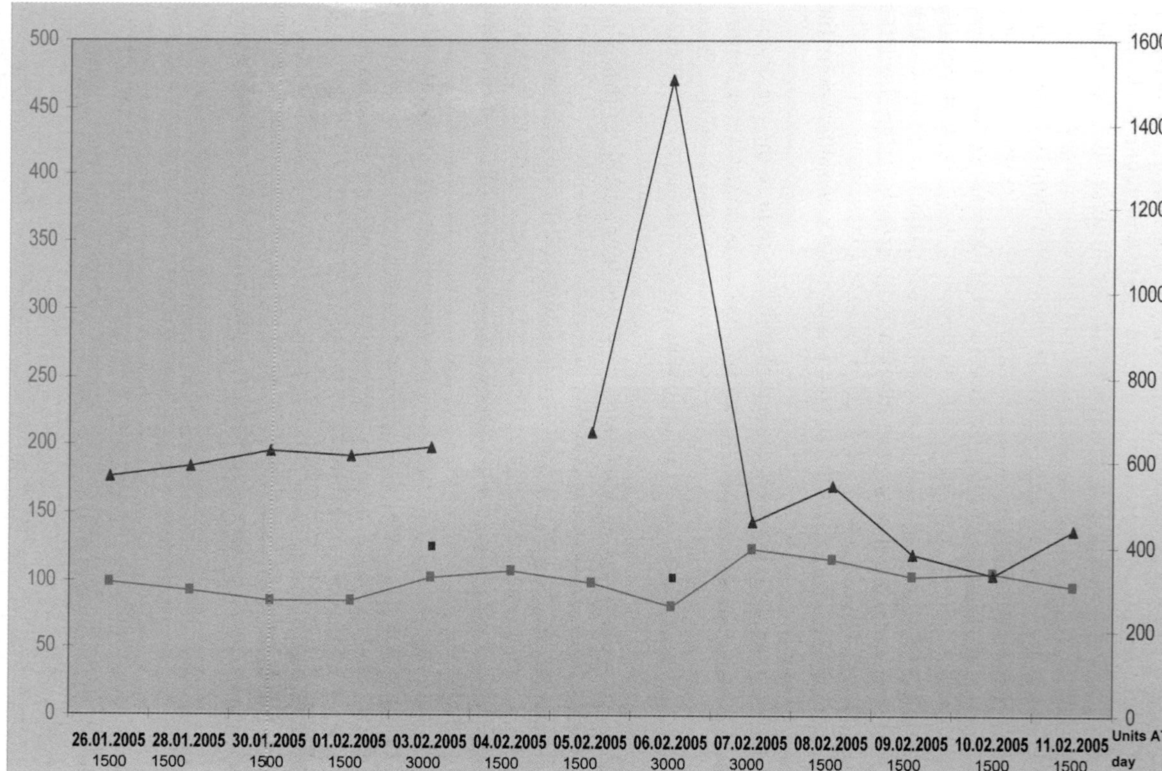

Fig. 1. Antithrombin activities (squares) and D-dimer concentrations (triangles) during the perinatal period. The additional squares denote antithrombin activities resulting from a second dose given on the same day. Ordinate left: Antithrombin activity (per cent), ordinate right: D-dimer concentration (μg/l). All values were obtained approximately 24 hours after the last antithrombin administration. Abscissa: Day of investigation (upper row), units of antithrombin administered per day (lower row).

father was not tested. We believe that the base exchange in the antithrombin gene of the patient represents a novel mutation. The existence of this mutation in the patient's baby supports the assumption of the antithrombin deficiency as a hereditary disorder.

The history of the patient is in accordance with the results obtained from other patients. In the patient described here it seems possible that the thrombotic potential originating from antithrombin deficiency was aggravated by the presence of the HR 2-haplotype within the factor V-gene. Up to now it is believed that the HR 2-haplotype potentiates the thrombotic risk in individuals with the factor V »Leiden«. However a recently published study shows a decrease of the bleeding symptoms in patients with factor VII deficiency and HR 2-haplotype [11]. The explanation of this phenomenon is the increased endogenous thrombin potential originating from the HR 2-haplotype.

It is well known that heparin and also LMWH are inefficient in the presence of low antithrombin activity. Therefore the effect of heparin administration in antithrombin deficient patients should be carefully monitored. In the cases of reduced or absent effects of heparin administration the addition of antithrombin is indicated.

The occurrence of a clinically silent thrombosis in the presence of antithrombin concentrations within the normal range and also during a prophylactic treatment with a LMWH confirms the high thrombotic risk existing during the perinatal and postnatal periods. Therefore, we recommend testing for D-dimers in short intervals in patients with antithrombin deficiency and also with other prothrombotic conditions.

The application of the chosen antithrombin concentrate was well tolerated and no side effects were observed, especially the transmission of viruses (hepatitis B, hepatitis C, HIV) could be excluded.

Further studies are necessary to find out the optimal therapeutic course to prevent thromboses in pregnant women with antithrombin deficiency and also to give the possibility of a normal fetal development.

References

1. van Boven HH, Lane DA. Antithrombin and its inherited deficiency states. Sem Hemat 1997; 34: 188–204
2. Blondel-Hill E, Mant MJ. The pregnant antithrombin III deficient patient: Management without antithrombin III concentrate. Thromb Res 1992; 65: 193–198
3. Brandt P. Observations during the treatment of antithrombin III deficient women with heparin and antithrombin concentrate during pregnancy, parturition, and abortion. Thromb Res 1981; 22: 15–24
4. Conard J, Horellou MH, van Dreden P, Samama M. Pregnancy and congenital deficiency in antithrombin III or protein C. Thromb Haemost 1987; 58:39
5. De Stefano V, Leone G, De Carolis S, Ferrelli R, Di Donfrancesco A, Moneta E, Bizzi B. Management of pregnancy in women with antithrombin III congenital defect: Report of four cases. Thromb Haemost 1988; 59: 193–196
6. Egeberg O. Inherited antithrombin deficiency causing thrombophilia. Thromb Diath Haemorrh 1965; 13: 516–530

7. Hellgren M, Tengborn L, Abildgaard U. Pregnancy in women with congenital antithrombin deficiency: Experience of treatment with heparin and antithrombin. Gynecol Obstet Invest 1982; 14: 127–141
8. Hiller E, Salat C, Kempter B. Antithrombin III deficiency and pregnancy – successful management with LMW-heparin. Ann Hematol 1992; 64 (Suppl.): A 111
9. Owen I. Antithrombin replacement therapy in pregnancy. Sem Hemat 1991; 28: 46–52
10. Schramm W. Thromboembolie. Die klinische Bedeutung des AT III. Internist 1984; 25: 88–92
11. Strey RF, Siegemund A, Siegemund T, Schubert C, Schuster G, Wulff K, Herrmann FH. Einfluss von Faktor V HR 2 auf die Thrombinbildung und die klinische Ausprägung eines Faktor VII-Mangels. 36. Hämophilie-Symposion Hamburg 2005
12. Tengborn L, Bengtsson T. Antithrombin III concentrate. Thromboprophylaxis during pregnancy in a patient with congenital antithrombin III deficiency. Acta Obstet Gynec Scand 1986; 65: 375–376
13. Thaler E, Lechner K. Antithrombin III deficiency and thromboembolism. Clin Hematol 1981; 10: 369–390

Successful Inhibitor-Elimination with Rituximab in Acquired Hemophilia A and a Patient with a Carrier Status for Hemophilia A: Two Case Reports

P. Lages, A. Huth-Kühne, and R. Zimmermann

Introduction

Acquired hemophilia (AH) is a rare bleeding disorder with an incidence of approximately 1.5 cases/million/year [1]. It is characterized by the development of autoantibodies depleting circulating Factor VIII (FVIII). These autoantibodies constitute the most common spontaneous inhibitor to any coagulation factor and are associated with spontaneous bleeds in patients with no previous history of a bleeding diathesis. In about 50% of patients an underlying medical condition is found, including autoimmune diseases, solid tumors and lymphoproliferative malignancies. Due to the highly variable phenotypic presentation, the severity of the hemostatic defect varies between life-threatening bleeds, which may be fatal and mild bleeding episodes requiring no treatment with hemostatic agents in about 30% of patients [1]. According to a recent review of 249 patients, the overall mortality is 20% with an 11% mortality directly related to the inhibitor. The high overall mortality has been attributed to complications of immunosuppressive therapy or co-morbidity [2]. Besides the effective control of bleeding, the ultimate goal is the elimination of the inhibitor. Immunosuppressive regimens applied to suppress autoantibody pro-

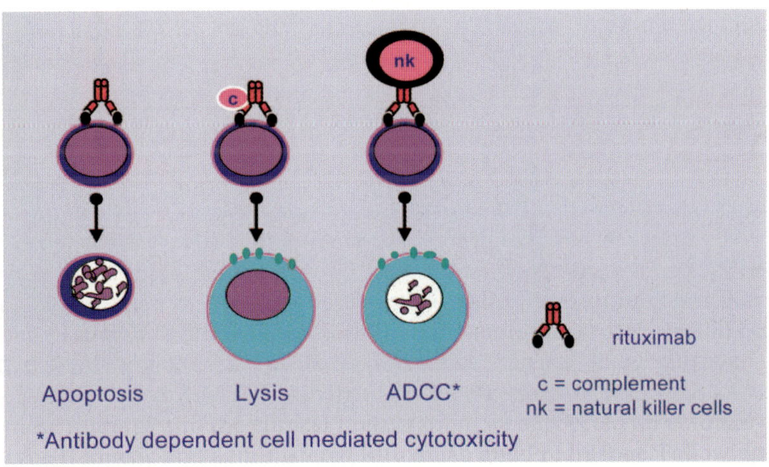

Fig. 1. Therapy with monoclonal antibodies

I. Scharrer/W. Schramm (Ed.)
36th Hemophilia Symposium Hamburg 2005

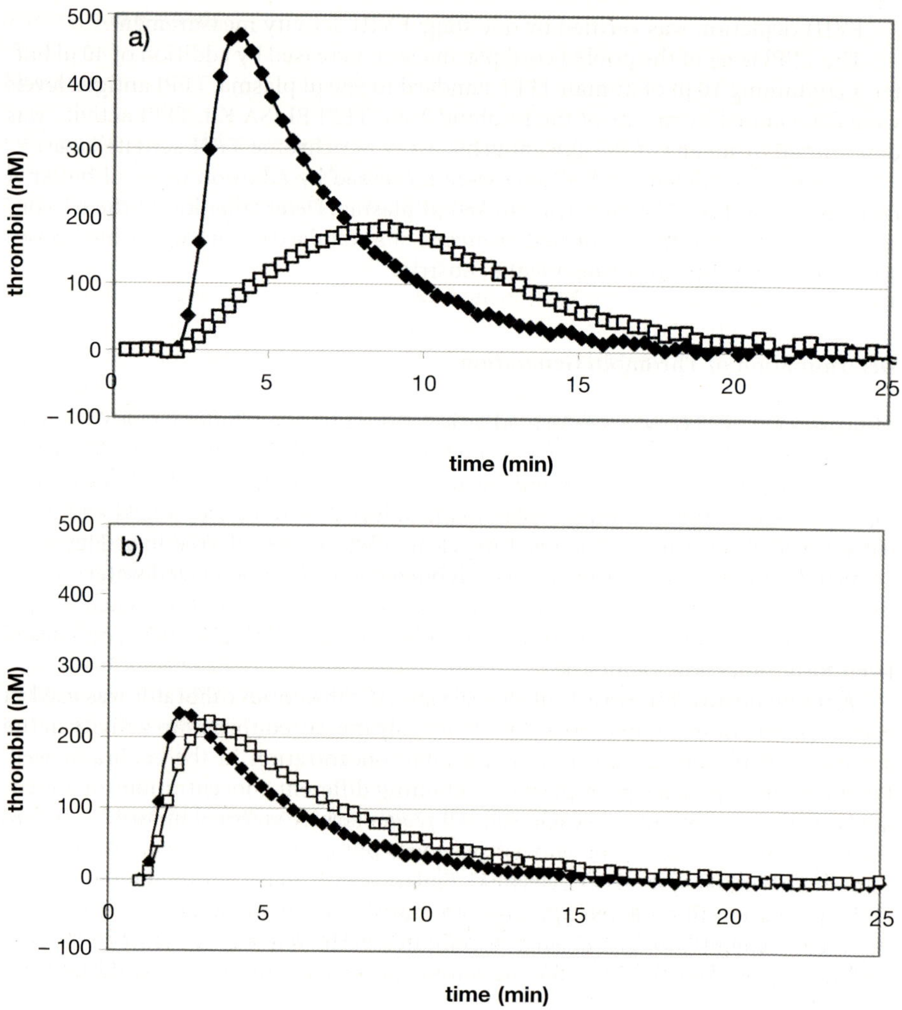

Fig. 1

Effect of AT and TFPI in FVIII-Deficient Plasma

In FVIII-depleted neonatal plasma raising the AT level to 105% did not result in a prolongation of the lag phase and the TTP. The peak height decreased by 40 % and the ETP by 69 %. There were nearly no differences in the changes of TG between normal and FVIII-depleted neonatal plasma.

In contrast, to the normal neonatal plasma, raising of TFPI in FVIII-depleted neonatal plasma resulted in a strong decrease of the peak height by 77 %, a more than 3 fold prolongation of the TTP of more than 8 minutes and also a prolongation of the lag phase of more than two minutes, and a decrease of the ETP by 40 %.

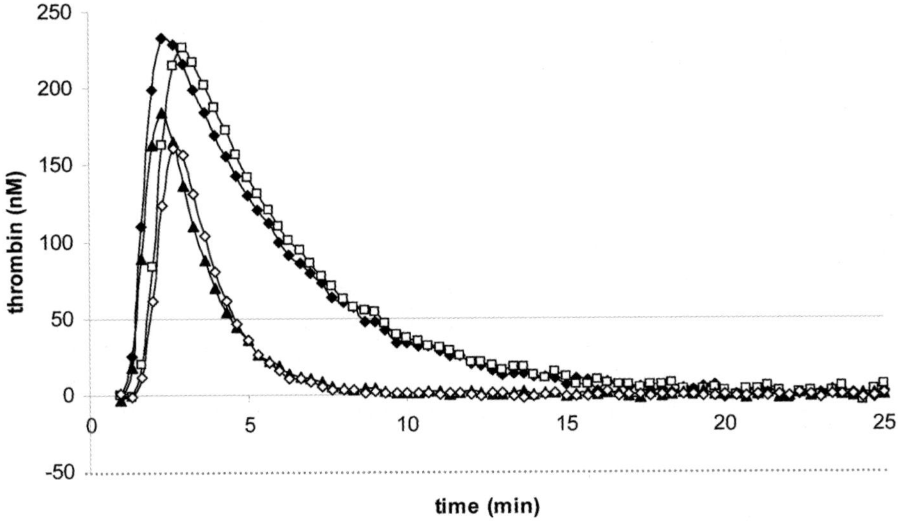

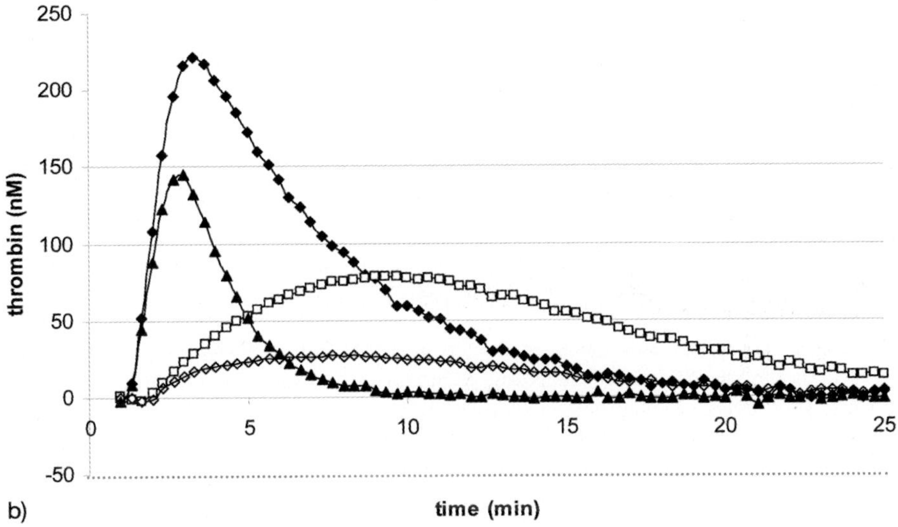

Fig. 2

The prolongation of the TTP in the FVIII-depleted neonatal plasma was 8 times longer than in normal neonatal plasma. In FVIII-depleted plasma raising AT and TFPI decreased the peak height by 90 %, prolonged the TTP more than 6 minutes and the lag phase more than 1 minute compared to unspiked FVIII-depleted neonatal plasma. The reduction of the peak height after raising both inhibitors in normal neonatal plasma was 35 %, whereas the reduction in the FVIII-depleted neonatal plasma was 90 % (Fig. 2).

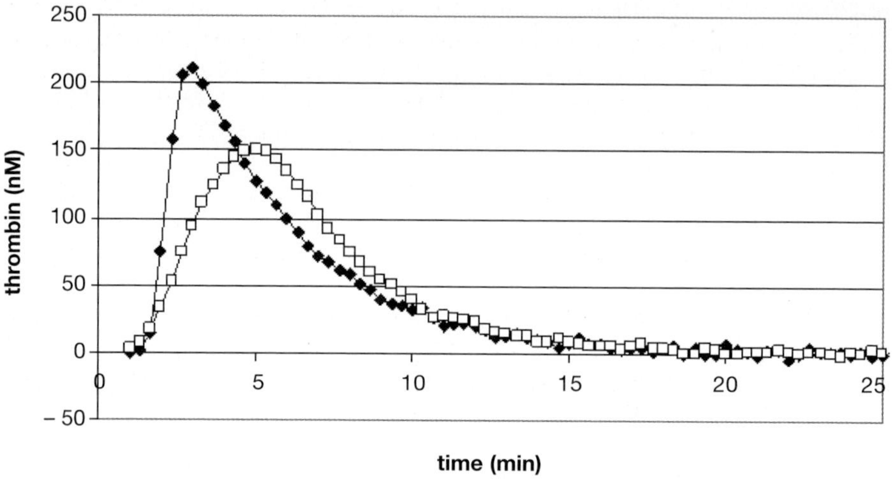

Fig. 3

TG in plasma of hemophilic newborn

One plasma sample of a hemophilic newborn was available. FVIII activity in this patient was < 1%. TG in this plasma showed only a small prolongation of the lag phase and the TTP and a decrease of the peak height by 25 % as compared to the TG of a plasma sample of a healthy newborn (Fig. 3).

Discussion

Recent investigations have focused on the problem that healthy neonates show no easy bruising, no increased bleeding during delivery and good wound healing, despite low levels of coagulation factors [3, 4]. It was shown that after activation with low concentrations of TF physiological low levels of natural inhibitors, like TFPI, AT and PC compensate for low concentrations of clotting factors and allow sufficient thrombin generation. Clinical data have shown that there is no higher bleeding tendency in hemophiliac neonates than in healthy [1, 2].

We showed that the TG in hemophilic plasma of the neonate is nearly as high as in normal plasma of the neonate, these findings are in correlation with the clinical observation of low bleeding incidence in hemophilic neonates. Raising the amount of TFPI to an adult level showed a reduction of the TG and a prolongation of the time to peak. Raising the amount of AT resulted in reduction of the TG, whereas time to peak showed no prolongation. After raising both inhibitors to adult concentration we saw a drastically debasement of the TG, what approves the synergistic effect of these inhibitors. We showed that raising the amount of the both stochiometric inhibitors, TFPI and AT, to adult levels led to a decrease of the TG and to a prolongation of the time to peak in both neonatal plasmas, what supports the theory the physiological low amounts of these inhibitors are responsible for the excellent hemostasis not only in normal neonates, but also in hemophilic neonates.

In previous work we already focused on the efficacy of TFPI and AT in the regulation of thrombin inhibition in neonates. It was explained by synergistic inhibition of the two phases of the thrombin generation- the »initiation phase« and the »propagation phase«. Van´t Veer et al. showed that high amounts of TFPI extends the »initiation phase« by delaying the Factor V activation, which normally builds the »prothrombinase (FXa/FVa)« complex and protects FX that way from the inactivation of AT. Thus TFPI and AT together are ~ 70 fold more potent than each of them alone [10].

Our findings could further be an explanation for the different clinical phenotypes of bleeding in hemophilic patients with the same FVIII levels. The measurement of TG in follow up investigations of hemophiliacs and in monitoring of FVIII therapy in presence of standardized test conditions could be an auxiliary option for therapy monitoring.

In conclusion, the activation of hemostasis done by low concentrations of TF, can be used for a sensitive detection of prothrombotic and inhibitory variables in plasma of hemophiliacs. Physiological low levels of TFPI and AT allow a hemostasis in plasma of hemophiliac neonates that is nearly as good as in the plasma of healthy neonates.

References

1. Ljung R, Lindgren AC, Petrini P, Tengborn L. Normal vaginal delivery is to be recommended for haemophilia carrier gravidae. Acta paediatr 1994; 83, 609–11
2. Kulkarni R, Lusher JM, Henry RC, Kallen DJ. Current practices regarding newborn intracranial haemorrhage and obstetrical care and mode of delivery of pregnant haemophilia carriers: a survey of obstetricians, neonatologists and haematologists in the United States, on behalf of the National Hemophilia Foundation´s medical and scientific advisory council. Haemophilia 1999; 5, 410–15
3. Cvirn G, Gallistl S, Muntean W. Effects of antithrombin and protein C on thrombin generation in newborn and adult plasma. Thromb Res 1999; 93: 183–90
4. Cvirn G, Gallistl S, Leschnik B, Muntean W. Low tissue factor pathway inhibitor (TFPI) together with low antithrombin allows sufficient thrombin generation in neonates. Journal of Thrombosis and Haemostasis; 1: 263–68
5. Baier K, Cvirn G, Fritsch P, Koestenberger M, Gallistl S, Leschnik B, Muntean W. Higher concentrations of heparin and hirudin are required to inhibit thrombin generation in tissue factor-activated cord plasma than in adult plasma. Pediatr Res. 2005; 57: 685–9.
6. Davie EW, Fujikawa K, Kisiel W, The coagulation cascade: Initiation, maintenance and regulation. Biochemistry 1991; 30: 10363–70
7. Butenas S, Van't Veer C, Mann KG. ›normal‹ thrombin generation. Blood 1999; 94:2169–78
8. Hemker HC, Giesen P, Al Dieri R et al. Calibrated automated thrombin generation measurement in clotting plasma. Pathophysiol Haemost Thromb 2003; 33: 4–15
9. Hemker HC, Giesen P, Al Dieri R et al. The calibrated automated thrombogram (CAT): an universal routine test for hyper- and hypocoaguability. Pathophysiol Haemost Thromb 2002; 32: 249–53
10. Van´t Veer C, Mann KG. Regulation of tissue factor initated thrombin generation by the stoichiometric inhibitors tissue factor pathway inhibitor, antithrombin III and heparin cofactor II. J Biol Chem 1997; 272: 4367-77

2. Human growth hormone (HGH) fragment (exons 3–4) was used as an internal PCR control.
3. Undeleted fragment(s) was/were also amplified as a second internal control. The heterozygous deletion identification was done on the bases of ratio calculation of the peaks' heights after superposing and normalization to the internal HGH control compared to a normal healthy control. Ratio between 0.4–0.5 presented large deletion.

Results and Discussion

Screening for large deletions of F8 was performed in 19 families where the index patients have severe hemophilia A and showed a large deletion. Twenty-four relative females, including 15 mothers, 7 sisters, 1 aunt and 1 grandmother, were investigated for carrier status of the corresponding observed deletion in the index patient (Table 1).

Table 1. FVIII large deletions in IP and carrier status of female relatives

Family #	Deletion in IP	Relationship	Carrier status
1	Ex 1	Sister	carrier
2	Ex 1	Mother	carrier
3	Ex 1	Mother	carrier
		Sister	noncarrier
4	Ex 1	Sister	carrier
5	Ex 6	Mother	carrier
		Sister	noncarrier
6	Ex 6	Mother	carrier
7	Ex 13	Mother	noncarrier
8	Ex 14.5-14.8	Mother	carrier
		Sister	noncarrier
9	Ex 14	Mother	carrier
10	Ex 14	Mother	carrier
11	Ex 21	Sister	carrier
12	Ex 22	Mother	carrier
13	Ex 26	Mother	carrier
14	Ex 26	Mother	carrier
15	Ex 1-6	Mother	carrier
16	Ex 15-18	Mother	carrier
17	Ex 15-22	Mother	carrier
18	Ex 23-24	Aunt	noncarrier
19	Ex 1-25	Grand Mother	noncarrier
		Mother	carrier
		Sister	noncarrier

Single exon deletions

In 14 families (17 females) the size of deletion in the index patients (IP) covered only one exon – exons 1, 6, 13, 14, 21, 22 and 26. In 13 female relatives a large deletion was confirmed in the same exon and they were identified as carriers (Table 1, Fig. 1a). The ratio in all deleted fragments was in the range of 0.3-0.5. In one case, where the boy represents the first case of hemophilia in the family due to a deletion

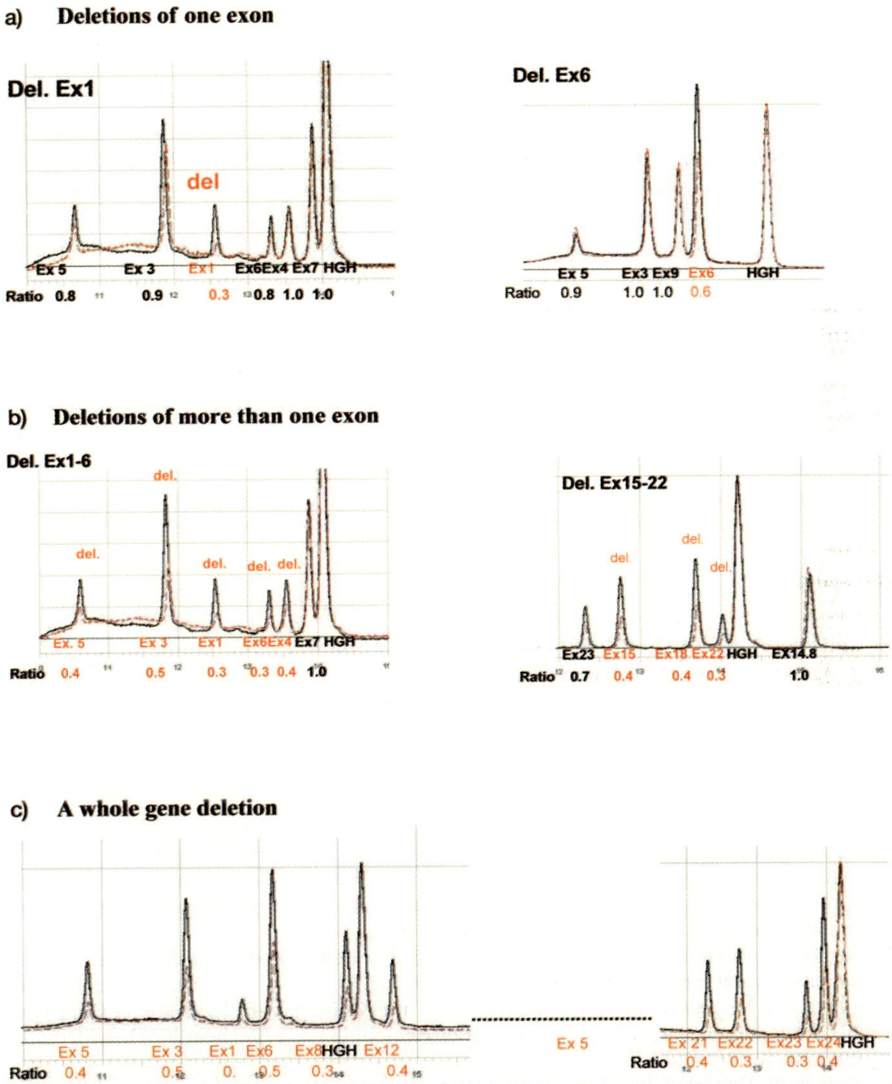

Fig. 1a–c. Chromatograms of representative families with different deletions. The black, straight line marks the referent control and the red punctured line – the investigated sample

Expression Analysis of C1-Inhibitor Mutants Confirms Causality of Missense Mutations for Hereditary Angioedema

T. Förster, C. R. Müller, and J. Oldenburg

Introduction

Hereditary angioedema (HAE) is an autosomal dominant disease due to mutations in the C1 inhibitor gene (C1INH). The C1INH protein is the sole inhibitor of the C1r and C1s components of the classical complement pathway and the major regulator of factors XI and XII and of plasma kallikrein in the contact system. HAE manifests as acute intermittent swellings of nearly every organ especially of the skin and the gastrointestinal tract. Laryngeal edema may cause suffocation and if not treated properly can be fatal.

Over the past years, we have established a genetic screening protocol for the genetic diagnosis of HAE in cooperation with the children's hospital in Frankfurt.

Methods

We chose C1INH mutations from our database in order to study their functional effect on C1INH activity by recombinant expression in HEK cells. Mutations were chosen on the basis of their phylogenetic conservation and likely functional impact (Fig. 1).

We successfully expressed the C1INH protein in human cells. The cDNA of C1INH was cloned into the expression vector pCEP4 and transfected into HEK 293 cells. Mutations were introduced into the cDNA construct by site-directed mutagenesis.

Two days after transfection the supernatants of the cells were harvested and were incubated with an excess of C1-esterase. Residual C1-esterase activity was measured photometrically. To control for the efficiency of transfection, C1INH antigen was determined by Western blotting and hybridization with an anti-C1INH-antibody (Fig. 2). Diluted human plasma was used as a control.

Results and Discussion

Wildtype C1INH protein showed activity and antigen comparable to diluted human plasma. Mock transfected cells featured neither activity nor antigen thus ruling out endogenous expression of C1-INH in HEK293 cells.

I. Scharrer/W. Schramm (Ed.)
36th Hemophilia Symposium Hamburg 2005

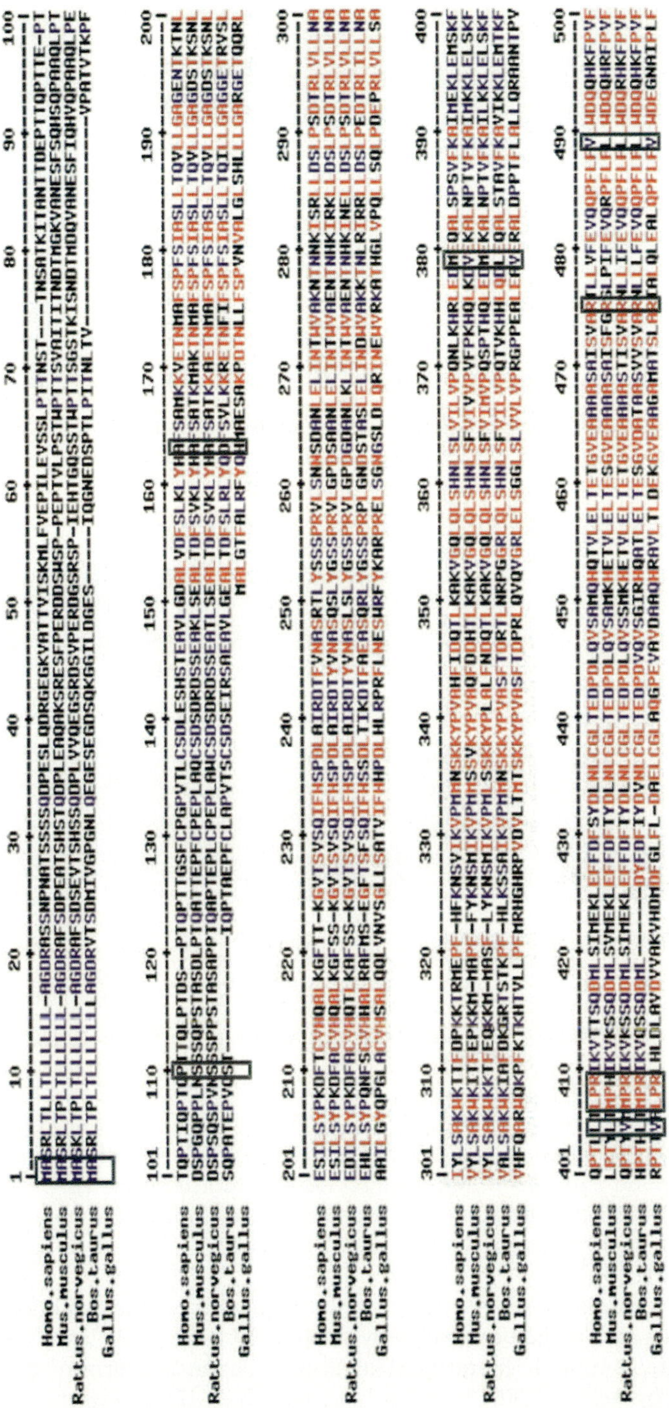

Fig. 1. Alignment of C1-Inhibitor protein sequences from different species. Amino acids that have been studied here are boxed

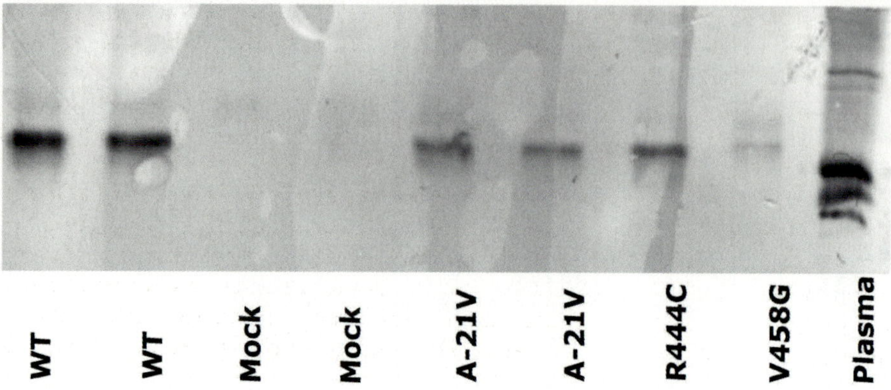

Fig. 2. Western Blot of supernatants from cells expressing recombinant C1INH

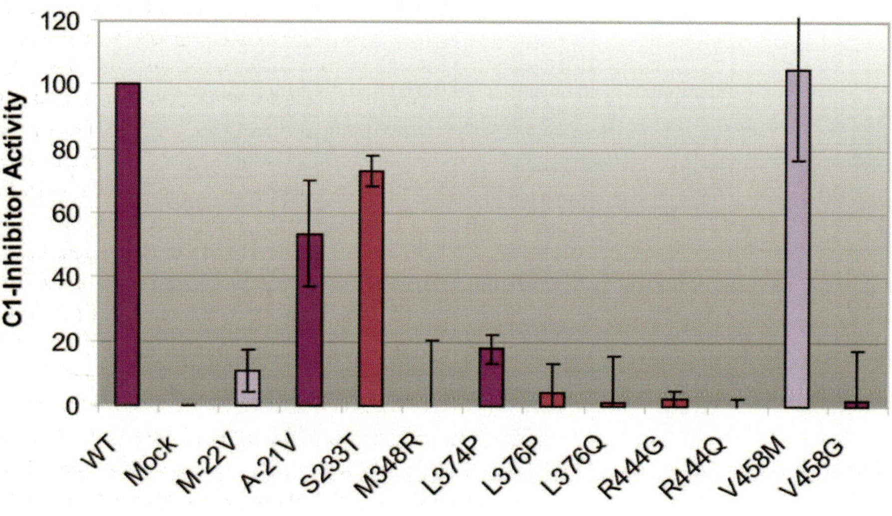

Fig. 3. Mutations in C1INH significantly decrease inhibition of C1-esterase activity

We studied the effects of mutations that had been identified in HAE patients by site-directed mutagenesis and expression. Most substitutions studied so far (M-22V, L374P, L376P, L376Q, V458G) resulted in a significant decrease of the activity of the recombinant proteins. Two mutations (A-21V, S233T) showed a reduced activity compared to wildtype (Fig. 3).

In particular, replacement of Arg444 either by glutamine or cysteine exhibited no activity while the antigen could be detected by Western blotting.

Both mutations are commonly found in HAE Type II patients, a form of the disease characterized by lacking C1INH activity but detectable C1INH antigen.

Expression of the variant V458M which is found in HAE patients but also in healthy persons resulted in activities comparable to wildtype protein. This confirms the assumption of this variant to be a polymorphism.

Conclusion

Recombinant expression of mutated C1INH protein is a useful tool to characterize the role of individual amino acid residues for C1INH activity and hereditary angioedema.

Expression of the γ-Glutamyl Carboxylase (GGCX) Containing the Arg485Pro Mutation Found in two Unrelated VKCFD1 Patients

S. Rost, A. Fregin, V. Mutucumarana, D. Stafford, C. R. Müller, and J. Oldenburg

Introduction

Familial multiple coagulation factor deficiency (VKCFD) is a very rare bleeding disorder, with only 15 cases described as yet. The clinical presentation is variable with respect to the residual activities of the affected proteins, the response to oral substitution of vitamin K and to the involvement of skeletal abnormalities. The phenotype may result either from a mutation within the γ-glutamyl carboxylase (GGCX) gene or a mutation affecting the vitamin K-epoxide reductase (VKOR) complex. So

Table 1. Levels of vitamin K-dependent coagulation factors of two VKCFD1 patients having the Arg485Pro mutation in common. Measurements were done before and after oral vitamin K substitution.

		Patient A		Patient B	
	normal range	before Vit. K	after Vit. K	before Vit. K	after Vit. K
APTT (sec)	30-45			38	28
Quick (%)	70-100	18-25	53	28	56
Fibrinogen (%)	2.0-4.5			2.8	
Factor II (%)	75-110	21	40	35	71
Factor V (%)	70-140			118	
Factor VII (%)	65-130	47	62	37	69
Factor VIII (%)	70-170			126	
Factor IX (%)	70-120			54	90
Factor X (%)	75-115	36	65	13	28
Antithrombin (%)	80-120			118	
Protein C (%)	70-120			56	63
Protein S (%)	60-140			37	48

I. Scharrer/W. Schramm (Ed.)
36th Hemophilia Symposium Hamburg 2005

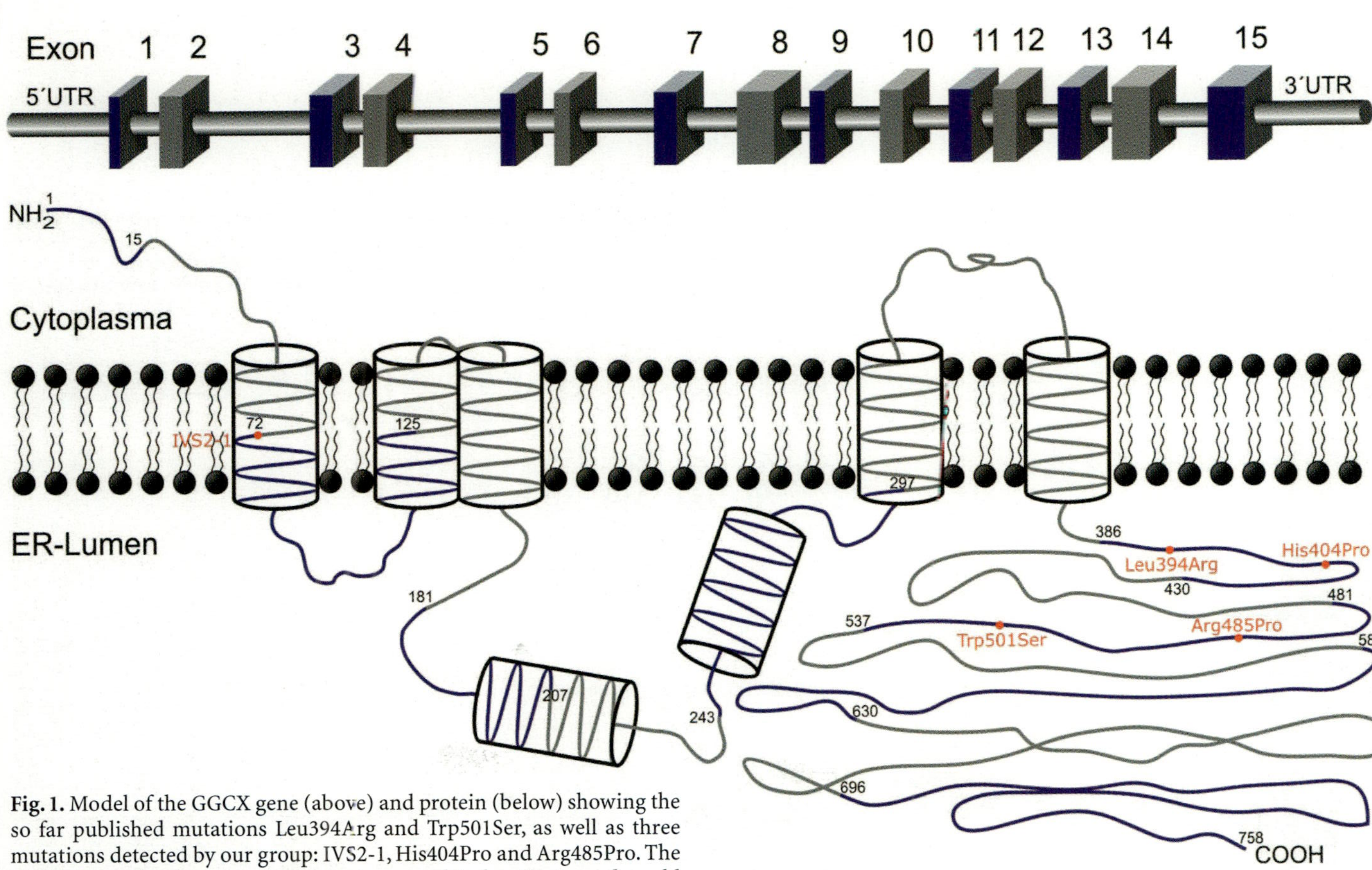

Fig. 1. Model of the GGCX gene (above) and protein (below) showing the so far published mutations Leu394Arg and Trp501Ser, as well as three mutations detected by our group: IVS2-1, His404Pro and Arg485Pro. The Arg485Pro mutation was found in two unrelated patients and could recently be shown to originate from a founder effect

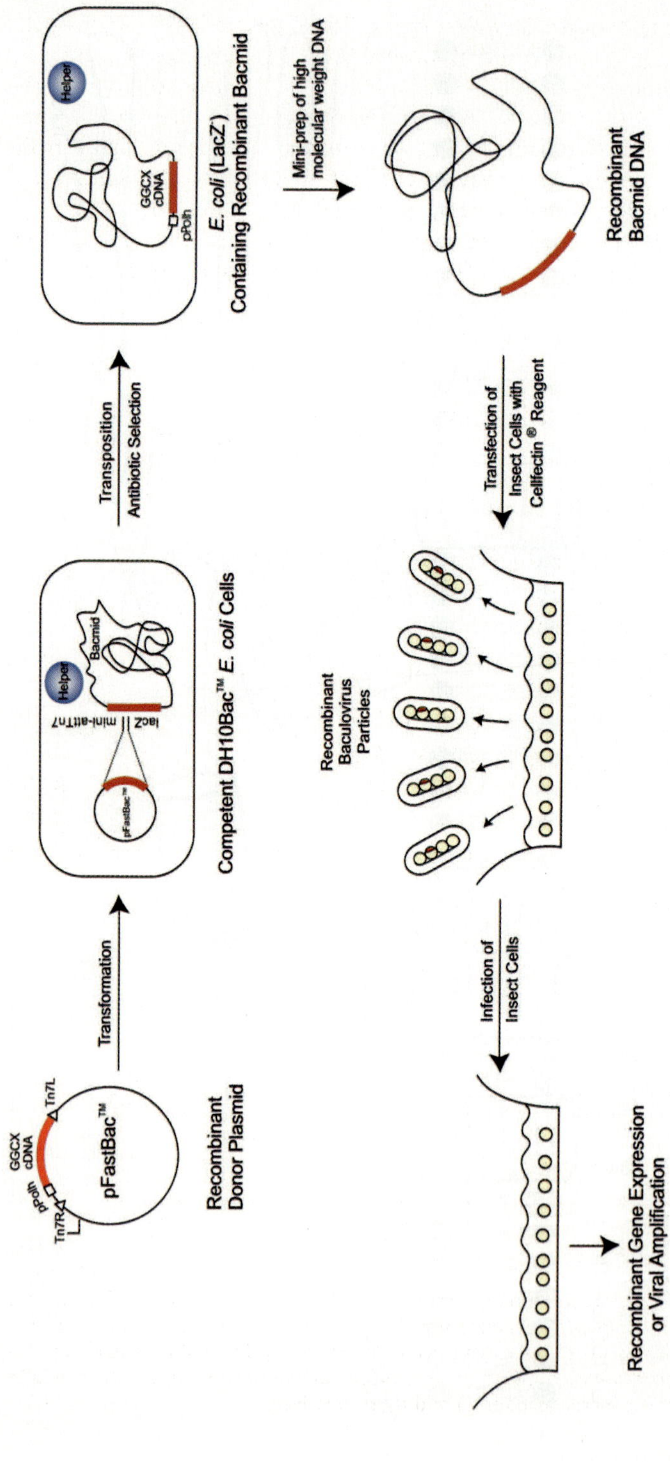

Fig. 2. Generation of recombinant baculovirus and GGCX gene expression with the Bac-to-Bac Expression System of Invitrogen

far, only two different mutations identified in the GGCX gene of two VKCFD patients (Leu394Arg and Trp501Ser) could be proven to be causative for the VKCFD1 phenotype by recombinant expression of the mutated GGCX in insect cells and subsequent measurement of the GGCX activity. In the present study we report on the expression of a GGCX variation comprising a substitution of arginine 485 by proline which has been detected in two unrelated patients (Fig. 1). Both patients showed mild deficiencies of all vitamin K-dependent coagulation factors with activities ranging from 20 to 40% of normal. Even high doses of intravenously administered vitamin K could not completely restore the factor activities (Table 1).

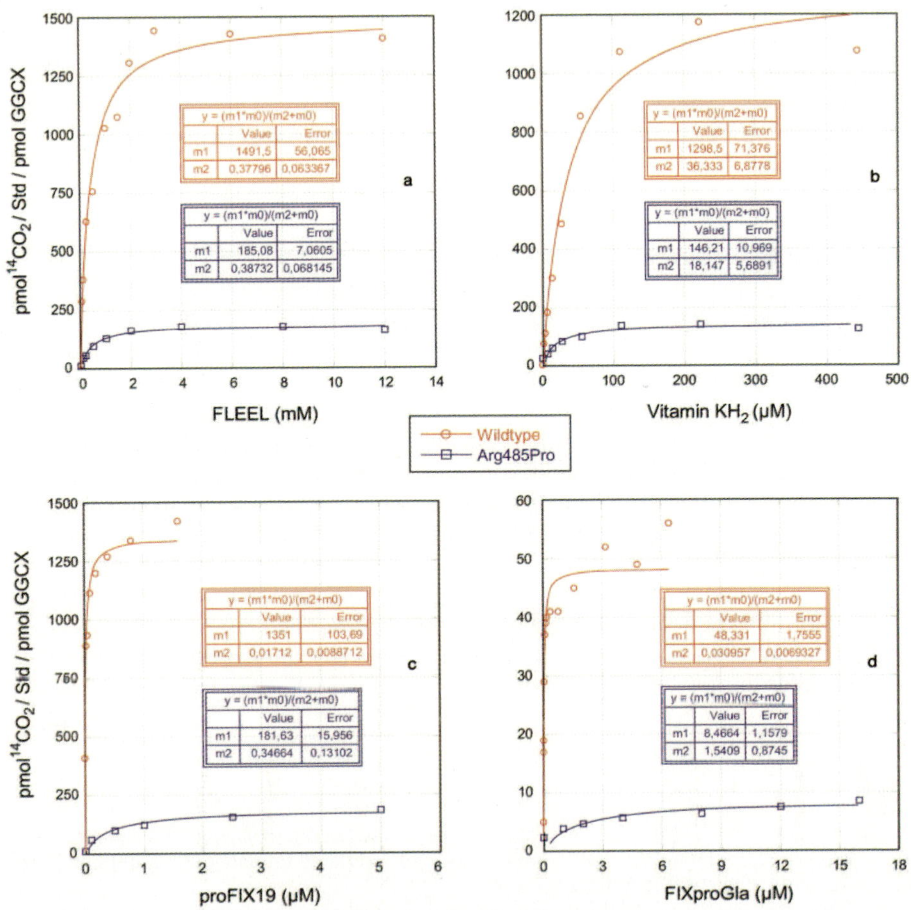

Fig. 3. Kinetic studies of the recombinant expressed GGCX wildtype protein (○) and the Arg485Pro variant (□). The software Kaleida Graph was used for determining V_{max} and K_M. FLEEL carboxylation with varying concentrations of the short peptide is shown in a), variations in vitamin K concentrations are shown in b). Concentrations of the propeptide proFIX19 and the substrate FIXproGla were varied in c) and d), respectively.

Methods and Results

The Arg485Pro variation and the GGCX wildtype were recombinantly expressed in Sf9 insect cells using the baculovirus system (Fig. 2). After purification of the GGCX proteins by affinity chromatography, GGCX activity was assayed by adding vitamin K hydroquinone, radioactive sodium hydrogen carbonate and either the small glutamate containing substrate FLEEL in combination with the propeptide ProFIX19, or FIXproGla as a more physiological substrate. Kinetic studies were carried out by adding various concentrations of one of these substrates or co-substrates while keeping the others constant. Maximal velocity (V_{max}) of GGCX activity of the Arg485Pro variant was always reduced compared to the wildtype protein independently from the substrate which was varied (Fig. 3). The Michaelis-Menten constant (K_M) for FLEEL carboxylation was similar for the mutant and the wildtype protein, even at different concentrations of vitamin K hydroquinone (Fig. 3a and b). However, the K_M values of the mutant were increased up to 20- and 50-fold for the kinetics with the cosubstrate ProFIX19 and for the substrate FIXproGla, respectively (Fig. 3c and d).

Discussion and Conclusion

The data show that the Arg485Pro mutation has no effect on FLEEL carboxylation and on vitamin K binding. But it strongly affects propeptide binding as demonstrated by the high K_M value for ProFIX19 and FIXproGla kinetics in the Arg485Pro variant. Reduced propeptide binding can also have a negative influence on glutamate binding because of allosteric effects in the enzyme's structure. Furthermore, the mutation is located in a highly conserved region of the GGCX between amino acid residues 438 and 507 which has previously been demonstrated to comprise the propeptide binding domain. It is situated close to the Trp501Ser mutation which also reduces obviously the affinity of the GGCX to the propeptide of vitamin K-dependent proteins.

Our results are in accordance with previously described reports on the location of the propeptide binding site of the GGCX and verify the Arg485Pro mutation as causative for the VKCFD1 phenotype.

References

1. Soute BA, Jin DY, Spronk HM, Mutucumarana VP, Lin PJ, Hackeng TM, Stafford DW, Vermeer C. Characteristics of recombinant W501S mutated human gamma-glutamyl carboxylase. J Thromb Haemost. 2004 Apr;2(4): 597-604.
2. Mutucumarana VP, Stafford DW, Stanley TB, Jin DY, Solera J, Brenner B, Azerad R, Wu SM. Expression and characterization of the naturally occurring mutation L394R in human gamma-glutamyl carboxylase. J Biol Chem. 2000 Oct 20;275(42): 32572-7.
3. Wu SM, Mutucumarana VP, Geromanos S, Stafford DW. The propeptide binding site of the bovine gamma-glutamyl carboxylase. J Biol Chem. 1997 May 2;272(18): 11718-22.

Concentration of Soluble Endothelial Protein C Receptor (EPCR) in Plasma in Relation to Age, Sex, BMI and Hemostasis Parameters

G. Siegert, P. Goez, H. Kostka, S. Gehrisch, E. Kuhlisch, and S. M. Schellong

Introduction

The Endothelial Protein C Receptor (EPCR) is a transmembrane glycoprotein, playing an important role in the activation process of protein C [1]. The complex between protein C and EPCR seems to play an important part for the non-hemostatic functions of activated protein C (APC) [2].

The proteolysis of EPCR results in the release of a 43 kDa form. This soluble EPCR (sEPCR) is able to bind protein C and APC with the same affinity. But, APC in complex with EPCR is, owing to the blockade of the point of binding on phospholipids, not in the position to have an anticoagulatoric effect. Concerning the clinical importance of high EPCR plasma concentration, as well as the dependence of other parameters, only little is known.

Aim of our study was to determine the sEPCR plasma concentration of healthy controls without thrombotic anamnesis and thrombotic risk factors and to find out the dependence on age, sex, body mass index (BMI), antithrombin, protein C, protein S, APC-response, factor VIII activity and D-dimer concentration.

Material and Methods

Controls were recruited from a prospective controlled study to assess the influence of venous thrombosis with long-haul flights [3]. 300 controls (170 males, 130 females) were selected by following criteria: No thrombotic history, no factor V Leiden mutation, no prothrombin mutation 20210, no deficiency of coagulation inhibitors antithrombin, protein C and protein S, negative results in lupus anticoagulant assay and D-dimer values within the normal range. The relationship between sEPCR plasma concentration and protein C activity as well as protein C concentration was intensively investigated in 152 samples of the males.

Sampling

Venous blood was sampled as part of routine checks. Plasma was separated and stored in aliquots at – 85 °C.

I. Scharrer/W. Schramm (Ed.)
36th Hemophilia Symposium Hamburg 2005

sEPCR and protein C plasma concentration

sEPCR plasma levels were measured by Enzyme-linked immuno-sorbent assay using the ELISA kit Asserachrom sEPCR. Protein C levels were measured by Enzyme-linked immuno-sorbent assay Protein C Antigen Test kit (Helena Biosciences).

Clotting Analysis

Clotting analysis was performed using the coagulation analyzer AMAX Amelung with the systems:

AT III COAMATIC (Chromogenix), COATEST APC (Chromogenix), COAMATIC Protein C (Chromogenix), Protein S clotting Assay (Helena), Auto D-dimer (Sigma), F VIII deficiency plasma (Helena) and DVV Test/DVV confirm (Axis Shield).

Genetic Analysis

10 ml of citrate-anticoagulated blood was collected and DNA was extracted using a salting out procedure [4]. The factor V Leiden mutation (1691G > A, Arg 506Gln) and the prothrombin mutation 20210 G > A were identified as described in literature. The A3 haplotype defined by Saposnik et al. [5] was identified through detection of EPCR 6936 A > G. The EPCR 6936 A > G was detected after amplification of genomic DNA. The digestion of the 6936 A allele results in fragments 210 bp and 17 bp.

Results

Plasma Levels of Determinants

The plasma concentration of sEPCR showed a bimodal distribution in the whole group of 300 healthy controls without thrombophilic risk factors (Fig. 1). The quartiles of the sEPCR plasma concentration were calculated with 80; 80-100; 101-138.5; 138.5 ng/ml. The median of the sEPCR concentration was 100.0 ng/ml (range 32-823). Values of other variables of the hemostasis as well as age and body mass index (BMI) are shown in Table 1.

The sEPCR plasma concentration was significantly ($p < 0.0001$) higher in men than in women. This sex difference was not caused by hormone drugs like oral contraceptives or hormone replacement therapy (Fig. 2).

We could not detect an age dependency of sEPCR plasma levels in men. In contrast, the sEPCR plasma concentration decreased with age in women. This result was caused by non hormone users only.

The sEPCR plasma concentration correlates significantly with protein C activity, however there was no relationship between sEPCR plasma concentration and activity of antithrombin, protein S and factor VIII, APC ratio, D-dimer as well as

Table1. Determinants of the healthy study population without thrombotic risk factors (median, range)

Genotype	All	6936 AA	6936 AG	6936 GG
n	300	244 (81%)	53 (18%)	3 (1%)
sEPCR (ng/ml)	100 (32–823)	92 (32–272)	283 (111–504)	412 (411–823)
Protein C activity (%)	116 (73–173)	112 (72–169)	127 (92–173)	152 (134–153)
Protein S activity (%)	100 (60–169)	100 (60–169)	100 (70–143)	95 (88–103)
APC-Ratio	2.36 (2.05–2.64)	2.36 (2.05–2.64)	2.36 (2.17–2.55)	2.47 (2.29–2.53)
Factor VIII activity (%)	122 (56–202)	122 (59–202)	122 (56–188)	112 (92–166)
D-dimer (μg/ml)	30 (16–154)	30 (16–154)	30 (16–94)	20 (18–42)
Age (years)	50.9 (19.5–79.2)	50.0 (19.5–79.2)	54.5 (21.5–66.9)	31.1 (29.4–59.6)
BMI (kg/m^2)	24.2 (17.7–30.1)	24.2 (17.7–30.1)	24.7 (19.6–29.7)	23.9 (20.5– 26.8)

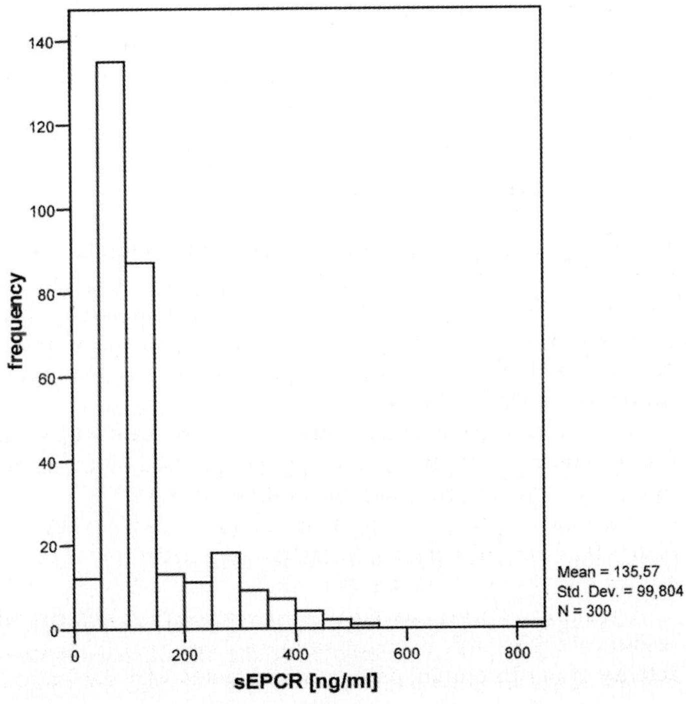

Fig. 1. Distribution of sEPCR plasma concentration

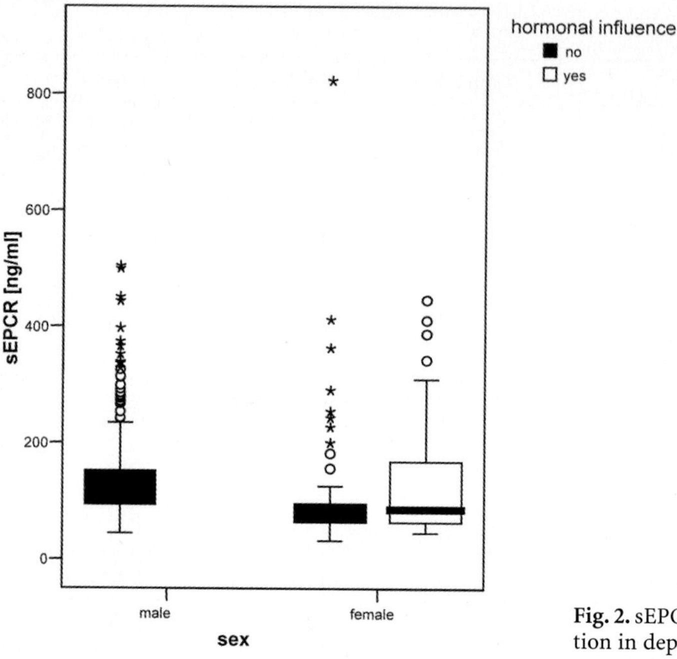

Fig. 2. sEPCR plasma concentration in dependence on sex

BMI. In the factor analysis the component 1 included age, BMI, protein S activity, factor VIII activity and APC ratio, component 2 included protein S activity, antithrombin, protein C activity and D-dimer, component 3 included sEPCR and protein C.

Frequency of the 6936 A>G Polymorphism

The frequency of the 6936 G allele was calculated with 0.098 (carriers 18.7%) in the healthy group without thrombophilic risk factors. 244 were genotype A6936A, 53 were A6936G and 3 were G6936G. The allelic frequencies were in Hardy-Weinberg equilibrium. There was no sex related difference of the G allele.

The 6936 A G polymorphism showed an important influence on the sEPCR plasma concentration. Carriers of the G allele showed significantly higher sEPCR plasma concentrations than the A allele carriers. The highest plasma levels were measured in the G6936G genotype (Fig. 3).

sEPCR and Protein C in a Male Subpopulation

In the subpopulation of males, protein C activity and protein C concentration correlate significantly and directly with the sEPCR plasma concentration. The frequency of the 6936G allele did not differ between the whole group and the sub-

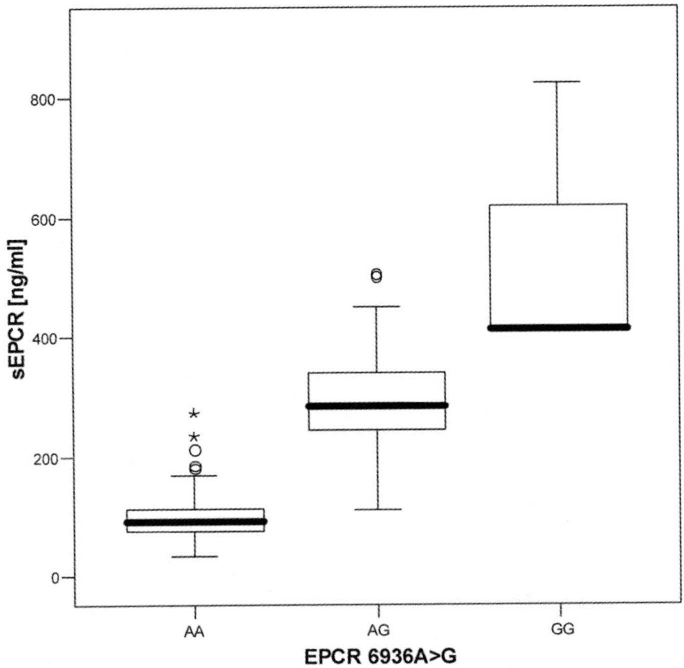

Fig. 3. sEPCR plasma concentration in dependence on EPCR genotype 6936 A>G

population. Protein C activity and protein C concentration as well as sEPCR plasma concentration were higher in A6936G than in A6936A genotype.

The ratio of protein C activity to protein C concentration showed no dependency on this EPCR genotype. The scatter diagrams showed a relationship between sEPCR plasma concentration and protein C in the A6936A genotype for protein C concentration only. In contrast protein C concentration as well as protein C activity was related to sEPCR plasma concentration in A6936 G genotype. In factor analysis component 1 was formed by antithrombin, BMI, D-dimer, protein C activity and age. sEPCR, protein C activity and protein C concentration were included in component 2.

Discussion

The protein C pathway is comprised of multiple proteins involved in different reactions. Thus, there are proteins affecting the activation of protein C by the thrombin-thrombomodulin-complex, cofactor proteins that modulate the proteolytic activity of APC and serine protease inhibitors that inactivate APC. The EPCR stimulates the thrombin-thrombomodulin-mediated activation of protein C on the endothelial surface. Endothelial cells play a critical role in the protein C pathway. They express two of the known receptors responsible for protein C activation: thrombomodulin and the endothelial protein C / APC receptor EPCR. EPCR is a receptor with homology to the CD1/MHC class 1 family. EPCR binds protein C and APC with similar affinity and facilitates protein C activation by presenting the protein C substrate to the thrombin-thrombomodulin activation complex.

sEPCR circulates in plasma, which retains its ability to bind protein C and APC, but does not enhance protein C activation. sEPCR is generated in vitro through proteolytic cleavage by metalloprotease activity inducible by thrombin and other inflammatory mediators. The physiological significance of sEPCR in vivo is unknown. Elevated plasma sEPCR levels might be associated with higher thrombotic risk, because plasma sEPCR inhibits both protein C activation and APC anticoagulant activity. Also high sEPCR might result in a low residual EPCR level on the membrane and thus indicate reduced protein C activation.

The general distribution as well as the sex related differences of sEPCR plasma levels in our study of the German population without thrombophilic risk factors was in a good agreement with the other studies in Europe using the same assay.

The allele frequency of the 6936 G-allele was in a good agreement with the Dutch, French and Spanish population. In all studies the 6936 G allele was associated with strongly elevated sEPCR plasma levels. Our study confirmed an association of the 6936 A>G polymorphism of the EPCR gene with strongly elevated plasma levels of sEPCR. The 6936 A>G EPCR gene polymorphism is not responsible for the sex related differences of the sEPCR plasma concentration.

The correlation of sEPCR plasma level with protein C activity and protein C concentration supports the assumption of a circulating protein C-sEPCR complex.

References

1. Fukudome K, Kurosawa S, Srearns-Kurosawa DJ. He X, Rezaie AR, Esmon CT. The endothelial cell protein C receptor. J Biol Chem 1996; 271(29):17491–98
2. Esmon CT. The protein C pathway. Chest 2003; 124 (3 Suppl):26S–32S
3. Schwarz T, Siegert G, Oettler W, Halbritter K, Beyer J, Frommhold R, Gerisch S, Lenz F, Kuhlisch E, Schroeder HE, Schellong SM. Venous thrombosis after long-haul flights. Arch Intern Med 2003; 163(22): 2759–64
4. Miller SA, Dykes DD, Polesky HF. A simple salting out procedure for extracting DANN from human nucleated cells. Nucleic Acids Res 1988; 16(3): 1215
5. Saposnik B, Reny JL, Gaussem P, Emmerich J, Aiach M, Gandrille S. A haplotype of the EPCR gen is associated with increased plasma levels of sEPCR and is a candidate risk factor for thrombosis. Blood 2004; 103(4): 1311–18

Thrombin Generation is Age-Dependent in Children as well as in Adults

H. HAIDL, C. CIMENTI, B. LESCHNIK, D. ZACH, and W. MUNTEAN

Background

Children have prolonged routine coagulation parameters like PT and aPTT, mainly due to lower concentrations of procoagulant clotting factors, but also inhibitory factors are reduced in children. These differences are pronounced in the early life years, but the raise to adult values lasts for all the time of childhood and adolescence [1].

Existing data of thrombin generation in childhood concentrate on the neonatal period. It was found that newborns are able to generate only 30–50 % of adult amounts of thrombin [2]. This was due to the use of high amounts of tissue factor (TF) – similar to the routine coagulation assay PT – to initialize coagulation. It has been shown that, using TF in lower quantities, the assay reflects probably the physiological conditions better [3]. We have shown that neonatal plasma can generate thrombin nearly at adult values when low amounts of tissue factor (<10 pmol) are applied, suggesting – in accordance to the clinical observation of excellent hemostasis in newborns – that the low levels of inhibitors compensate for low procoagulant protein levels [4, 5].

With the calibrated automated thrombography (CAT) an instrument was developed, that allows simultaneous analysis of several samples, contrary to the time consuming subsampling method. Importance of thrombin generation measurement lies in the key enzyme role of thrombin, so this method may become a new tool better reflecting overall hemostasis than global tests such as PT and aPTT or specific factor assays. Effects of different pro- and anticoagulants have been shown to be detected with thrombin generation measurement [6].

Parameters of thrombin generation measured by CAT show an intraindividual stability for healthy adults, but a wide interindividual scatter [7]. To our knowledge no data have been published about the age dependency of thrombin generation measured with CAT.

Materials and Methods

Collection of blood samples

Samples of 121 children who were screened for the routine coagulation parameters before minor elective surgery such as tonsillectomy, adenoidectomy, phimosis, or

I. Scharrer/W. Schramm (Ed.)
36th Hemophilia Symposium Hamburg 2005

oral surgery were – with consent of the children and their parents – additionally assayed for thrombin generation parameters. The children were clinically well, had no serious acute illness and no known inherited coagulation deficiency. Age ranged from 0.5 to 17 years. Additionally, blood from a group of 86 obviously healthy adult volunteers consisting of students and medical staff who were not taking coagulation disturbing medication was studied. The aPTT of each tested person was within the normal range.

This study was approved by the local ethics committee (Nr. 17-078 ex 05/06) and informed consent was obtained.

Blood was collected into plastic tubes containing sodium citrate (0.1 M end concentration) using S-Monovette tubes from Sarstedt (Nümbrecht, Germany). Platelet-poor plasma was obtained by centrifugation for 10 minutes at 2800xg at room temperature and stored at – 70 °C degree until further examination.

Reagents and Devices

Fluorbuffer contained 20 mM HEPES and 60 mg/ml bovine serum albumin (BSA) (both Sigma, St. Louis, Mo., USA). Working buffer consisted of 140 mM NaCl (Merck, Darmstadt, Germany), 20 mM HEPES and 5 mg/ml human serum albumin (HSA) (both Sigma, St. Louis, Mo., USA). The fluorogenic substrate Z-Gly-Gly-Arg-amino-methyl-coumarin (AMC) was purchased from Bachem, Bubendorf, Switzerland, and was solubilized in pure dimethylsulfoxide (DMSO), which was purchased from Sigma, St. Louis, Mo., USA. Calcium chloride was purchased from Merck, Darmstadt, Germany.

The platelet-poor plasma (PPP) reagent with a content of 5 pM tissue factor and 4 μM phospholipids and the thrombin calibrator was purchased from Thrombinoscope BV, Maastricht, Netherlands.

Assays were performed by means of Fluoroskan Ascent plate reader (Thermo Labsystems, Helsinki, Finland) and Thrombinoscope software (Thrombinoscope BV, Maastricht, the Netherlands) as described by the producer.

Analysis

Statistical analyses were performed with help of SPSS 8.0. Correlation between age and the thrombin generation values was calculated using Pearson's correlation. In addition, parameters of children were compared to adults using Mann-Whitney-U-Test. P-values less than 0.05 were considered to be significant.

Results

Children were divided into three age groups (0.5 to 6, 7 to 11 and 12 to 17 years) and compared with adults, also divided into two groups (›younger‹ and »older« adults fixing the age limit of 35 arbitrary). The mean values (± 2-fold SD) and the standard

Table 1. Results of thrombin generation measurement in different age groups. Mean values (± 2-fold SD) of lag time and time to peak (ttpeak) in minutes, endogenous thrombin potential (ETP) in nmol.min and peak in nmol and the respective standard errors of mean (SEM). Significant differences from the »younger« adults (18 to 35 years) are marked with #, from the »older« adults (> 35 years) with †.

	1/2–6 years (n=52)	7–11 years (n=20)	12–17 years (n=49)	18–35 years (n=51)	> 35 years (n=35)
lag time	2.15 (1.61–2.69) #†	2.20 (01.662.74) #†	1.95 (1.13–2.77)	2.05 (1.49–2.61) †	1.87 (1.35–2.39)
SEM	0.04	0.06	0.06	0.04	0.04
ETP	1413 (963–1863) #†	1594 (1048–2140) #†	1508 (958–2058) #†	1820 (1102–2538) †	2241 (1745–2737)
SEM	31	61	40	50	42
peak	425 (315–535) #†	462 (338–586) †	446 (318–574)	482 (336–628) †	551 (433–669)
SEM	55	62	64	73	59
ttpeak	3.82 (3.18–4.46) #†	3.86 (3.16–4.56) †	3.51 (2.59–4.43) #	3.67 (3.07–4.27) †	3.53 (2.75–4.31)
SEM	0.04	0.03	0.05	0.04	0.03

errors of mean (SEM) of ETP, lag time, peak and time to peak of each age group are listed in Table 1. ETP of all children was significantly lower than ETP of adults. Lag time was significantly longer in children up to 11 years compared to adults. Peak values of the youngest children were significantly lower than adult's and their time to peak values were significant longer, whereas lower peak values and longer time to peak values of the 7 to 11 year old children differ significantly only from the »older« adults. »Younger« adults differ in all parameters significantly from »older« adults.

Endogenous thrombin potential (ETP) (r = 0.702) and peak (r = 0.533) correlated significantly with the age of the investigated subjects. A negative correlation was found between age and lag time (r = – 0.266) and between age and time to peak (r = – 0.214) (Fig. 1a–d).

Discussion

Our results clearly show that thrombin generation is age dependent and age has to be considered, if thrombin generation measurement should be used as a routine method in clinical assessment of bleeding or thrombosis, as is true for other coagulation parameters. Beyond this, there is some evidence that high ETP might reflect risk of thrombosis [8]. If so, the steadily increase of ETP might be interpreted as the accumulation of risk factors through life time and so it would be in accordance to the increase in incidence of thromboembolic disease with higher age. Especially in venous thrombosis our findings may help to explain the increase of incidence with age that is not so well understood as in arterial thrombosis.

The first intent of this study was to investigate thrombin generation parameters of children and potential differences from adults, but regression analysis showed a steady increase in thrombin generation with increasing age also beyond the juvenile period.

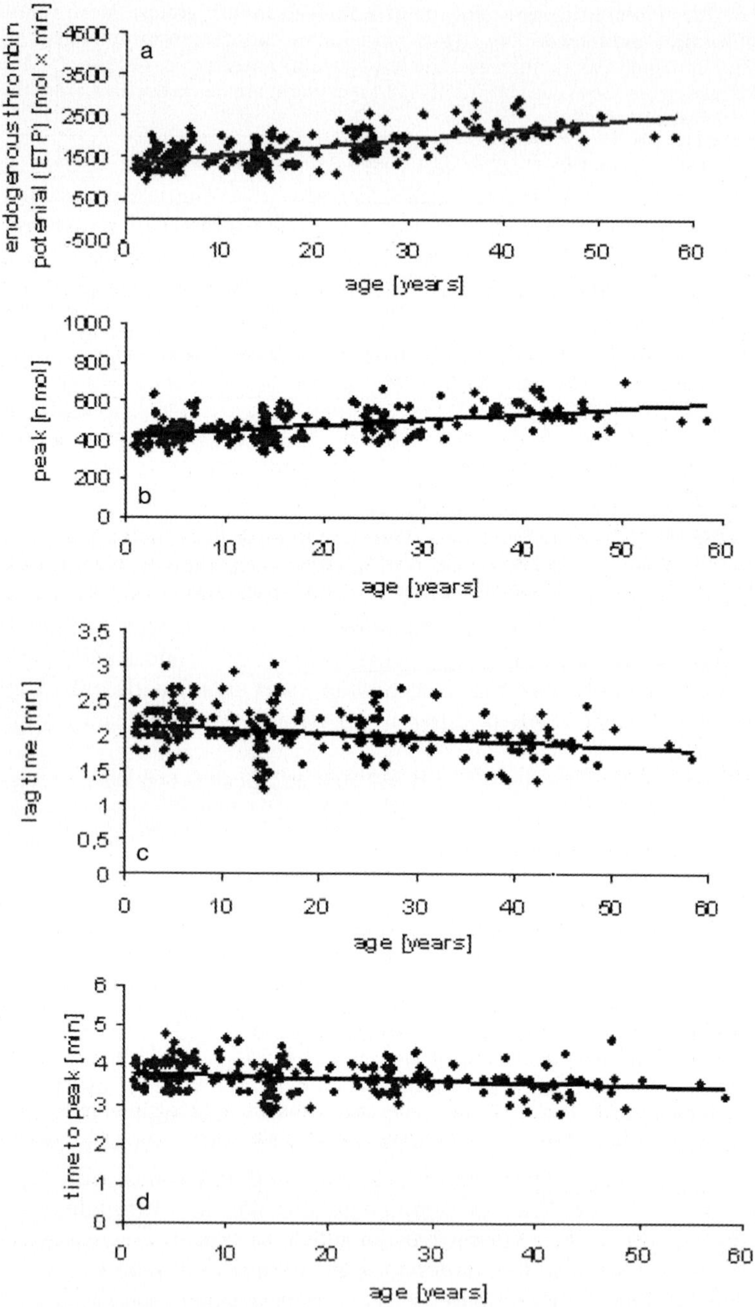

Fig. 1a–d. Correlation between age and (a) endogenous thrombin generation (ETP) (r = 0.702), (b) peak of thrombin generation (r = 0.533), (c) lag time of thrombin generation (r = – 0.266) and (d) time to peak of thrombin generation (r = – 0.214).

Childrens' values showed differences in all parameters – most distinct in the group of 1/2 to 6 year old children – compared to adults: longer lag times and times to peak, lower peak values and a decreased ETP. In children, these results do not surprise, because differences exist in several factors that have influence on thrombin generation. Since the studies of Andrew [1] we know about the lower amounts of most of the coagulation factors, and among these prothrombin, of children and their tendency for higher antithrombin (AT) levels. Butenas [6] found, that the most limiting factors for the ETP are the levels of prothrombin and AT. Gallistl [9] also showed that prothrombin levels have the highest impact on thrombin potential in the presence of APCC. So the physiological low levels of prothrombin and higher levels of AT very likely are one reason for lower ETP of children. The interindividual wide physiological scatter of all these factors in all ages could explain the wide range also in thrombin generation parameters.

Several inherited or acquired disorders of coagulation can be recognized in changed patterns of thrombin generation [7]. For this study we did not make a preselection, except known inherited disorders or coagulation disturbing medication. That means, that these data represent the wide range of risk or protective factors like family predisposition, obesity, oral contraception and others, which may have impact on bleeding or thrombosis incidence. The influence of life style on the ETP could be shown by our group comparing severely obese children with normal weighted [10].

References

1. Andrew M, Vegh P, Johnston M, et al. Maturation of the hemostatic system during childhood. Blood 1992;80:1998–2005.
2. Andrew M, Schmidt B, Mitchell L, et al. Thrombin generation in newborn plasma is critically dependent on the concentration of prothrombin. Thromb Haemost 1990;63:27–30.
3. Davie E, Fujikawa K, Kisiel W. The coagulation cascade: initiation, maintenance and regulation. Biochemistry 1991;30:10363–10370.
4. Cvirn G, Gallistl S, Leschnik B, et al. Low tissue factor pathway inhibitor (TFPI) together with low antithrombin allows sufficient thrombin generation in neonates. J Thromb Haemost 2003;1:263–268.
5. Cvirn G, Gallistl S, Rehak T, et al. Elevated thrombin-forming capacity of tissue factor-activated cord compared with adult plasma. J Thromb Haemost 2003;1:1785 1790.
6. Butenas S, van't Veer C, Mann KG. „Normal" Thrombin Generation. Blood 1999;94:2169–2178.
7. Hemker HC, Giesen P, Al Dieri R, et al. Calibrated Automated Thrombin Generation Measurement in Clotting Plasma. Pathophysiology of Haemostasis and Thrombosis 2003;33:4.
8. Mann KG, Brummel K, Butenas S. What is all that thrombin for? J Thromb Haemost 2003;1:1504–1514.
9. Gallistl S, Cvirn G, Leschnik B, et al. Respective roles of factors II, VII, IX, and X in the procoagulant activity of FEIBA. Blood Coagulation & Fibrinolysis 2002;13:653–655.
10. Cimenti C, Mangge H, Leschnik B, et al. Thrombin generation in severely obese children. In: Scharrer I, Schramm W, editors. 36th Hemophilia Symposium Hamburg 2005. Berlin Heidelberg New York: Springer. p. in press.

Effects of PFA-100 in Preoperative Screening for von Willebrand Disease in 310 Patients

B. Roschitz, C. Weitzer, M. Lindinger, A. Wirnsberger, S. Gindl, M. Köstenberger, and W. Muntean

Introduction

The purpose of any screening test is to identify disease early enough for therapeutic intervention to be effective. Therefore preoperative coagulation studies are employed in order to identify the 2–4% of all patients undergoing surgery who experience hemorrhagic complications. However, the predictive value of preoperative laboratory coagulation screening is questionable [1, 2]. The best screening tool for von Willebrand disease (vWD) is still the bleeding time (BT) which is problematic in the pediatric setting. We wanted to assess the role of the PFA-100, which provides a global measure for primary hemostasis [3], in screening for vWD in children before surgery.

Patients and Methods

We investigated 310 children consecutively seen in our outpatient service before surgery. Bleeding history of the patients and their parents was assessed by a questionnaire. Blood cell count, aPTT, PFA-100 closure times (Collagen/ADP, Collagen/Epinephrine) were done in all patients. If abnormalities were found, the patient was seen in our specialized hemostasic service. A questionnaire and physical examination were done, vWF:Ag, R:Cof, factor VIII, IX, X, XI, XII were analyzed.

Results

24% of all patients showed pathologic screening values. 1 patient with low vWF:Ag and RCof was detected by prolonged aPTT, 3 by prolonged PFA-100 closure times, and 4 by prolonged aPTT and PFA-100. No VWD was found by questionnaire.

Conclusions

The debate for the need of systematic coagulation screening tests in pediatric patients undergoing elective surgery is still open. In pediatric patients the reliability of the history may be poor since there may not have been any hemostatic challenge in the

I. Scharrer/W. Schramm (Ed.)
36th Hemophilia Symposium Hamburg 2005

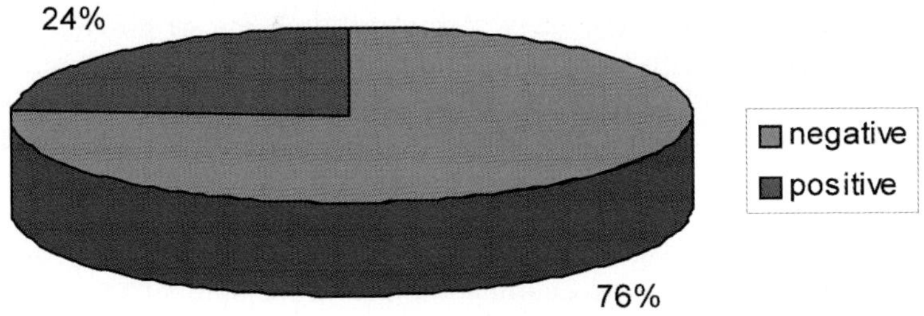

Fig. 1. Distribution of normal (negative) and abnormal (positive) coagulation screening

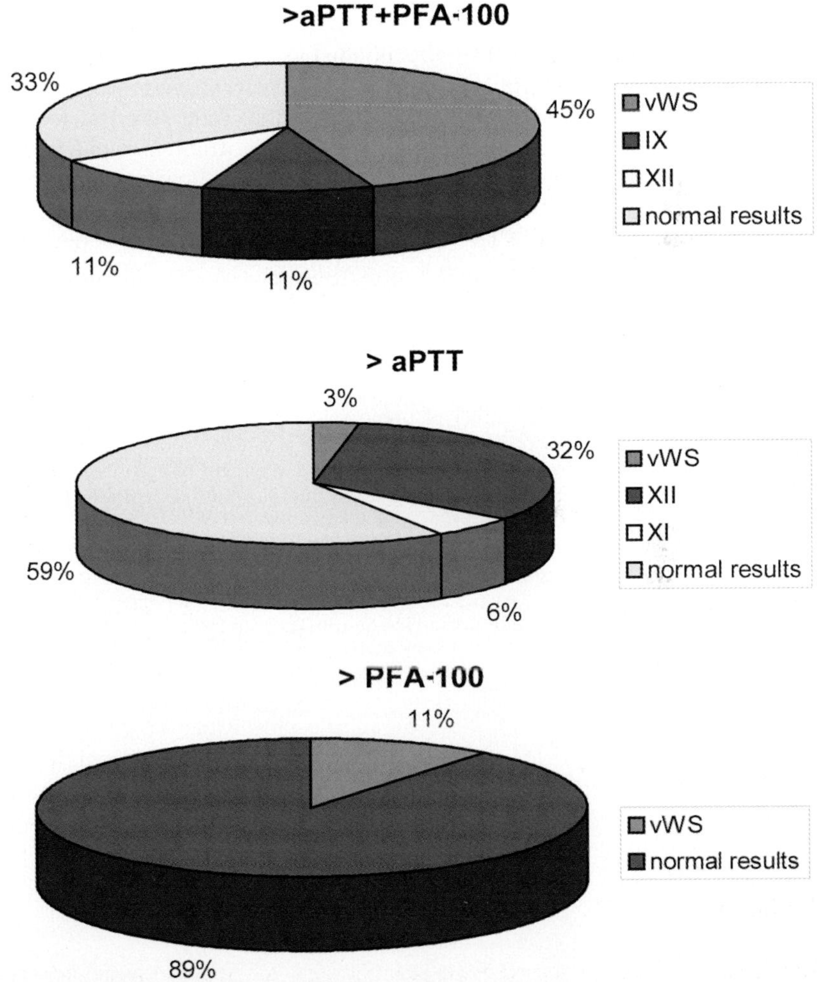

Fig. 2–4. Distribution of vWF-Ag < 60% (vWS), factor XII- (XII), factor XI- (XI) deficiency in patients with prolonged aPTT/ PFA-100

past. The assessment of hemorrhagic risk in children can be difficult. Questionnaires often miss their effectiveness due to the young age of the patient. Tonsillectomy with or without adenoidectomy is the most common major surgical procedure performed in the pediatric patient and often is the first hemostatic challenge in children.

Although preoperative PT/PTT will occasionally identify an unsuspected von Willebrand`s or other coagulopathy, the prevalence of bleeding disorders in patients with negative history and examination is low enough that PTT has essentially zero predictive value for surgical bleeding. On the other hand many situations not related to hemorrhage are associated with perturbations of the PPT, a prolonged PTT is not strongly predictive of hemorrhage nor does a normal PTT provide shelter against hemorrhagic risk [1, 2, 4]. The most common hereditary bleeding disorder is the vWD. The BT is known to be very reliable in detecting vWD but very difficult to perform and impossible to be handled as a preoperative screening laboratory method [5]. The PFA-100, designed as an in vitro measure of primary hemostasis under conditions of high shear, is a potential screening test for assessing patients with primary platelet disorders and vWD. It is a simple, rapid, non-invasive test, easy to perform in the pediatric setting. Our results show that the PFA is a very sensitive tool for the detection of vWD, but seems to have poor specifity. In our routine setting inclusion of PFA-100 increased the false positive screening results from 4 to 12 %.

References

1. Zwack GC, Derkay CS. The utility of preoperative hemostatic assessment in adenotonsillectomy. Int J Pediatr Otorhinolaryngol. 1997;39(1):67–76.
2. Manning SC, Beste D, McBride T, Goldberg A. An assessment of preoperative coagulation screening for tonsillectomy and adenoidectomy. Int. J. Pediatr. Otorhinolaryngol. 1987;13: 1237–44.
3. Favaloro EJ. Clinical application of the PFA-100. Curr Opin Hematol 2002; 9:407–15.
4. Kitchens CS. To bleed or not to bleed? Is that the question for the PTT? J Thromb Haemost. 2005;3(12):2607–11.
5. Sutor AH. The bleeding time in pediatrics. Semin Thromb Hemost. 1998;24(6):531–43.

Control of Aspirin Effect in Chronic Cardiovascular Patients Using two Whole Blood Platelet Function Assays: PFA-100 and Multiple Electrode Aggregometry

K.-W. von Pape, M. Dzijan-Horn, J. Bohner, M. Spannagl, H. Weisser, and A. Calatzis

Acetylsalicylic acid (ASA) reduces the occurrence of arterial thromboembolism during primary and secondary prophylaxis [1]. However, a considerable number of patients still experience recurrent ischemic events during ASA therapy. Lack of compliance, insufficient absorption or altered pharmacodynamics might contribute to recurrence in spite of anti-platelet therapy in these patients. In this study platelet function was tested in 76 ASA treated patients using two different monitoring methods based on whole blood.

Methods

In vitro bleeding time and whole blood aggregometry were determined in 76 patients under chronic ASA treatment. In addition whole blood aggregometry was assessed in 57 healthy blood donors who reported no aspirin intake during the 2 weeks before testing.

In vitro bleeding time [2] was determined using the PFA-100 analyzer (Dade-Behring, Marburg, Germany) using the collagen/epinephrine cartridge and citrated blood (3.8%, Sarstedt blood collection vials).

Whole blood aggregometry was performed using the Multiplate analyzer (Dynabyte medical, Munich, Germany) [3]. The instrument has 5 channels for parallel determinations and an internal computer system for real time analysis and documentation. Pipetting is performed by means of an attached, software controlled electronic pipette, which enables the user to perform the analysis according to standardized operating procedures.

The system uses a single use test cell, which incorporates 2 independent sensors consisting of a total of 4 metal electrodes. The electrodes have a diameter of 0.3 mm and a length of 3 mm. They are covered with a thin silver layer to avoid oxidation from blood elements or drugs.

For the analysis 300 µl of saline and 300 µl of blood anticoagulated with a thrombin inhibitor (TI blood collection vials, Dynabyte) were pipetted into the test cell and stirred using a magnetic stirrer. After an incubation period of 3 minutes, which ensures appropriate warming of the sample, the agonist is added and the recording starts. During the following 6 minutes the ability of platelets to adhere to the metal sensors is detected. The adhesion and aggregation of platelets is measured by the electrical resistance change between two sensor wires. Because of the use

I. Scharrer/W. Schramm (Ed.)
36th Hemophilia Symposium Hamburg 2005

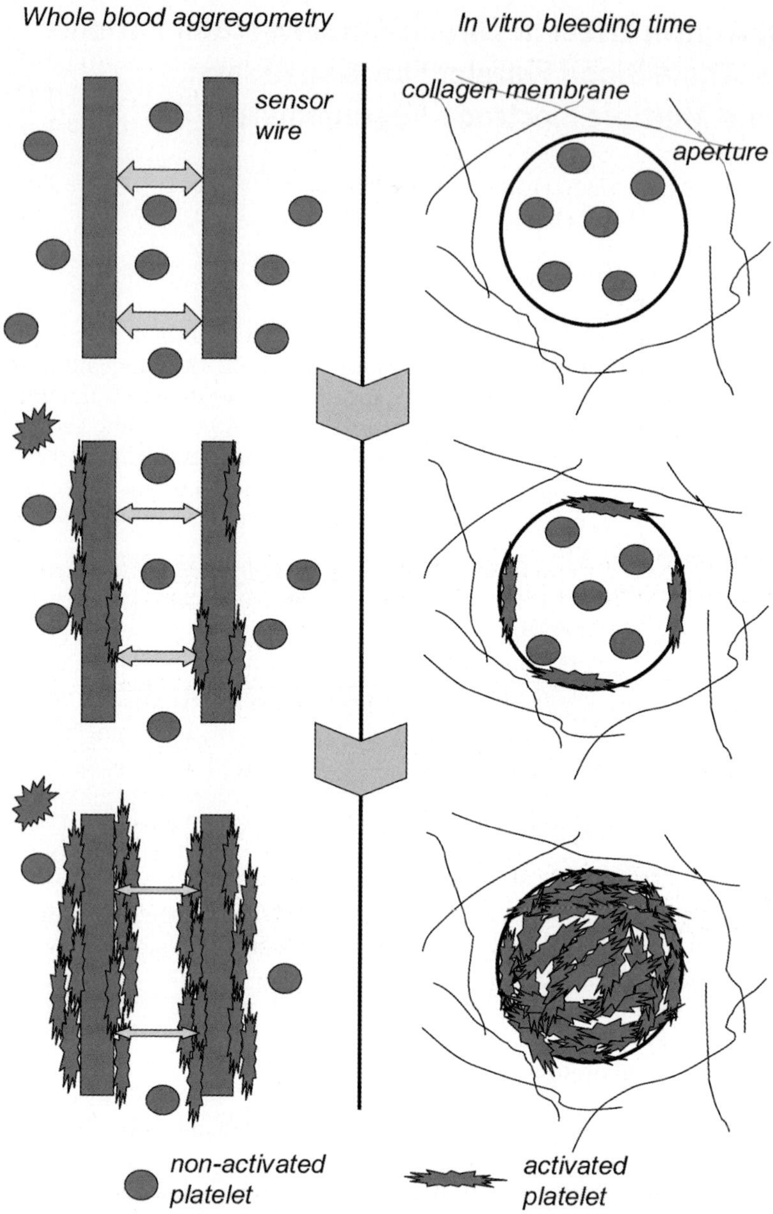

Fig. 1. Principle of whole blood aggregometry (left) and in vitro bleeding time (right): platelets get stimulated by either arachidonic acid, ADP, collagen or TRAP-6 (whole blood aggregation), or by a combination of shear stress, contact with collagen and ADP or epinephrine (in vitro bleeding time). In whole blood aggregometry platelets adhere and aggregate on metal sensor wires via their GPIIb/IIIa receptor and enhance the electrical resistance between them. In IVBT activated platelets adhere and aggregate on the collagen membrane surrounding the aperture and gradually reduce blood flow, until the closure time is reached.

of an alternating current for the detection the term »impedance« is applied. The impedance change by the adhesion of the platelets onto the sensor surfaces is expressed in arbitrary »aggregation units« and plotted against time. For this study the area under the aggregation curve (AUC) was used to quantify the aggregation response. As mentioned the analysis is measured simultaneously on 2 sensor units. The results shown represent the mean value of the 2 determined AUC values (automatically calculated by the analyzer). Impedance aggregometry was originally presented by Cardinal et al [4].

The detection principles of the 2 platelet function methods compared here are shown in Figure 1 and Table 1.

Aggregation was triggered according to manufacturer's instructions using arachidonic acid (final concentration 0.5 mM, ASPItest), collagen (3.2 µg/ml, COLtest), or TRAP-6 (thrombin receptor activating peptide, 15 µM, TRAPtest). The instrument and all reagents are commercially available.

Table 1. Determinants of in vitro bleeding time (PFA-100 and whole blood aggregometry (Multiplate)

	In vitro bleeding time	**Whole blood aggregometry**
Signal reaction	Adhesion and aggregation of platelets on an aperture of a collagen membrane	Adhesion and aggregation of platelets on metal sensors
Parameter	Closure time	Impedance change
Sample material	Whole blood	Whole blood
Shear stress	High	Low
Activation stimulus	Shear stress + contact of blood with collagen + ADP or epinephrine	Mainly activation by the activator reagent (TRAP / arachidonic acid / ADP / collagen)
Effect of von Willebrand factor	High	Absent (only in Ristocetin induced aggregation)
Sensitivity to vWS	High	Low
Sensitivity to Aspirin	High	High
Sensitivity to Clopidogrel	Low	High

Results

In vitro bleeding time : Distribution of closure time, hematocrit and platelet count in the aspirin patients is shown in Figure 2 and Table 2. Based on the local cut-off of 175 sec (determined by the analysis of normal subjects without aspirin ingestion) 71 of 76 patients can be stratified as aspirin responders and 5 of 76 patients can be attributed as aspirin non-responders.

Whole blood aggregation: Distribution of TRAPtest, COLtest and ASPItest in the aspirin patients and blood donors is shown in Figure 3 and Table 2. Comparable aggregation responses are found using TRAPtest in the two sample groups, while

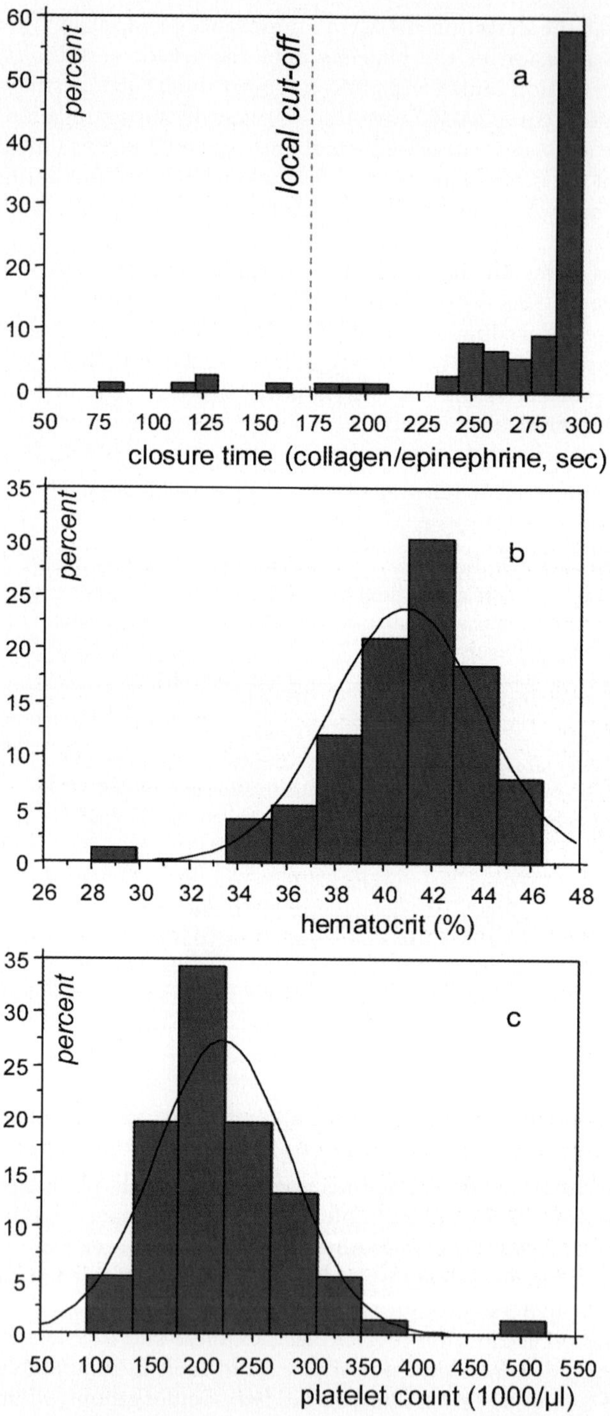

Fig. 2. Results of PFA-100 analysis, hematocrit and platelet count of the aspirin patients (n=76).

Table 2. Mean values, standard deviations, as well as the 5 and 95 percentile of the determined parameters.

		mean	sd	5 percentile	95 percentile
Aspirin patients n=76	platelet count (1000/μl)	220	63	139	311
	hematocrit (%)	41	3,1	35,4	44,9
	closure time (collagen – epinephrine, sec)	273	49	148	300
	TRAPtest	1150	273	711	1504
	COLtest	401	209	112	790
	ASPItest	146	112	47	254
blood donors n=57	TRAPtest	1232	207	939	1562
	COLtest	821	217	534	1166
	ASPItest	997	255	745	1361

aggregation is significantly inhibited in the aspirin patients. All but 3 ASPItest values determined in the aspirin patients were below 300 aggregation units, which was applied as a potential cut-off for response/non-response to aspirin. No such clear distinction between the normal subjects and aspirin patients is detected in COLtest. Therefore the 5 percentile (543 aggregation units) of the COLtest aggregation value of the blood donors was used as a cut-off for aspirin non-response. This resulted in 17 patients being allocated as non-responders and 59 as responders. As expected TRAPtest showed comparable results in both groups.

Correlating the three aspirin-sensitive methods, a high degree of non-concordance is seen when looking to classify patients as »aspirin non-responders«.

Discussion

In this study two whole blood based methods for the analysis of platelet function were used for monitoring aspirin effects in a group of patients on chronic aspirin therapy. PFA-100 analysis is based on a co-stimulation of platelets by shear stress and the contact of platelets with a membrane coated with collagen and epinephrine [1].

The results of the PFA-100 analysis revealed a rate of 6.6% of non-response of aspirin, when a cut-off of 170 sec was applied (Fig. 2a). This was the locally accepted upper threshold of the normal range.

This rate of non-response is relatively low compared with literature [5–7], which may be explained by a high rate of compliance in the tested group of patients. Persons tested were members of a sports group for individuals with cardiac disease

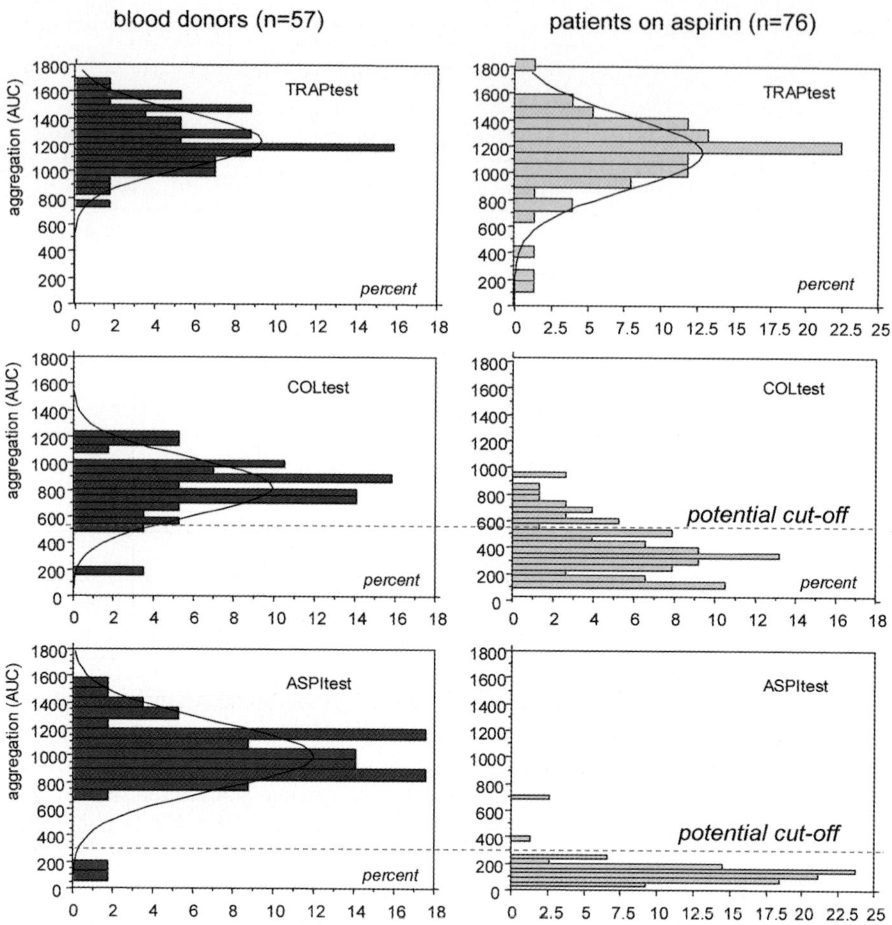

Fig. 3. Distribution of results of whole blood aggregometry (Multiplate).

and were informed that they would be tested on this day in advance. Therefore a high level of compliance could be expected [8].

Analysis of platelet aggregation by whole blood aggregometry on the Multiplate device is based on a more singular stimulation of platelets by either collagen (COLtest), arachidonic acid (ASPItest) or the peptide TRAP-6 (TRAPtest). During the analysis only low shear stress acts on the platelets by the stirring.

In TRAPtest a low sensitivity of the analysis towards the effects of aspirin is found, as shown by the similar distribution of the results of patients and controls (Fig. 3). This can be explained by the strong stimulation of the thrombin receptor, which does not need additional positive feedback stimulation by the platelet cyclooxygenase for achieving platelet activation. Collagen- and arachidonic acid-stimulated aggregation was strongly inhibited in the aspirin group (Fig. 3). Arachidonic acid is the substrate of the cyclooxygenase and is by itself not a plate-

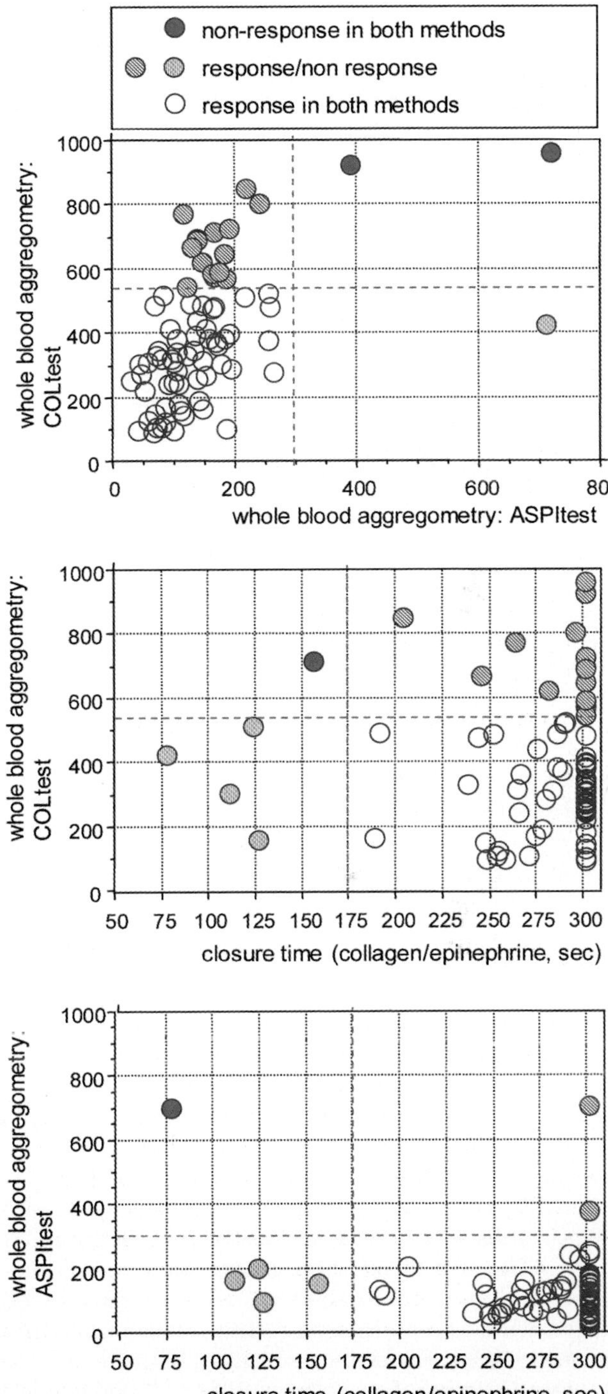

Fig. 4. Correlation of closure times, ASPItest and COLtest values in the aspirin patients.

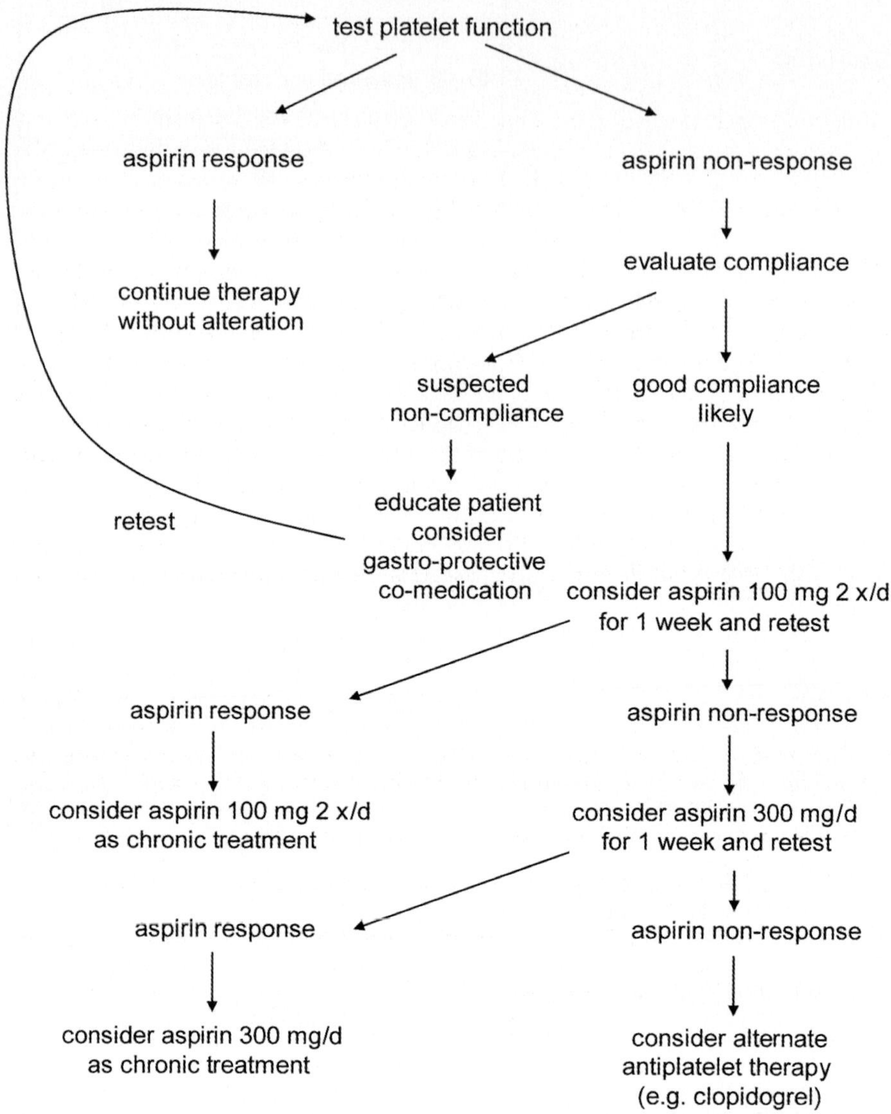

Fig. 5. Potential algorithm for individualization of aspirin therapy in high-risk patients.

let activator. Only after conversion to Thromboxane A2 it triggers platelet activation. In COLtest the platelet cyclooxygenase converts endogenously released arachidonic acid into thromboxane A2, while in ASPItest exogenous arachidonic acid added in the reagent. Therefore ASPItest is more specific towards the effects of aspirin, which was reflected by the smaller number of non-responders in ASPItest compared to COLtest.

Rate of aspirin non-response in Multiplate analysis was 4% in ASPItest and 22% in COLtest.

The results of aggregometry and PFA-100 analysis in respect to the diagnosis »ASA non-response« showed a high level of discordance between PFA-100 and aggregation, but also between ASPItest and COLtest. Also in previous studies a high level of discordance between aggregometric determination of aspirin non-response to the results of PFA-100 was found. Clinical studies are required to show which parameter of platelet function correlates best with an elevated risk for thromboembolism in patients stratified as ASA non-responders in a laboratory assay. By now most studies have applied optical platelet aggregometry testing (9–10], which is quite laborious and therefore not available for the monitoring of large cohorts.

If the clinical predictivity of a platelet function test can be shown, then a personalization of the chronic therapy is imaginable. A potential algorithm is shown in Figure 5. Obviously such therapeutic approaches require prospective validation.

In conclusion our results confirm that a proportion of aspirin-treated patients show in vitro a platelet aggregation potential which is comparable to non-treated patients. Therefore it appears imaginable to optimize treatment in these subjects, by improved patient training, adaptation of the dosing regime or change to an alternate medication. Further studies are required to establish diagnostic and therapeutic algorithms.

References

1. Antithrombotic Trialists Collaboration. Collaborative meta-analysis of randomized trials of antiplatelet therapy for prevention of death, myocardial infarction, and stroke in high risk patients. BMJ. 2002; 324:71–86.
2. Kratzer MA, Born GV. Simulation of primary haemostasis in vitro. Haemostasis. 1985;15(6):357–62.
3. Calatzis A, Wittwer M, Krueger B. A new approach to platelet function analysis in whole blood - The Multiplate Analyzer. Platelets. 2004;15:479–517.
4. Cardinal DC, Flower RJ. The electronic aggregometer: a novel device for assessing platelet behavior in blood. J Pharmacol Methods. 1980;3:135–158.
5. Grotemeyer KM. Effects of acetylsalicylic acid in stroke patients. Evidence of nonresponders in a subpopulation of treated patients. Thromb Res. 1991; 63:587–593
6. Pappas JM, Westengard JC, Bull BS. Population variability in the effect of aspirin on platelet function. Implications for clinical trials and therapy. Arch Pathol Lab Med. 1994; 118:801–804.
7. Gum PA, Kottke-Marchant K, Poggio ED et al. Profile and prevalence of aspirin resistance in patients with cardiovascular disease. Am J Cardiol. 2001; 88: 230–235.
8. K.-W. von Pape, G. Strupp,T. Bonzel, J. Bohner Effect of compliance and dosage adaption of long term aspirin on platelet function with PFA-100 in patients after myocardial infarction. Thrombosis and Haemostasis 2005; 94: 889–891.
9. K.H. Grotemeyer, H.W. Scharafinski and I.W. Husstedt, Two-year-follow-up of aspirin responder and aspirin non responder. A pilot-study including 180 post-stroke patients. Thromb Res 71 (1993), pp. 397–403.
10. Gum PA, Kottke-Marchant K, Welsh PA, White J, Topol EJ. A prospective, blinded determination of the natural history of aspirin resistance among stable patients with cardiovascular disease. JACC. 2003; 41: 961–965.

Difficulties in the Interpretation of the Term »Patient-Related« in the Scope of the Introduction of a Remuneration of Additional Payments According to the OPS

K. H. Beck, P. Dirschedl, M. Mohrmann, and B. Waibel

Background

Since 2005 the catalogue of case-based lump sums, beside the DRG, also provides additional payments (AP) for expensive medical drugs. AP 34 and 35 (8-800..) are reserved for the calculation of the remuneration of thrombopheresis concentrates (TAC). AP 35 refers to »patient-related« TAC.

The OPS-301 (version 2004) defines (8-800.6): *»patient-related platelet concentrates means specifically prepared TAC for patients with suspicion of or proof of HPA- or HLA-antibodies«*. The Health Insurances examine the proper account calculated by the various medical institutions. Deviations from correct calculation were found in the account of AP 35.

Methods

- Medical service inquiry by the health insurances.
- Procurement of the patient documentation.
- Questioning of three regional and four local blood donation services regarding the label handling on platelet concentrates and the pertinent release notes with respect to »patient-related«.
- Estimation of the additional expenditure for AP 35 on the basis of the difference of AP in € from 34.01 to 34.08, and 35.01 to 35.08.
- Estimation of the annual loss for the health insurances by using the § 21 transfusion law related platelet concentrate consumption amounts.

Results

Most of the AP examined so far by the medical service showed normal TAC and were not »patient-related« as calculated by the medical institution. It remains unclear if the preference for TAC instead of platelet-pool-concentrates for transfusion, in order to minimize transfusion-related risks, was interpreted as »patient-related«.

By questioning the blood banks it was found that the labeling procedure on blood concentrates and release notes was missing or not clearly expressed regar-

I. Scharrer/W. Schramm (Ed.)
36th Hemophilia Symposium Hamburg 2005

ding the term »patient-related«. This fact causes mistakes for the coding procedure by the physician.

Meanwhile, one blood donation unit (DRK) has introduced the new term »patient-related« on platelet concentrates and the pertinent release notes.

The average additional expenditure amounts to 111 €. According to data published by the Paul-Ehrlich-Institute *(www.pei.de)* referring to the time interval of 2000–2002 the overall consumption of TAC in Germany was 163,266.

Using these data based on an assumed incorrect accounting of 20% to 30% an annual deficit of 3.6–5.4 million Euros would result for the German health system as a consequence.

Discussion

The term »patient-related« leaves much room for interpretation, despite its unambiguous definition in the OPS. Quite obviously, also the irradiated concentrates were accounted as »patient-related« in the same way. There is no consistent labeling on TAC or pertinent release notes. Nor does the legislator stipulate this. Consequently, a clear marking on TAC and release notes for the coding physician is lacking, and this causes coding errors.

In order to avoid additional erroneous accounts of AP 35 it is necessary to train the staff in medical institutions who are responsible for transfusions. The standardized marking of TAC and/or pertinent release notes should preferably be regulated by law.

Factor VIII as Positive Regulator of Activated Platelets

A. Sturm, A. Obergfell, U. Walter, and R. Grossmann

Abstract

Deficiency of factor VIII (FVIII) as an important cofactor in the tenase coagulation factor complex causes severe bleeding, whereas high FVIII levels seem to be associated with venous and arterial thromboembolism. Resting platelets do not bind FVIII, but activated platelets bind inactivated FVIII if vWF is not present. In this study the influence of platelet bound FVIII on platelet function itself was investigated as a direct effect of FVIII on platelets has not been shown so far. Methods: The influence of platelet bound FVIII on platelet function was investigated by flow cytometric analysis of P-selectin expression (CD62P) and PAC-1 binding before and after submaximal stimulation with TRAP-6 (5 μM final concentration) and by confocal microscopy. Blood was incubated with human recombinant FVIII concentrate (Helixate, ZLB Behring, Marburg, Germany) for 5 minutes at 37 °C. Results: There were no significant changes in P-selectin expression or PAC-1 binding respectively in FVIII-pretreated platelets. Stimulation of platelets with TRAP-6 increased the expression of P-selectin (445 %) and PAC-1 binding (934 %) as expected. These effects were significantly further increased when platelets were stimulated with TRAP-6 and FVIII (P-selectin 499 %, PAC-1 1626 %; Student's t-test, $p < 0.05$. Values were expressed in %, related to unstimulated, Helixate buffer treated platelets). The assessment of platelet spreading by the means of confocal microscopy showed an increased spreading on fibrinogen matrix after stimulation with TRAP-6 and FVIII. This effect was higher, compared to platelets stimulated with TRAP-6 alone. Conclusions: TRAP-co-stimulated platelets seem to be positively regulation by additional FVIII. Thus a FVIII-induced increase in platelet activation might contribute to venous and even more arterial thrombus formation in patients with high FVIII levels.

Introduction

Deficiency of factor VIII (FVIII) as an important cofactor in the tenase coagulation factor complex causes severe bleeding symptoms, whereas high FVIII levels seem to be associated with venous and arterial thromboembolism [1–4]. Resting platelets do not bind FVIII, whereas platelets activated by thrombin, epinephrine or polymerized fibrin bind inactivated FVIII if vWF is not present. Both, FVIII and activated factor VIII (FVIIIa) binding to platelets were shown to be specific, reversible and

I. Scharrer/W. Schramm (Ed.)
36th Hemophilia Symposium Hamburg 2005

saturable and seemed to be affected by the FVIII B-domain and the presence of soluble von Willebrand factor (vWF) [5, 6, 8].

Presently only few data exist about direct effects of FVIII on platelet function: whereas porcine FVIII seemed to be able to activate human platelets, possibly due to residual porcine vWF in the porcine FVIII preparation, human FVIII did not [5, 6]. The aim of this study was to investigate the influence of human recombinant FVIII on platelet function by flow cytometry (P-selectin (CD62P) expression, PAC-1 binding), platelet aggregometry and confocal microscopy.

Material and Methods

Flow cytometry analysis

Blood from healthy volunteers (n = 5) was anticoagulated with citrate and washed human platelets were obtained as described previously [7]. Briefly, prostaglandine I2 (1 µM final) and Apyrase 1 µl/ml were added to platelet rich plasma. After centrifugation the pellet was resuspended in CGS buffer (120 mM sodium chloride, 12.9 mM trisodiumcitrate, 30 mM D-glucose, pH 6,5). Prostaglandine and Apyrase were added and samples were centrifuged once more. The pellet was resuspended in Tyrode's buffer (150 mM sodium chloride, 5 mM potassium chloride, 1 mM magnesium chloride, 10 mM D-glucose, 10 mM hepes, pH 7,4) and the platelet concentration was adjusted to 150.000/µl.

20 µl of washed platelets were incubated with either 10 µl Tyrode's buffer or 10 µl TRAP-6 (thrombin receptor activated peptide) (5 µM final) (Bachem Distribution Services GmbH, Weil am Rhein, Germany) and/or Factor VIII concentrate (Helixate, ZLB Behring, Marburg, Germany) for 5 minutes. FVIII concentrations of about 200 % were aspired. Then 10 µl of FITC-labeled anti-CD62P (P-selectin), PAC-1 or the appropriate isotype control were added. The samples were incubated at room temperature for 10 minutes, and 500 µl PBS was added. In all samples, 10,000 platelets gated by FSC and SSC characteristics were analyzed in a FITC (Fl1) histogram on a Becton Dickinson FACScan flow cytometer (Becton Dickinson, Heidelberg, Germany) using CellQuest Software. Binding of each antibody was expressed in % of mean fluorescence intensity (MFI) relative to MFI in buffer-incubated platelets. In all experiments the FVIII concentration was adjusted to approximately 200–250 %, the final TRAP-6 concentration was 5 mM. All antibodies were purchased from Becton Dickinson, Heidelberg, Germany.

Confocal microscopy

Washed human platelets were obtained as described above and plated on fibrinogen-coated coverslips for 45 min at room temperature. Buffer, TRAP-6 and/or FVIII was added to the platelets. Adherent cells were fixed in 3.7% formaldehyde, permeabilized with 0.1% Triton X-100, and F-actin was stained with Rhodamine-phalloidin. Single images were acquired with a Nikon fluorescence microscope equipped with a laser scanning confocal system (MRC 1024; Bio-Rad Laboratories, Hercules, CA, USA). Images were processed in Adobe photoshop. Surface areas of at least 100 platelets per sample were measured using Image-Pro Plus software (Media Cybernetics, Inc. Silver Spring, MD, USA). Platelet spreading was expressed in % of platelet surface pixels relative to buffer-incubated platelets (± SD). Fibrinogen was purchased from Enzyme Research Laboratories, South Bend, IN, USA.

Data Analysis

Differences between mean fluorescence intensity values for comparisons were determined by paired Student's t test. P-values for differences of platelet surface areas were calculated by unpaired Student's t test. P-values < 0.05 were considered statistically significant.

Results

FACS Analysis

To investigate platelet activation washed platelets were incubated with buffer, FVIII, and/or TRAP-6. Incubation with FVIII did not increase P-selectin expression (Fig. 1) or PAC-1 binding (Fig. 2). PAC-1 binds to the activated integrin $\alpha_{IIb}\beta_3$, the receptor for fibrinogen and vWF. Platelet stimulation with TRAP-6 increased the expression of P-selectin (445 %) (Fig. 1) and PAC-1 binding (934 %) (Fig. 2) as

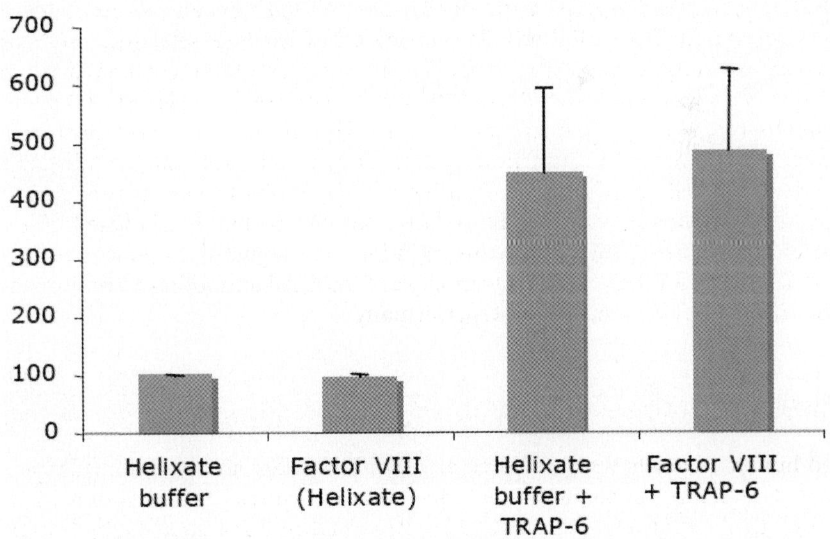

Fig. 1. P-selectin expression after adding TRAP-6 and/or FVIII concentrate relative to platelets incubated with buffer in percent. * $p < 0.05$. (Student's t-test, n = 5)

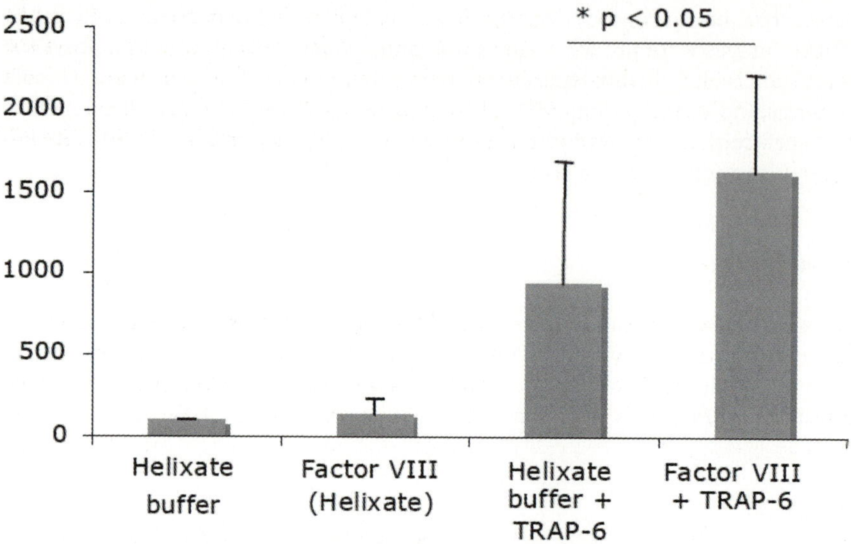

Fig. 2. PAC-1-binding after adding TRAP-6 and/or FVIII concentrate relative to platelets incubated with buffer in percent. * $p < 0.05$ (Student's t-test, n = 5)

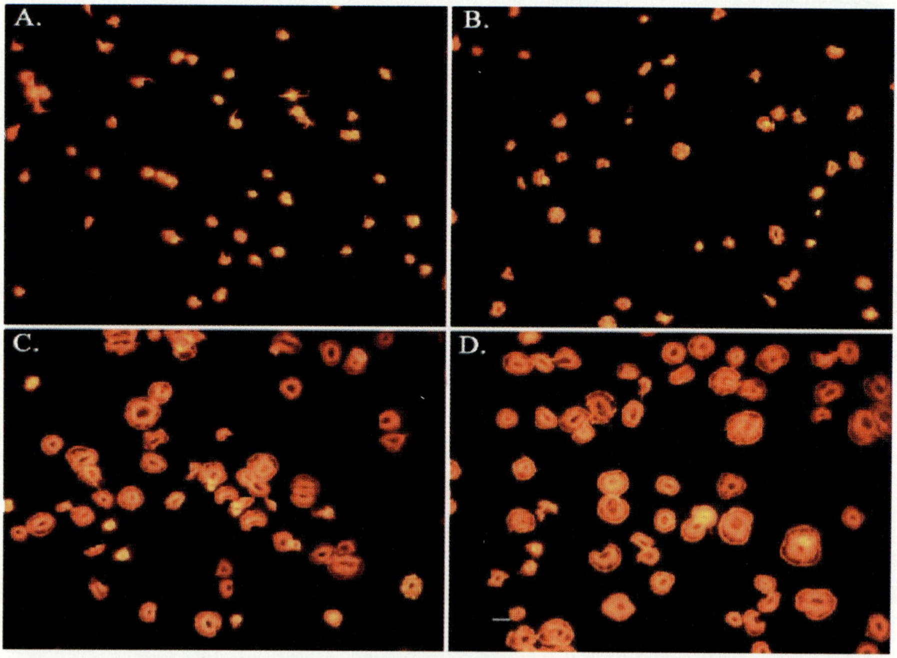

Fig. 3. Confocal images of platelets adherent on fibrinogen showed an increased spreading after co-stimulation with FVIII compared to stimulation with TRAP-6 only. F-actin is stained red (bar = 10 µm). A. unstimulated platelets, B. platelets and FVIII, C. platelets stimulated with TRAP-6, D. platelets stimulated with FVIII and TRAP-6

expected. Values were expressed in %, related to platelets incubated with buffer only. This buffer was identical to the buffer used in the FVIII concentrates. The observed effects with TRAP-6 were further increased when platelets were stimulated with TRAP-6 and FVIII (P-selectin 499 %) (Fig. 1), (PAC-1 1626 %) (Fig. 2). This increase in PAC-1 binding was significant compared to platelets stimulated with TRAP-6 only ($p < 0.05$).

Confocal microscopy

Platelet spreading on fibrinogen assessed by confocal microscopy (Fig. 3) showed increased spreading in FVIII-co-stimulated platelets compared to platelets activated with TRAP-6 only. Platelets were stained for F-actin (red). Computerized image analysis confirmed that the average surface area of the platelets treated with TRAP-6 and FVIII was significantly greater than that of platelets treated with TRAP-6 only ($p < 0.05$). The average pixel size was 368 vs. 307 respectively (Fig. 4).

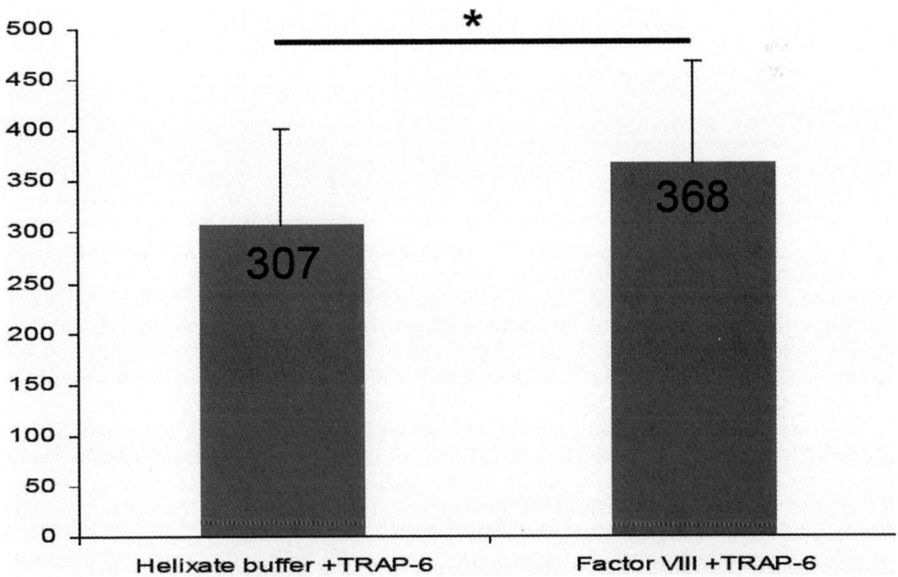

Fig. 4. Average platelet pixel amount after stimulation by TRAP-6 ± FVIII measured by confocal microscopy as shown in Fig. 3. * $p < 0.05$ (Student's t-test, n = 4)

Discussion

As FVIII plays a key role in hemostasis and FVIII binds to platelets, we investigated the effect of FVIII on platelet function by flow cytometry and confocal microscopy. We found an increase in P-selectin expression and PAC-1-binding in TRAP-6-

activated platelets co-stimulated with recombinant FVIII. This means that co-stimulation of platelets with FVIII increases α-degranulation and the activation of the integrin $\alpha_{IIb}\beta_3$, which is recognized by the PAC-1-antibody. Spreading of fibrinogen-adherent TRAP-6-activated platelets co-stimulated with FVIII was increased as well.

There was no influence of factor VIII on any investigated parameter of resting platelets. This might be explained by the fact, that unstimulated platelets do not bind significant amounts of FVIII molecules. In any case, blocking of FVIII binding or direct platelet activation by vWF could be excluded due to the use of recombinant FVIII, which does not contain any vWF.

In conclusion, FVIII appears to be a positive regulator of platelet function in TRAP-co-stimulated platelets. FVIII increases alpha-granule secretion and activates $\alpha_{IIb}\beta_3$ receptors, thus inducing platelet spreading, which can be visualized by confocal microscopy.

We conclude that FVIII enhances platelet-dependent hemostasis. Thus FVIII substitution in hemophilia might as well support primary hemostasis. Furthermore increased platelet activation might contribute to arterial and venous thromboembolism in patients with chronically elevated levels of FVIII.

References

1. Hoffman M, Monroe DM. A cell-based model of hemostasis. Thromb Haemost. 2001; 85: 958–65.
2. Catto AJ, Carter AM, Barrett JH, Bamford J, Rice PJ, Grant PJ. Von Willebrand factor and factor VIII:C in acute cerebrovascular disease. Relationship to stroke subtype and mortality. Thromb Haemost. 1997; 77: 1104–08.
3. Schambeck C, Grossmann R, Zonnur S, Berger M, Teuchert K, Spahn A, Walter U. High factor VIII levels in venous thromboembolism: role of unbound FVIII. Thrombosis Haemostasis. 2004;92:42–46.
4. Bank I, Libourel EJ, Middeldorp S, Hamulyak K, van Pampus EC, Koopman MM, Prins MH, van der Meer J, Buller HR. Elevated levels of FVIII:C within families are associated with an increased risk for venous and arterial thrombosis. J Thromb Haemost. 2005; 3: 79–84.
5. Gilbert GE, Sims PJ, Wiedmer T, Furie B, Furie BC, Shattil SJ. Platelet derived microparticles express high affinity receptors for FVIII. JBC. 1991; 266: 17261–268.
6. Ahmad SS, Scandura JM, Walsh PN. Structural and functional characterization of platelet receptor-mediated factor VIII binding. JBC. 2000; 275: 13071–81.
7. Obergfell A, Eto K, Mocsai A, Buensuceso C, Moores SL, Brugge JS, Lowell CA, Shattil SJ.: Coordinate interactions of Csk, Src, and Syk kinases with [alpha]IIb[beta]3 initiate integrin signaling to the cytoskeleton. J Cell Biol 2002 Apr 15;157(2):265–75.
8. Li X, Gabriel DA. The physical exchange of factor VIII (FVIII) between von Willebrand factor and activated platelets and the effect of the FVIII B-domain on platelet binding. Biochemistry. 1997; 36: 10760–767.

Characterization of Three Novel Mutations in the Sodium Binding Site of Coagulation Factor X

R. F. Strey, K. Wulff, W. Schröder, and F. H. Herrmann

Abstract

In this study we characterized the novel mutations FX_{G325R}, FX_{E329G} and FX_{G410R} by biochemical methods as well as by protein modeling. For the biochemical analysis the proteins have been expressed in HEK 293 cells. The antigen activities (determined using sandwich ELISA) of the mutations FX_{G325R} and FX_{E329G} have been reduced compared to the wild type, whereas FX_{G410R} did not lead to reduced expression. The amidolytic and prothrombinase activities (determined using fluorogenic substrates) of all three mutants have been drastically reduced compared to the wild type. This is in accordance with reduced factor X activities in the (heterozygous) patients.

The protein modeling suggests an impaired function of the sodium loop as a result of the mutations FX_{G325R}, FX_{E329G} or FX_{G410R}. Although only Gly410 is located in the sodium loop of factor X, all three mutations lead to a shift of the electrostatic potential in the sodium loop from the acid to the basic range. This could lead to reduced sodium or substrate binding and therefore to an impaired catalytic function of the mutants.

Additionally to their influence on the electrostatic potential the mutations FX_{G325R} and FX_{G410R} may lead to steric conflicts as a result of the replacement of the small glycine by the bulky arginine. In the case of FX_{G325R} the side chain of Arg325 inhibits the salt bridge between Ile195 and Asp378, which is important for the formation of the catalytic active conformation of factor Xa. In the mutant FX_{R410} the side chain of Arg410 may fill the binding site of the sodium ion or of the P1 residue of substrates.

Introduction

Factor X is a vitamin K dependent serine protease of vital importance for the blood coagulation system [1]. The gene coding for factor X is located on chromosome 13 and consists of 8 exons. In vivo the protein is expressed in liver cells as a single chain protein. A cleavage during or after secretion leads to a heavy chain of 42 kDa connected via a disulfide bridge to a light chain of 16 kDa [2, 3]. A cleavage of the activation peptide at the N-terminus of the heavy chain between Arg194 and Ile195 by the tissue factor – factor VIIa complex (TF·FVIIa) or by the tenase complex (FVIIIa·FIXa) leads to activation of the zymogen factor X to activated factor Xa [4].

I. Scharrer/W. Schramm (Ed.)
36th Hemophilia Symposium Hamburg 2005

The change from the zymogen to the catalytic active conformation of factor X involves the formation of a salt bridge from the remaining N-terminal Ile195 to Asp378 between the sodium loop and the autolysis loop into the catalytic center [2].

Because only activated factor Xa and mainly the prothrombinase complex (FVa·FXa) may activate prothrombin (FII) to thrombin (FIIa) in significant amounts, factor X deficiency often lead to severe bleeding symptoms in homozygous patients [5].

We characterized the three novel mutations FX_{G325R}, FX_{E329G} and FX_{G410R} which have been found in heterozygous patients without or only with mild bleeding symptoms (muscle hematomas) but with significant reduced factor X activities.

Patients

The mutation FX_{G325R} has been found in three heterozygous patients within one family. The factor X activity has only been reported for one of these patients with FX:C=40%. All three patients are asymptomatic.

The mutation FX_{E329G} has been found in one heterozygous patient with a factor X activity of FX:C=32 %. This patient shows no bleeding symptoms.

The mutation FX_{G410R} has been found within one family in three heterozygous patients with factor X activities of FX:C=23%, 27% and 46%. Additionally the factor IX activities are reduced (FIX:C=43%, 30% and 50%), but a sequencing of the factor IX gene did not show factor IX mutations. One of these patients shows only mild bleeding symptoms (muscle hematomas). The other two patients are asymptomatic.

Methods

Protein Expression

For the protein expression we used HEK 293 cells and the expression vector pCMV4.hFX (R. Camire, University of Vermont). The mutations have been inserted into the cDNA insert of the vector using side directed mutagenesis. Media and lysated cells have been harvested 24 hours after the transfection.

Antigen Activity

The FX antigen activities of cell lysate and media have been determined using a FX ELISA kit (Haemochrom Diagnostica, Essen, Germany).

Amidolytic Activity

For the determination of the amidolytic activity of Xa each 10 µl sample was activated by a mixture of 10 µl 4.8 nM FVIIa and 10 µl Innovin (Dade Behring, Marburg,

Germany) as a source of tissue factor and incubation at 37°C for 5 minutes. Immediately after addition of 55 µl 0.3 mM spectrozyme FX fluorogenic substrate (American Diagnostica GmbH, Pfungstadt, Germany) in HBS/Ca buffer the conversion of the substrate have been recorded by a BMG Fluorostar Galaxy (BMG Lab Technologies GmbH, Offenburg, Germany) at 37°C. The obtained initial conversion rates have been taken as a measure of the activity of factor Xa. The amidolytic activity of wild type FXa has been set to 100%.

Prothrombinase Activity

For the determination of the prothrombinase activity of FXa each 5 µl sample was incubated with 4 µl FX depleted plasma at 37°C. Immediately after addition of 30 µl Innovin (Dade Behring, Marburg, Germany) as a source of tissue factor and 46 µl 0.3 mM Thrombin Substrate III (Merck Biosciences GmbH, Bad Soden, Germany) the conversion of the fluorogenic substrate has been recorded by a BMG Fluorostar Galaxy (BMG Lab Technologies GmbH, Offenburg, Germany) at 37°C. The prothrombinase activities of the samples have been determined by comparison of the conversion rates of the samples with conversion rates of a dilution series of wild type factor X. The prothrombinase activity of wild type FXa has been set to 100%.

Protein Modeling

The homology modeling using the Swiss-PdbViewer (http://www.expasy.org/spdbv/) based on the x-ray structure of the active-site-inhibited human FXa [6], solved at 2.3-Å resolution (Protein Data Bank (PDB) entry 1XKA). For the visualization of the obtained structures we used the POV raytracer (http://www.povray.org/).

Results

Factor X Activity

The mutations FX_{G325R}, FX_{E329G} and FX_{G410R} are characterized by reduced catalytic activities of factor X both *in vivo* and *in vitro* (see Fig. 1 and 2).

A significant reduction of the FX antigen values has been observed only for the mutation FX_{G325R}, which is characterized by FX:Ag values between 50% and 60% in comparison to the wild type. The Mutation FX_{E329G} leads to a marginal reduction of the FX antigen activity and the mutation FX_{G410R} has no influence on the FX:Ag values (see Fig. 3).

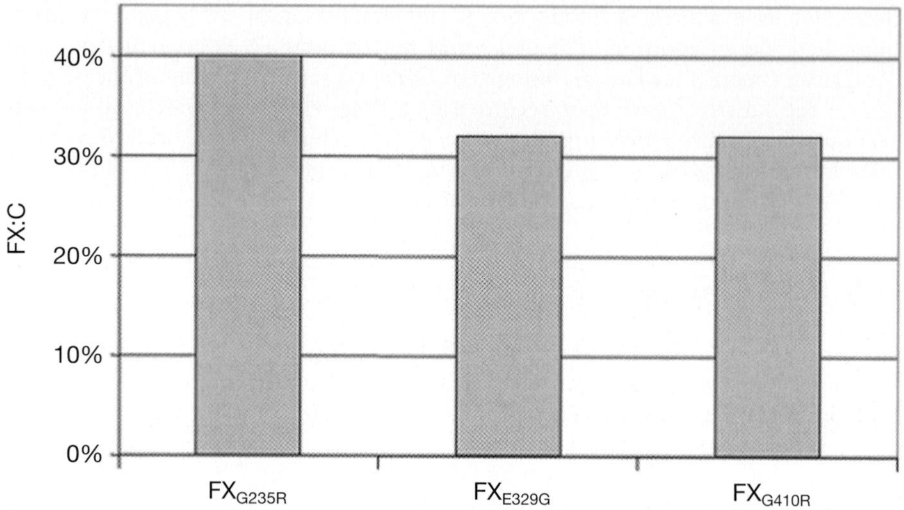

Fig. 1. FX activities in heterozygous patients (70%–120% = normal range [7])

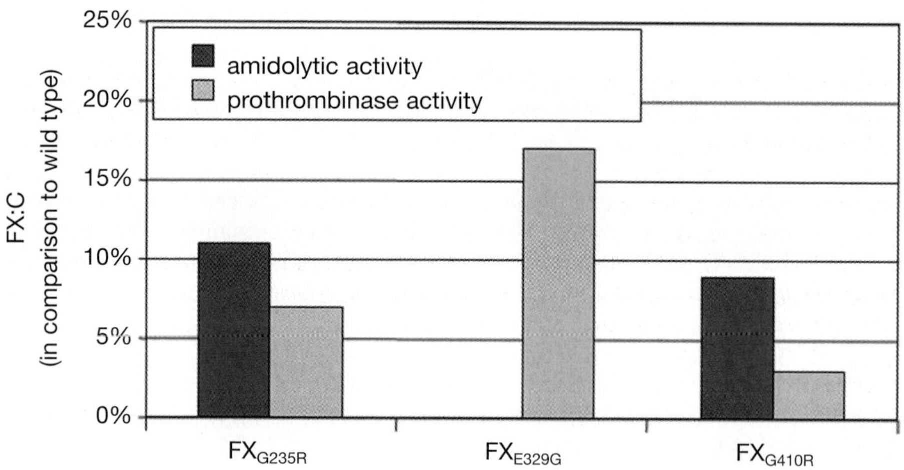

Fig. 2. Catalytic activities of FX in the expression study

Electrostatic Potential

Although only the mutation FX_{G410R} is located in the sodium loop, the protein modeling of all three mutations FX_{G325R}, FX_{E329G} and FX_{G410R} lead to extensive changes of the electrostatic potential in the sodium loop. The replacement of the non polar glycine by the basic arginine in the mutations FX_{G325R} and FX_{G410R} as well as the replacement of the acid glutamate by the non polar glycine leads to a shift of the electrostatic potential of the sodium loop from the acid to the basic range (see Fig. 4).

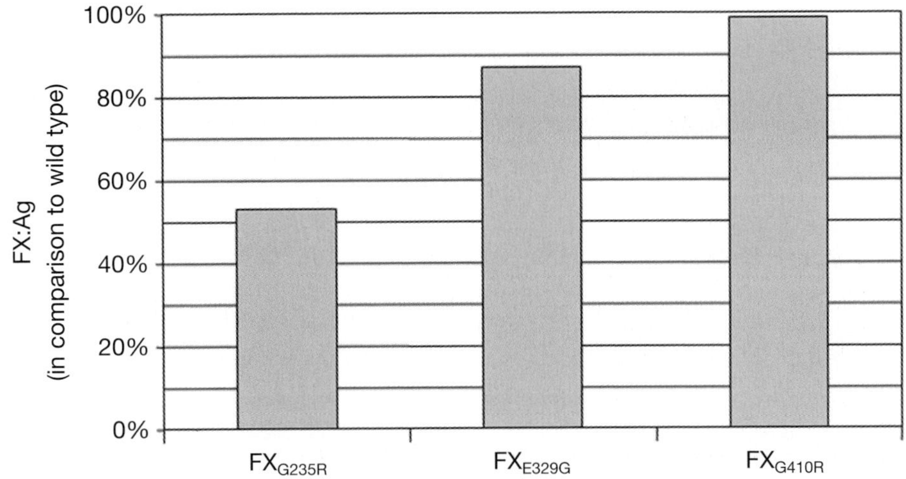

Fig. 3. FX antigen activities in the expression study

Steric Conflicts

After cleavage of the activation peptide in wild type factor X the N-terminal residues Ile195, Val196, Gly197 and Gly198 of the heavy chain bind into a hydrophobic cavity between the autolysis loop and the sodium loop. In this process Ile195 forms a salt bridge to Asp378 in the catalytic center (see Fig. 5). This plays a key role in the conversion from the zymogen form of factor Xa to its catalytic active conformation [8].

Gly325 is located at the origin of the autolysis loop in the adjacency of this salt bridge. As a result of the replacement of Gly325 by Arginine the access of Ile195 to Asp378 can be blocked by the bulky side chain of Arg325 (see Fig. 5). This would inhibit the formation of the salt bridge and therefore interfere with the formation of the catalytic active conformation of factor Xa.

Gly410 is located in the sodium loop of factor X. In wild type factor X this loop contains a cavity which is filled with water, Na^+ and the P1 residue of the substrate. Because this cavity may absorb the bulky side chain of Arg410, the mutation FX_{G410R} leads only to marginal structural changes in the computer model. Nevertheless this mutation leads to steric conflicts. Dependent on the orientation of the side chain of Arg410 the sodium binding site or the site of factor Xa may be blocked by the mutation FX_{G410R}. Figure 6 shows a computer model of FX_{R410} with the side chain of Arg410 directed to the S1 site. In this case the access of the P1 residue of the substrate to Asp373 would be blocked.

In addition to its influence on the electrostatic potential, Glu329 seems to have a structural function in factor X. It is not only part of a b-turn type I consisting of the residues His328, Glu329, Lsy330 and Gly331 which connects the two b strands of the autolysis loop but it is also connected via hydrogen bonds to Cys403 and Arg405 in the sodium loop. Surprisingly the computer model of the mutant FX_{G329} shows no significant structural changes compared to the wild type (see Fig. 7).

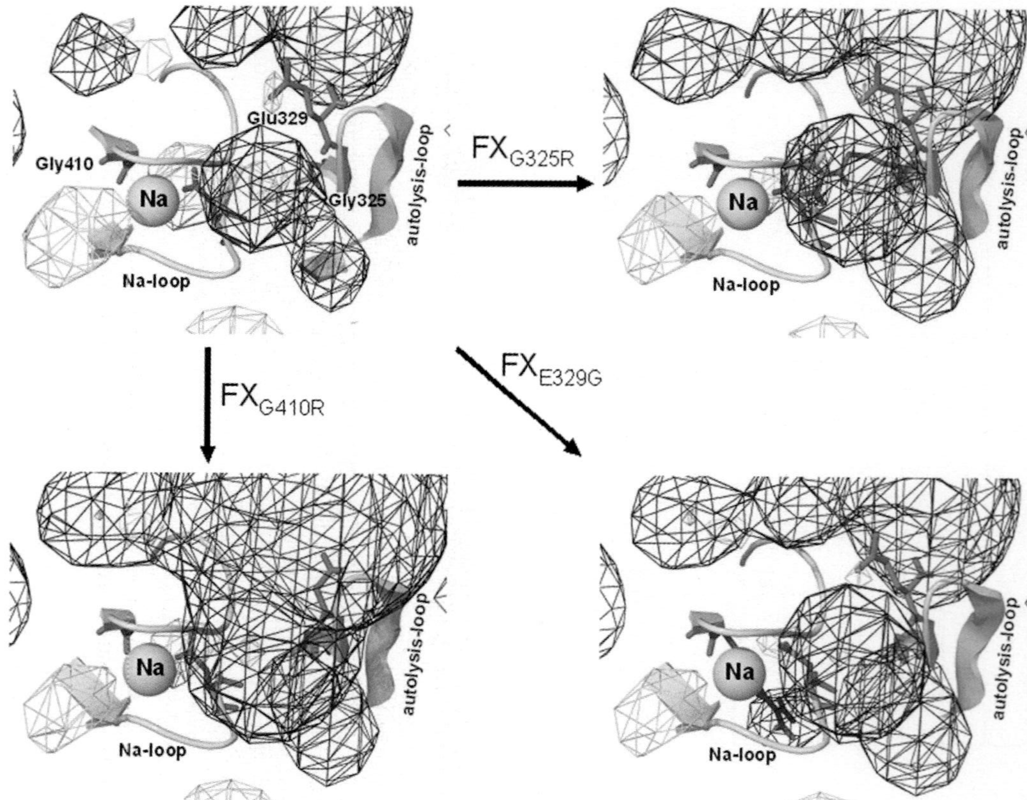

Fig. 4. By the mutations FX_{G325R}, FX_{E329G} and FX_{G410R} the electrostatic potential in the environment of the Na-loop will be changed from the acid to the basic range. This may lead to impaired binding of Na^+ or substrates. Positive charged areas are represented by dark grids and negative charges by bright grids

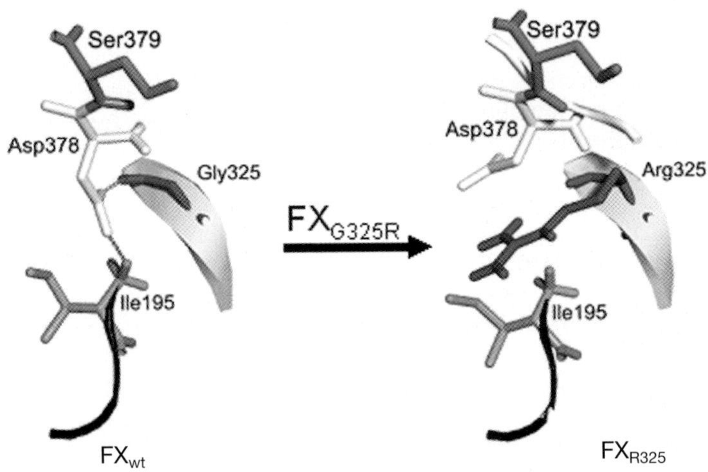

Fig. 5. In the mutant FX_{R325} the salt bridge between Ile195 and Asp378 is blocked by the side chain of Arg325

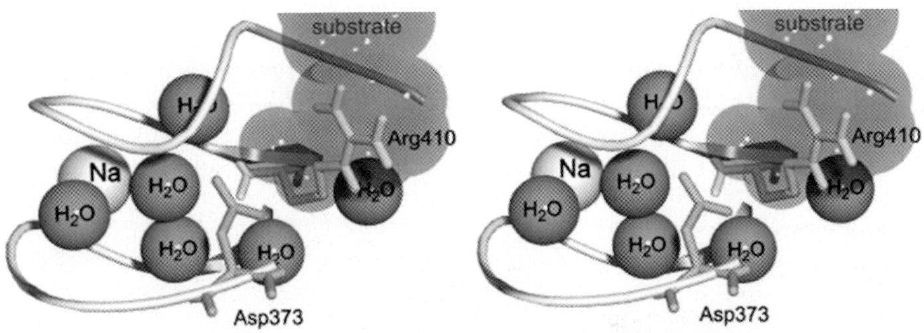

Fig. 6. Stereo image of the sodium loop of FX_{R410}; In this computer model of the mutant FX_{R410} the access of the substrate (transparent) to the SI site (Asp373) is blocked by the residue of Arg410

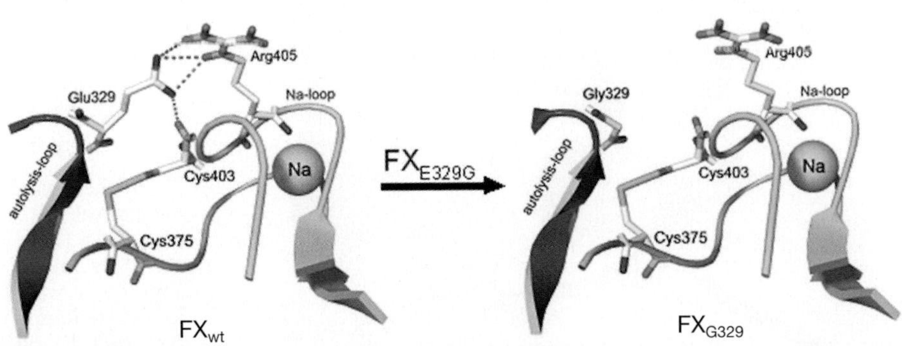

Fig. 7. Regardless of several broken hydrogen bonds between autolysis-loop and Na-loop, the mutation FX_{E329G} leads only to marginal structural changes in the computer model

Discussion

Similarities of the mutations FX_{G325R}, FX_{E329G} and FX_{G410R}

All three mutations FX_{G325R}, FX_{E329G} and FX_{G410R} lead to a significant change of the electrostatic potential of the sodium loop. The sodium loop of factor X provides a Na+ binding site and the S1 site for selective substrate binding. According to Underwood et al. (2000) in the Na^+ binding site of factor Xa, Na^+ is octahedric coordinated by the backbone carbonyl groups of the amino acids Tyr367, Asp368, Arg405 and Lys408 as well as by two water molecules [9]. The S1 site consists in the acid side chain of Asp373. The binding of sodium as well as of the P1 residue of substrates depend on the acid character of the sodium loop. By changing the electrostatic potential from acid to basic by the mutation FX_{G325R}, FX_{E329G} or FX_{G410R} the binding of Na^+ or substrates may be impaired. This would explain the reduced catalytic activities of the mutants *in vivo* and *in vitro*.

Additionally to their influence on the electrostatic potential the mutations FX_{G325R} and FX_{G410R} have different individual effects on the function of factor X.

As a result of the mutation FX_{G325R} the salt bridge between Ile195 and Asp378 is blocked by the bulky side chain of Arg325. Because this salt bridge is important for the catalytic active conformation of factor Xa, this would reduce the catalytic activity of the mutant. A similar effect has been observed in the case of the mutation FX_{G323S}. Actually both mutations are characterized by strongly reduced catalytic activities. In case of FX_{G323S} even heterozygous patients show bleeding symptoms.

Because the side chains of Val321 and Ala374 are also directed to the salt bridge between Ile195 and Asp378 (see Fig. 8), mutations at these positions should also lead to reduced catalytic activities. This is also suggested by the genetic conservation of these amino acids.

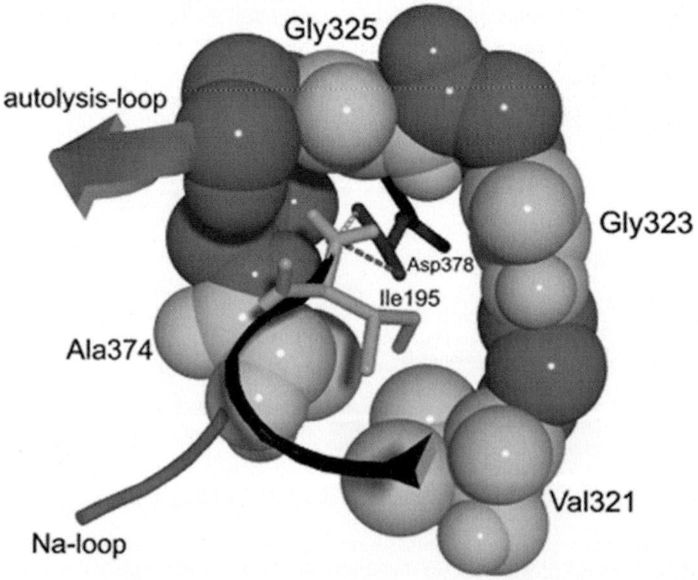

Fig. 8. The replacement of Val321, Gly323, Gly325 or Ala375 by bulky amino acids would lead to steric conflicts with the salt bridge between Ile195 and Asp378

Although the mutation FX_{G410R} leads only to the marginal conformational changes, the replacement of the small glycine by the bulky arginine may lead to steric conflicts interfering the sodium or substrate binding. This would reduce the catalytic activity of the factor Xa mutant additionally to the change of the electrostatic potential.

The mutation FX_{E329G} results in several broken hydrogen bonds between autolysis loop and sodium loop, but the energy minimization using the GROMOS96 implementation of the Swiss-Pdbviewer did not lead to significant structural changes. Therefore the reducing effect of this mutation on the catalytic activity of factor Xa can only be explained by the change of the electrostatic potential.

References

1. Jackson CM, Johnson TF, Hanahan DJ. Studies on bovine factor X. I. Large-scale purification of the bovine plasma protein possessing factor X. Biochemistry 1968; 7: 4492-17
2. Fair DS, Bahnak BR. Human hepatoma cells secrete single chain factor X, prothrombin, and antithrombin III. Blood. 1984; 64(1): 194-204
3. Duffy EJ and Lollar P. Intrinsic pathway activation of factor X and its activation peptide-deficient derivative, factor Xdes-143-191. J Biol Chem 1992; 267: 7821-7
4. Venkateswarlu D, Perera L, Darden T, Pedersen LG. Structure and Dynamics of Zymogen Human Blood Coagulation Factor X. Biophys J. 2002; 82(3): 1190-206
5. Peyvandi F, Mannucci PM, Lak M, Abdoullahi M, Zeinali S, Sharifian R, Perry D. Congenital factor X deficiency: spectrum of bleeding symptoms in 32 Iranian patients. British Journal of Haematology 1998; 102: 626-628
6. Kamata, K, Kawamoto H, Honma T, Iwama T, Kim S-H. Structural basis for chemical inhibition of human blood coagulation factor Xa. Proc. Natl. Acad. Sci. U.S.A. 1998; 95: 6630-35
7. Monagle P, Andrew M. Hemorrhagic and thromboembolic complications during infancy and childhood. In: Colman RW, Hirsh J, Marder VJ, Clowes AW, George JN, eds. Hemostasis and thrombosis. Philadelphia: Lippincott Willams & Wilkins; 2001: 1053-1070
8. Oppenheimer HL, Labouesse B, Hess GP. Implication of an Ionizing Group in the Control of Conformation and Activity of Chymotrypsin. J. Biol. Chem. 1966; 241: 2720-30
9. Underwood MC, Zhong D, Mathur A, Heyduk T, Bajaj SP. Thermodynamic Linkage between the S1 Site, the Na+ Site, and the Ca2+ Site in the Protease Domain of Human Coagulation Factor Xa. Studies on catalytic efficiency and inhibitor binding. J. Biol. Chem. 2000; 275: 36876-84

Characterization of a Mutation in the 5′ Flanking Region and a Novel IVS7 Splice site Mutation in a Patient with Severe FVII Deficiency

W. Schröder, K. Wulff, R. Tech, R. Grempler, A. Ruiz-Saez, and F. H. Herrmann

Abstract

The molecular basis of a factor VII deficiency was investigated in a Venezuelan patient. The five-year-old boy with a residual FVII:C of 1.7% and FVII:Ag < 8% suffered from epistaxis and easy bruising since birth. By sequence analysis a mutation –60T>C in the 5' flanking region of the FVII gene and the novel mutation at the IVS7 donor splice site IVS7+1G>A were detected. The mutated splice site is located within the first repeat of a minisatellite region. Each repeat in this region contains a normally silent pseudo splice site. By an electrophoretic mobility shift assay (EMSA) the decrease of the binding of the nuclear factor HNF-4 by the promoter mutation –60T>C could be shown. To characterize the consequence of the mutated splice site IVS7+1G>A we constructed wildtype and mutated minigens spanning exons 7 to 8. HEK 293 cells were transfected with these constructs. In cells transfected with the mutant transcript no normal splicing occurred. Three different cryptic splice sites were used in vitro, all predicting a premature termination.

Introduction

Factor VII (FVII) is a vitamin K-dependent coagulation protease essential for the initiation phase of normal hemostasis. In the Greifswald FVII deficiency study the molecular basis of inherited FVII deficiency is studied [1, 2, 5, 6, 16–20]. More than 126 different causative mutations were characterized by sequence analysis up to now. Among them 67% were missense mutations, 6.3% nonsense mutations, 7% small deletions and 0.7% insertions. 11% of the mutations affected splice sites and 8% of the mutations were located in the 5' flanking region of the FVII gene.

Accurate splicing requires highly conserved sequences at the 5' donor- and 3' acceptor splice sites at the exon-intron borders and an weakly conserved branch point sequence, located about 20–40 base pairs upstream the acceptor splice site. Mutations in the 3' or 5' splice sites usually result in exon skipping or activation of cryptic splice sites.

Intron 7 (IVS7) of the factor VII gene is characterized by the presence of 3 to 9 37 bp-repeats. The repeated elements provide multiple identical 5' splice junctions, normally silent [4, 8].

I. Scharrer/W. Schramm (Ed.)
36th Hemophilia Symposium Hamburg 2005

Within the first 400 bp of the promoter region of the FVII-gene four protein binding regions have been characterized by DNAse I footprint analysis and several proteins that regulate FVII gene expression have been identified. The liver specific hepatocyte nuclear factor 4 (HNF 4) which plays an important role in the regulation of liver specific proteins binds to the region at –63 to –58 [10]. Disturbing the specific binding of nuclear proteins mutations in this region can be a reason of a FVII deficiency.

Patients and Methods

Patient

The patient G-11012, a 5 year-old Venezuelan (Mestizo) boy, is the son of healthy non consanguineous parents. There was no familial history of bleeding. At the age of 4 months the patient first time was presented with bleeding diathesis with epistaxis.

Coagulation Tests

FVII coagulant activity was determined by a one stage method using FVII deficient plasma as substrate and a commercial human thromboplastin preparation. FVII antigen (FVII:Ag) level was measured using an enzyme-immunoassay (Affinity Biological incorporated, Hamilton, Canada).

Molecular Analysis

DNA was isolated from leucocytes by standard salting out method [7]. Exons, exon-intron bounds and the 5'flanking region were amplified by polymerase chain reaction (PCR) and sequenced with an ABI 377 sequencer (Perkin Elmer Applied Biosystems, Warrington, UK) [16].

For splice analysis the genomic region spanning nucleotides nt 9568 (exon 7) to nt 10652 (exon 8; primer 2 and 5 as earlier described in [9]) of the patient and a normal subject was amplified and cloned by TA-cloning into the expression vector pCR3.1 (Invitrogen Corp, Carlsbad, CA). All coding sequences and splice junctions were sequenced.

RT-PCR and first strand PCR were performed with the superscript one-step RT-PCR system (Invitrogen) with 20 ml of the total RNA extract. For one–step RT-PCR and a subsequent nested PCR primers 3 and 5 [9] were used. Non purified PCR products were subsequently cloned into the pCR3.1 vector by TA-cloning and sequenced.

Transfections

For characterization of the splice site mutations HEK 293 cells have been grown in DMEM/F10 supplemented with 10% fetal calf serum. Transfections of wildtype and mutant-minigenes were performed with Lipofectamine2000 (Invitrogen). Cells were seeded in a 6 well plate at a density of 4 x 10^5 cells/ml. At 80% confluence cells were transfected with 4 µg DNA and 10 µl Lipofectamine/well. 24 hours after transfection total RNA was extracted from the cells using the Nucleospin RNAII kit (Macherey-Nagel).

Electrophoretic Mobility Shift Assay (EMSA)

The double-stranded oligonucleotides containing the wildtype (5'-CTT GGA GGC AGA GAA CT**T** TGC CCG TCA GTC C -3') or mutated sequence (5'-CTT GGA GGC AGA GAA CT**C** TGC CCG TCA GTC C-3') spanning from nt –77 to nt –47 of the FVII promoter were end labeled with γ-^{32}P-ATP (30000Ci/mM, Hartmann Analytik) using T4 polynucleotide kinase (Roche Applied Sciences). For the EMSA nuclear extracts (10 µg protein) isolated from HepG2 cells [13] were incubated in a total of 20 ml with the labeled oligonucleotide (25,000 cpm) [12]. Additionally nuclear extracts were preincubated for 15' with either 2 µg of HNF-4 antibody (Santa Cruz Biotechnology) or the indicated molar excess of unlabelled oligonucleotide competitor. Bound and free probe were resolved on 6% non-denaturating polyacrylamide gels prior to autoradiography.

Results and Discussion

The FVII residual activity of the severe affected patient was less than 2.5%, antigen < 8% of the normal. By sequence analysis a mutation –60T>C in the 5' region of the FVII gene and a novel splice site mutation IVS7+1G>A have been detected. Polymorphisms characterized in the 5' region of the promoter –401G>T, -323 ins and –122T>C [3, 4, 8, 15] which are known to influence the promoter activity were homozygous wt in the patients DNA.

–60T>C

An EMSA was used to investigate the influence of the mutation –60 T>C on the binding of the nuclear factor HNF-4. It could be indicated, that the wt oligonucleotide binds specifically to a protein of the Hep G2 nuclear extract. By preincubation of the wt oligonucleotide with an HNF-4 antibody a supershift of the protein band specific for HNF-4 was observed (not shown). Mutated oligonucleotide binds to a much lower extend to the nuclear extract compared to the wt (Fig 1). The promoter mutation –60T>C leads to a significant loss of ability of the nuclear protein HNF-4 to bind and transactivate the FVII-gene promoter. These results are in concordance

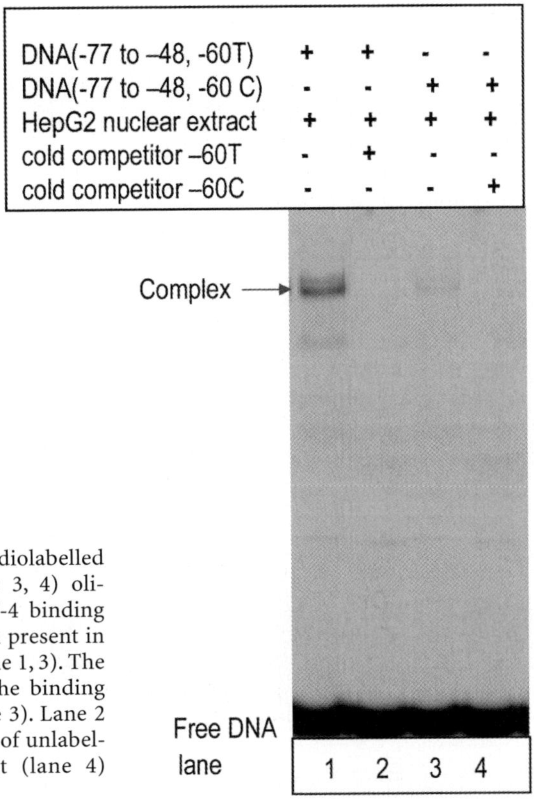

Fig. 1. Electromobility shift assay. A radiolabelled wildtyp (lane 1, 2) or mutant (lane 3, 4) oligonucleotide encompassing the HNF-4 binding site show specific binding to a protein present in nuclear extracts from HepG2 cells (lane 1, 3). The mutation -60T>C strongly reduces the binding capacity to about 30% of the wt (lane 3). Lane 2 and 4: Incubation with a molar excess of unlabelled wild-type (lane 2) and mutant (lane 4) sequences

with a previously reported strongly reduced promoter activity in a reporter gene assay for this mutation [14].

IVS7+1G>A

Analysis of the RT-PCR-Product from cells transfected with the wildtype construct showed a correct splicing of the transcripts in all cases whereas the mutation prevents a normal splicing. Sequence analysis of cloned RT-PCR fragments from the mutant constructs revealed the occurrence of three different fragments (Fig. 2). Cryptic splice sites at position +5, +38 and +75 of the IVS7 were used. To estimate the percentage of the different mRNAs we cloned the RT-PCR products from wildtype and mutant transfected cells and analyzed 100 individual inserts from each product. The most frequent was the one spliced at position +37 (63%). The cryptic splice site at +4 was used in 10% and the one at +75 in 28%. For the wt-construct no usage of one of the cryptic splice sites was observed.

The mutated splice site is located in the first repeat of a minisatellite characterized by 5-8 repeated 37 bp elements. Each of this elements contains a normally silent

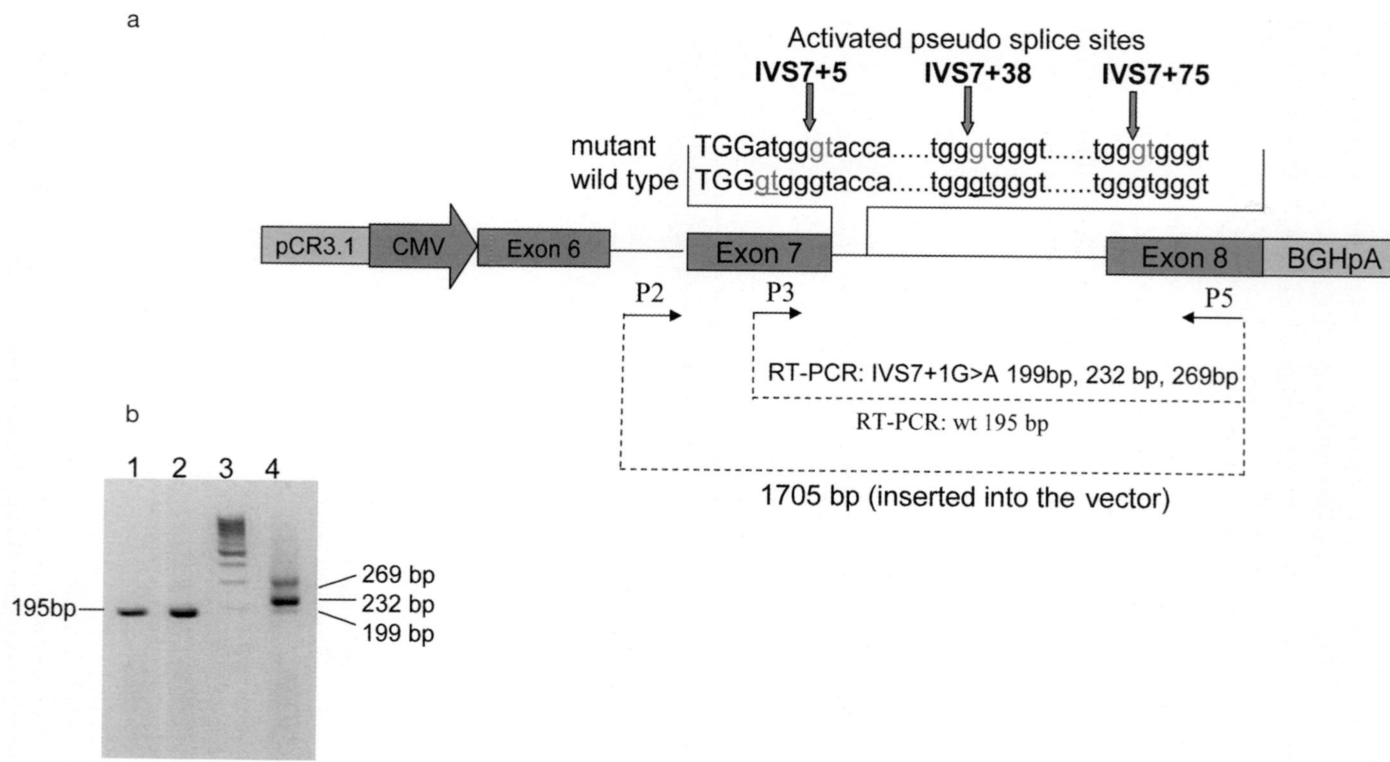

Fig. 2. In vitro expression of FVII mRNA. a) Schematic diagramme of the construct with the FVII wt and mutant gene region. Primers P2 and P5 used for vector construction, primers P3 and P5 used for RT-PCR. b) RT-PCR amplification of FVII mRNA expressed in cells transfected with constructs containing wt sequence or mutation IVS7+1G>A. lane 1, 2: wt, lane 3: 100 bp ladder, lane 4 IVS7+1G>A

pseudo–splice site. The authentic splice wt site as well as the cryptic splice sites at +38 and +75 have identical consensus values (CV) of 74.7 [11]. The cryptic site at position +5 has a lower CV of 58.6. This explains the less frequent use of this site, though it is located closest to the authentic site. All insertions result in a reading frameshift and predict premature termination of protein synthesis. The mechanism in the wt allele selecting the correct splice site among the multiple identical sites is not yet revealed and still in discussion.

All polymorphisms in the 5' region which are known to modulate promoter activity are wildtype in both of the patients alleles. Assuming that the in vitro results mimic the in vivo situation, both mutations are causative for the FVII deficiency and contribute to the severe phenotype of the patient. The residual FVII antigen and activity detected in the patients plasma probably results from a low residual activity of the mutant allele with the –60 C>T mutation.

References

1. Herrmann FH, Wulff K, Auberger K, Aumann V, Bergmann F, Bergmann K, Bratanoff E, Franke D, Grundeis M, Kreuz W, Lenk H, Losonczy H, Maak B, Marx G, Mauz-Körholz CH, Pollmann H, Serban M, Sutor A, Syrbe G, Vogel G, Weinstock N, Wenzel E, Wolf K. Molecular biology and clinical manifestation of hereditary factor VII deficiency. Seminars in Thrombosis and Hemostasis 2000; 26: 393–400
2. Herrmann FH, Wulff K. Gerinnungsfaktoren VII, VIII, IX und X.Ausgewählte Aspekte zur Molekulargenetik und Gendiagnostik Hämostaseologie 2004; 24:94–107
3. Kudaravalli R, Tidd T, Pinotti M, Ratti A, Santacroce R, Margaglione M, Dallapicola B, Bernardi F, Fortina P, Devoto D, Pollack E. Polymorphic changes in the 5' flanking region of factor VII have a combined effect on promoter strenght. Thromb Haemost 2002; 88:763–767
4. Marchetti G, Gemmati D, Patraccini P, Pinotti M, Bernardi F. PCR detection of a repeat polymorphism within the F7 gene. Nucleic Acids Res 1991:19(16) 4570
5. Mariani G, Herrmann FH, Bernardi F, Schved JF, Auerswald G, Ingerslev J. Clinical manifestations, management and molecular genetics in congenital factor VII deficiency: the International Registry on Congenital Factor VII deficiency (IRF7). Blood (letter) 2000; 96: 374
6. Mariani G, Herrmann FH, Dolce A, Batorova A, Etro D, Peyvandi F, Wulff K, Schved JF, Auerswald G, Ingerslev J, Bernardi F. Clinical phenotypes and factor VII genotype in congenital factor VII deficiency. Thromb Haemost 2005; 93: 481–7
7. Miller M, Dykes DD, Polesky HF. A simple salting out procedure for extracting DNA from human nucleated cells. Nucleic Acids Res 1988; 16:121
8. O'Hara PJ, Grant FJ. The human factor VII gene is polymorphic due to variation in repeat copy number in a minisatellite. Gene. 1988:66:147–158
9. Pinotti M, Toso R, Redaelli R, Berrettini M, Marchetti G, Bernardi F. Molecular mechanisms of FVII deficiency: Expression of mutations clustered in the IVS7 donor splice site of factor VII gene. Blood 1998:92 (5):1646–1651
10. Pollak E, Hung H-L, Godin W, Overton GC, High KA. Functional characterization of the human factor VII 5'-flanking region.; J Biol Chem 1996; 271(3):1738–1747
11. Shapiro MB, Senapathy P. RNA splice junctions of different classes of eukaryotes: sequence statistics and functional implications in gene expression. Nucleic Acids research 1987; 15(17):7155–7174
12. Schmoll D, Walker K, Alessi DR, Grempler R, Burchell A, Guo S, Walther R, Unterman TG. Regulation of Glucose-6-phosphatase Gene Expression by protein kinase Ba and the Forkhead Transcription Factor FKHR. J Biol Chem 2000; 275 (46): 36624–36333

13. Schreiber E, Matthias P, Müller M M, Schaffner W. Rapid detection of octamer binding proteins with ›mini-extracts‹, prepared from a small number of cells. Nucleic Acids Research 17 (15); 6419
14. Tidd T, Kudaravalli R, Beaverson K, DiMichele DM, Highs KA, Pollak ES. Two novel point mutations identified in the human coagulant protein factor VII gene. Thromb Haemost Suppl 1999; 467; 1476
15. Van't Hooft F, Silveira A, Tornvall P, Illiadou A, Ehrenborg E, Eriksson P, Hamstern A. Two common Functional polymorphisms in the promoter region of the coagulation Factor VII gene determining plasma FVII activity and mass concentration. Blood 1999; 10; 3432-3441
16. Wulff K, Herrmann FH. Twenty-two novel mutations of the FVII gene in factor VII deficiency. Hum Mutat. 2000; 15(6):489–496)
17. Wulff K, Glenschek C, Auberger K, Aumann V, Bergmann F, Bergmann K, Bratanoff E, Grundeis M, Kreuz W, Lenk H, Losonczy H, Maak B, Marx G, Mauz-Körholz U, Scheel H, Serban M, Sutor H, Syrbe G, Vogel G, Weinstock N, Wenzel E, Wolf K, Herrmann FH. Analyse von Genmutationen bei hereditärem Faktor-VII-Mangel. In: I. Scharrer, W. Schramm (ed.) 29. Hämophilie-Symposion Hamburg 1998; Springer-Verlag, (2000) 112–117
18. Wulff K, Herrmann FH. Twenty-two novel mutations of factor VII gene in factor VII deficiency. In: I. Scharrer/W. Schramm (Hrsg.) 30. Hämophilie-Symposion Hamburg 1999 Springer-Verlag Berlin Heidelberg (2001), S. 235–239
19. Wulff K, Herrmann FH and the study group. Greifswald Study Congenital Factor VII Deficieny. In: F.H. Herrmann (ed.) Gene Diagnosis of Inherited Bleeding Disorders. Verlag Pabst Science Publishers Lengerich, Berlin, Bremen (2002) S. 127–134
20. Wulff K, Batorova A, Herrmann FH. Mutation Analysis of Factor VII Deficiency in Slovakia. In: F.H. Herrmann (ed.) Gene Diagnosis of Inherited Bleeding Disorders. Verlag Pabst Science Publishers Lengerich, Berlin, Bremen (2002) S. 162–168

On the Molecular Basis of Warfarin Resistance in Rats

M. Hünerberg, S. Rost, A. Fregin, H. J. Pelz, C. R. Müller,
and J. Oldenburg

Introduction

For 60 years, coumarin drugs (e.g. warfarin) are in use for the treatment of thromboembolic events in humans and for the treatment of coagulation via inhibition of the vitamin K epoxide reductase complex (VKOR), and in high doses lead to spontaneous fatal bleedings. VKOR recycles vitamin K 2,3-epoxide to vitamin K hydrochinone, an essential cofactor for the post-translational gamma-carboxylation of several blood coagulation factors.

Resistance to warfarin and its more potent derivatives (e.g. difenacoum, bromadiolon) has been reported for several wild populations of rats and mice. The recent identification of the VKORC1 gene, a key component of the VKOR, allowed for the characterization of the molecular basis of warfarin resistance (Rw).

Methods

The VKORC1-gene of resistant rats from laboratory life stocks were analyzed by sequencing. Rats were tested before for warfarin resistance with the blood-clotting response method. VKOR enzymatic activity was measured in HEK293 cells transfected with VKORC1 cDNA constructs and its inhibition by warfarin was determined.

Results and Discussion

Four mutations in the rat VKORC1 gene have been identified in Rw animals from Denmark, Germany and the UK. While Danish and German rats share an Y139C mutation of supposedly common origin, three different mutations were observed in British rats. All mutations cluster in the hydrophobic domain of the protein. Upon recombinant expression, all Rw mutations conferred resistance to warfarin at the expense of a lower basal activity. We could show that mutations in the VKORC1-gene are associated with warfarin resistance in rats. The lower basal activity is in line with previous reports on the reduced fitness of Rw rats in the absence of warfarin selection.

I. Scharrer/W. Schramm (Ed.)
36th Hemophilia Symposium Hamburg 2005

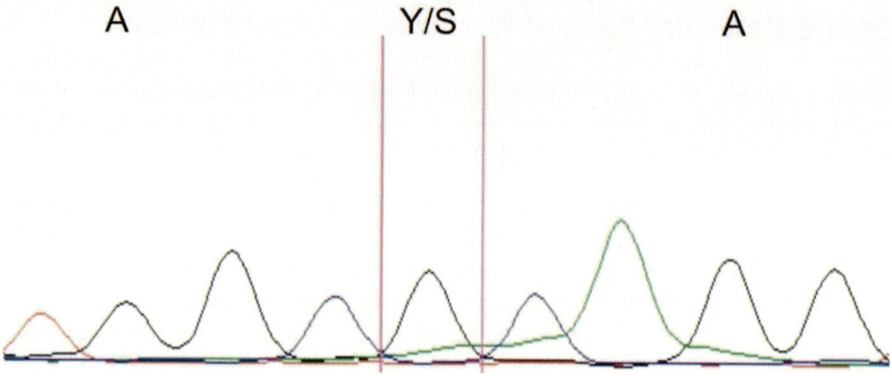

Fig. 1a. Y139S mutation

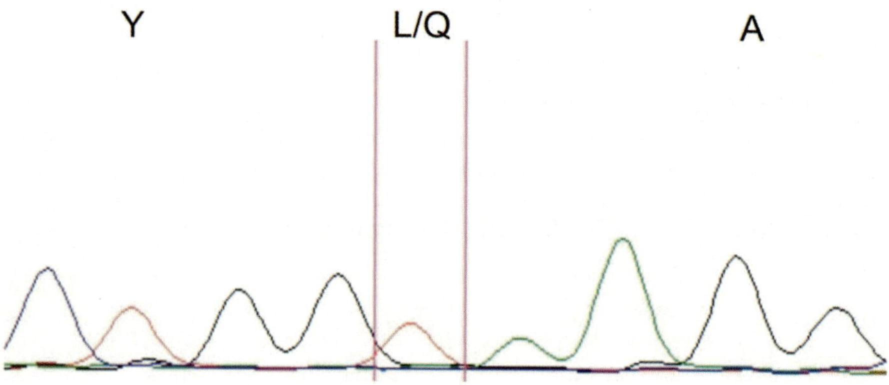

Fig. 1b. L120Q mutation

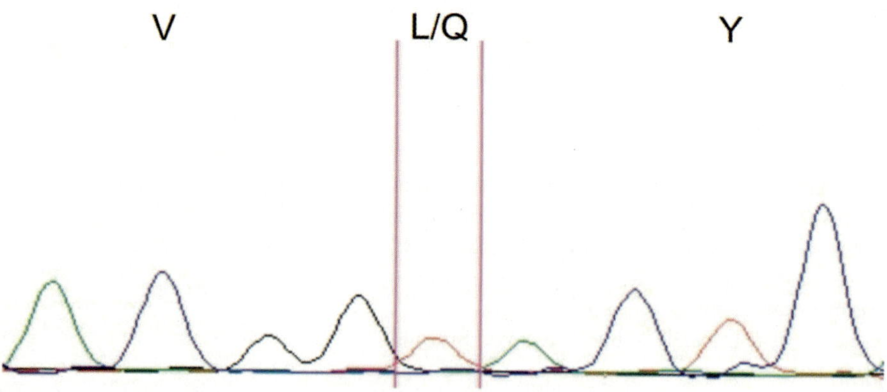

Fig. 1c. L128Q mutation

Fig. 1a–c. Sequence analysis of exon 3 of the VKORC-1gene in British rats

Conclusion

VKORC1 mutations alone, however, do not explain the observed differences in sensitivity against second generation coumarins. Apparently, other modulating factors are required for multiple anticoagulant resistants.

In stocks from the British main island three different mutations were identified: Tyr139Ser (a), Leu120Gln (b) and Leu128Gln (c). Recently, leucine (CTG) 128 had been found mutated to arginine (CGG) in a human patient resistant to coumarin treatment for thrombosis. Likewise, two mutations have altered codon 139 (TAT = tyrosine) to either serine (TCT) or cystein (TGT). Resistant rats from Denmark were found to carry this Tyr139Cys mutation that had been described before in rats from north-west Germany (Münsterland).

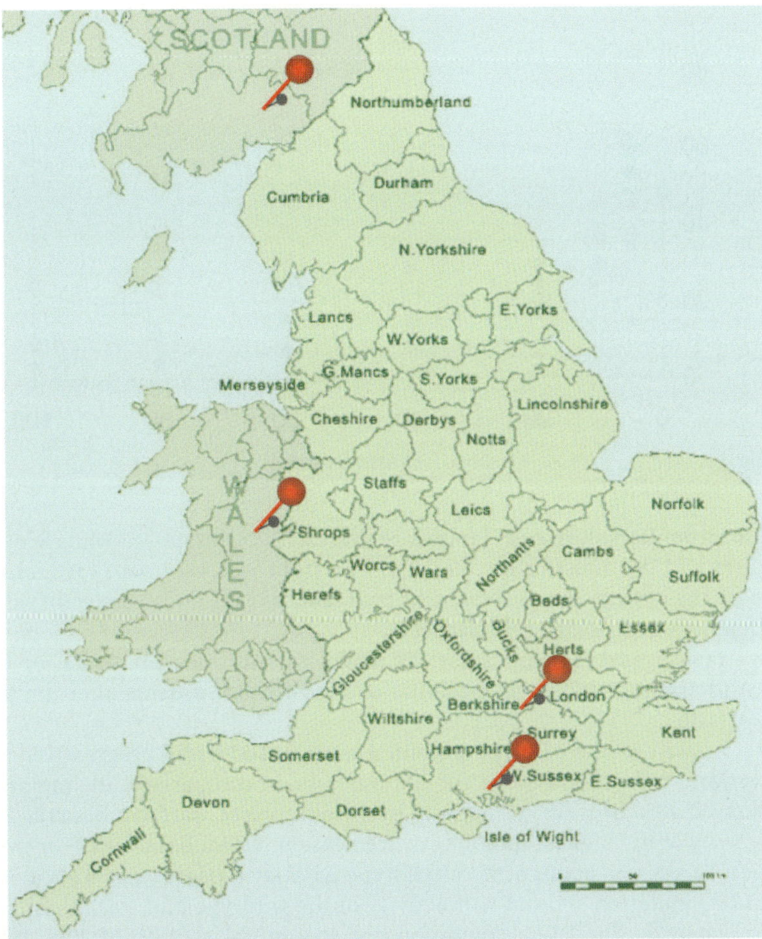

Fig. 2. Distribution of the three detected mutations in British rats

Table 1.

	activity (%)				
Warfarin (μM)	**WT**	**Y139C**	**Y139S**	**L128Q**	**L120Q**
0	100	47.57	56.62	50	20.09
5	52.98	37.42	45.47	34.33	14.68
10	29.69	36.09	46.47	28.26	10.6
20	24.06	29.25	42.82	20.31	6.84
40	15.67	28.48	34.22	14.46	8.72
60	7.4	30.91	40.07	14.9	7.61
80	4.42	23.84	35.1	11.81	9.16
100	3.86	25.17	32.67	9.49	8.83

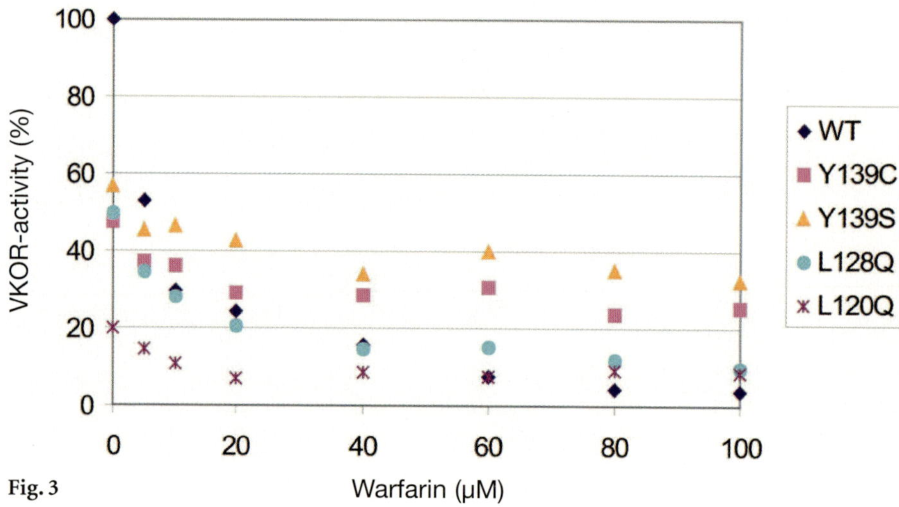

Fig. 3

Rats from Berkshire and Hampshire share a L120Q mutation while Scottish animals carry a L128Q substitution. Resistant rats from Wales show a Y139S mutation which is on the same position like the known mutation Y139C in resistant rat strain from Denmark and north-west Germany.

Table 1 and Figure 3 show the VKOR activity measurements for the wildtype (WT) and four independent mutations in resistant rodents after the inhibition by warfarin.

Activity of the wildtype protein was set to 100% and progressively inhibited by warfarin to less than 5% at 100 μM warfarin. In comparison, the mutation Tyr139C showed 48% of wildtype activity in the absence of warfarin but still 25% residual activity at the highest inhibitor concentration tested. Basal VKOR activity of mutation Y139S was about 57% of wildtype without warfarin and 33% at 100 μM. The L128Q mutation showed half activity of the wildtype and was inhibited at 100 μM to just 10%. The L120Q mutation had low initial activity of 20% of normal but showed with 9% more activity at 100 μM warfarin than the wildtype.

References

1. Goodstadt L, Ponting CP, 2004 Vitamin K epoxide reductase: homology, active site and catalytic mechanism. Trends Biochem. Sci. 29: 289–292
2. Li T, Chang CY, Jin DY, Lin PJ, Khorova A et al., 2004 Identification of the gene for vitamin K epoxide reductase. Nature 427: 541–544
3. Pelz H-J, Rost S, Hünerberg M, Fregin A et al., 2005 The Genetic Basis of Anticoagulants in Rodents. Genetics, 170: 1839–1847
4. Rost S, Fregin A, Ivaskevicius V, Conzelmann E, Hoertnagel K et al., 2004 Mutations in VKORC1 cause warfarin resistance and multiple coagulation factor deficiency type 2. Nature 427: 537–541

Influence of Factor V_{HR2} on Endogenous Thrombin Potential and Clinical Phenotype in Factor VII Deficiency

R. F. Strey, A. Siegemund, T. Siegemund, C. Schubert, G. Schuster, K. Wulff, and F. H. Herrmann

Abstract

We investigated the influence of the factor V haplotype R2 (FV_{HR2}), defined by the mutation FV_{H1299R}, on the thrombin generation in plasma as well as on the clinical expression of bleeding symptoms in patients homozygous for $FVII_{A294V}$. Due to its impaired interaction with activated protein C (APC) FV_{HR2} increases the thrombin generation. Measurements of the endogenous thrombin potential in presence of high APC concentrations showed significant increased ETP values in plasma containing FV_{HR2} compared to references with factor V wild type. In our measurements this effect is comparable to the increase of thrombin generation caused by FV_{Leiden}. This suggests FV_{HR2} to be a risk factor for thrombosis similar to factor V_{Leiden}.

On the basis of these findings, we investigated the influence of FV_{HR2} on the clinical expression of bleeding symptoms in factor VII deficient patients. A moderating effect of FV_{Leiden} to bleeding symptoms in hemophilia A and B as well as in case of FII_{Lazio} has already been reported by other authors. This effect is explained by the increased APC resistance of FV_{Leiden}. Based on the APC resistance we expected a similar effect for FV_{HR2}. This was confirmed for four patients homozygous for the mutation $FVII_{A294V}$. Two of these patients did not carry FV_{HR2} and show bleeding symptoms. The two asymptomatic patients are heterozygous or homozygous for FV_{HR2} respectively. This indicates a moderating effect of FV_{HR2} to bleeding symptoms in patients homozygous for the mutation $FVII_{A294V}$.

Introduction

The most important genetic cause of venous thromboses consists in an activated protein C (APC) resistance caused by the point mutation FV_{R506Q} (FV_{Leiden}) [1–8]. The factor V haplotype R2 (FV_{HR2}), defined by the mutations FV_{M385T}, FV_{H1299R}, FV_{M1736V} and FV_{D2194G}, is also associated with an APC resistance, but it is not clearly shown to be a risk factor for venous thromboses too [9]. Another clinical effect of the APC resistance of FV_{Leiden} consists in a moderating effect on the clinical expression of bleeding disorders. But this effect has been studied by several groups with inconsistent results [10]. The APC resistance of factor V_{HR2} is mainly caused by an impaired APC cofactor activity of factor V resulting in a reduced degradation of fac-

I. Scharrer/W. Schramm (Ed.)
36th Hemophilia Symposium Hamburg 2005

tor VIIIa [11]. An alternative mechanism based on a changed ratio of the isoforms FV1 and FV2 in plasma [12].

In this study we present indications of an association between increased endogenous thrombin potential (ETP) values and the expression of FV_{Leiden} as well as FV_{HR2}. The association between different clinical manifestations in individuals with FVII deficiency on the one hand and ETP and the presence of FV_{HR2} on the other hand is studied.

Patients and References

For all individuals included in this study the plasma concentrations of fibrinogen, antithrombin, homocystein, protein C, protein S as well as factor XII have been found in normal range and lupus anticoagulant testing for antibodies against plasma proteins have been negative in all cases.

Samples with factor V_{Leiden} mutation or factor V haplotype R2 (FV_{HR2}) have been collected from 7 patients with and 8 patients without thromboses. In case of the thromboses patients the samples have been collected at least six months after the last thrombotic event. The mutations of persons without thromboses have been identified by family anamnesis or by a corresponding screening. As a marker for FV_{HR2} we used the mutation FV_{H1299R} [13, 14]. The FV_{Leiden} mutation has been determined according to Bertina et al. [5].

Plasma samples with the homozygous $FVII_{A294V}$ mutation [15] were taken from four patients of the »Greifswald Factor VII Deficiency Study« [16]. Two of these patients had spontaneous bleeding symptoms and the other two patients had never spontaneous bleeding symptoms related to the FVII deficiency (further referred to as »asymptomatic«).

Informed consent was obtained from all patients and donors of reference samples.

Experimental Determination of Thrombin Generation

The measurement of the endogenous thrombin potential (ETP) has been performed in a final volume of 75 µl containing 50 µl sample, 0.6 ng/ml recombinant tissue factor (2.5 µl 0.1x Innovin, Dade Behring, Marburg, Germany), 2.7 µg/ml activated protein C (1 µl 0,1x Xigris, Lilly & Co., Giessen, Germany), 0.8 ng/ml phospholipids, isotonic saline, $CaCl_2$, tris buffer and fluorogenic substrate (Z-Gly-Gly-Arg-AMC from Bachem, Heidelberg, Germany) [17, 18]. The calibration has been performed without recombinant tissue factor but with fondaparinux (Arixtra, Sanofi-Synthelabo, France) as a coagulation inhibitor and a dilution series of up to 20 nM thrombin. The initial conversion rate of the calibration measurements is linear correlated to the initial thrombin concentration.

Fluorescence intensity was detected using fluorimetric detection (Fluoroscan Ascent, Labsystem Helsinki, Finland) at wavelength of 340 nm (excitation) and 440 nm (emission).

Mathematical Evaluation

The calculation of the endogenous thrombin potential is based on a mechanism proposed by Hemker and Béguin [19] for the generation of the α_2-macroglobulin complex α_2M·FIIa and for the conversion of the fluorogenic substrate by free as well as α_2M bound thrombin. According to this mechanism the formation of the α_2M·FIIa complex as well as the conversion of the substrates by free and α_2M bound thrombin are 1st order reactions. This leads to the differential time equation

$$\frac{\partial}{\partial t}[F] = k_c \cdot \left([FIIa] + k_b \int [FIIa]dt + A_0\right) \cdot \left([S]_0 - [F]\right) \tag{1}$$

for the formation of the fluorogen *F*, where A_0 represents a background activity of the reaction mixture (mainly caused by activated protein C), $[S]_0$ the initial concentration of the fluorogenic substrate, k_b the rate constant for the formation of the α_2M·FIIa complex and k_c the rate constant of the conversion of the fluorogenic substrate. Assuming a linear correlation between the concentration *[F]* of the fluorogen and the measured signal *f*, this leads to

$$\frac{\dot{f}}{k_c \cdot (f_\infty - f)} = [FIIa] + k_b \int [FIIa]dt + A_0 \tag{2}$$

With an approximation of the integrals by trapezoidal rule the concentration *[FIIa]* of free thrombin results from the measured curve by an implicit formula. The constants A_0, f_∞ und k_c have been determined by calibration with a dilution series of thrombin and k_b have been estimated by a nonlinear optimization procedure (golden section algorithm) according to

$$\sum_{i=e}^{n} [FIIa(k_b, t_i)]^2 \Rightarrow Min. \tag{3}$$

Condition (3) results from the formation of the α_2M·FIIa complex which consumes all free thrombin after the end of the thrombin formation, leading to a final concentration of $[FIIa]_\infty = 0$ for free thrombin.

Statistical analysis has been performed by paired t-test.

Influence of Oral Anticoagulants

The method used in this study is characterized by a high sensitivity against oral anticoagulants. Two patients homozygous for FV_{HR2} have been treated with oral anticoagulants (phenprocumon) during collection of the first plasma sample. The ETP values of these samples have been found below the detection limit. Even four weeks after the end of treatment the ETP values remained significant below the reference values. Six weeks after the end of treatment the ETP reached its final value (see Fig. 1).

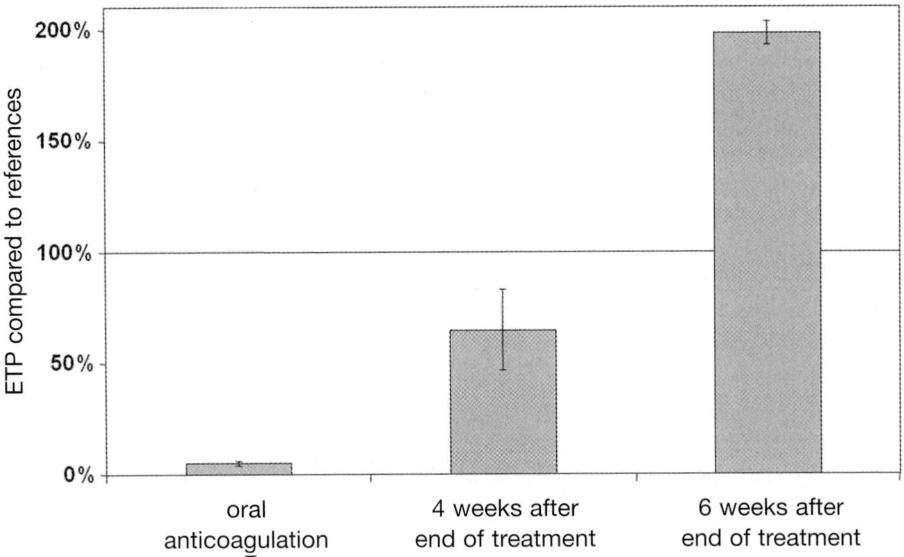

Fig. 1. Influence of oral anticoagulants to ETP

Influence of Factor V Genotype to ETP

In accordance to results of other authors [11, 20], without addition of APC, the ETP values of references as well as of samples with the factor V mutations FV_{Leiden} or FV_{HR2} did not show significant differences.

In presence of high APC concentrations (as specified in the experimental determination of thrombin generation), the average of ETP values of all samples with

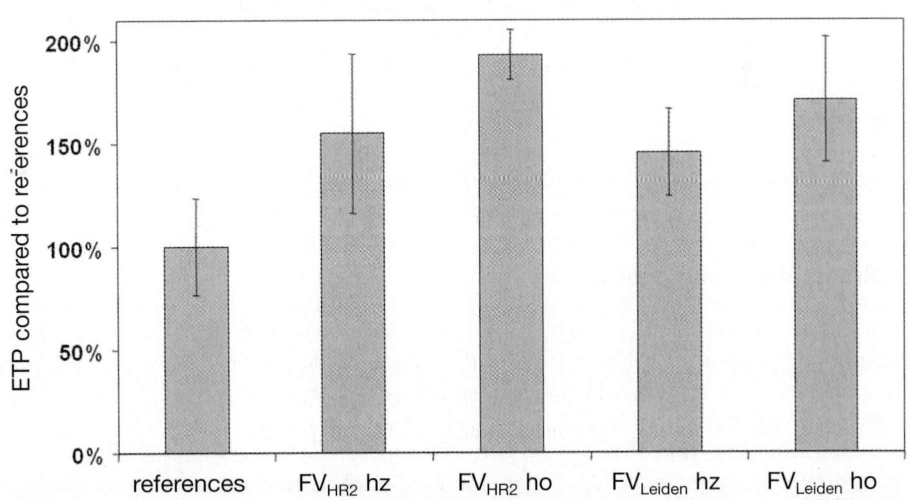

Fig. 2. Dependence of the ETP on the factor V genotype

Table 1. p-values for different combinations of factor V genotypes

	hz FV_{HR2}	ho FV_{HR2}	hz FV_{Leiden}	ho FV_{Leiden}
reference	0.0 %	0.0 %	0.0 %	0.0 %
hz FV_{HR2}		0.6 %	47 %	30 %
ho FV_{HR2}			0.0 %	6.9 %
hz FV_{Leiden}				4.8 %

FV_{Leiden} or FV_{HR2} have been found significant above the reference values (see Fig. 2). The differences between ETP values of heterozygous and homozygous samples of FV_{Leiden} and FV_{HR2} as well as between homozygous FV_{HR2} and heterozygous FV_{Leiden} have been significant, too.

Table 1 shows the p-values for the different combination of genotypes determined by two-sided t-tests. p-values below 5% have been chosen as a criterion for significant differences between ETP values of the corresponding genotypes.

Additionally to the differences, the measurements also showed similarities between the homozygous forms of FV_{Leiden} and FV_{HR2} and between the particular heterozygous forms. This is characterized by similar increased ETP values in case of the haplotype R2 and factor V_{Leiden}.

Combined Influence of FV_{HR2} and $FVII_{A294V}$

Additionally to the isolated influence of FV_{HR2} and FV_{Leiden} to the endogenous thrombin potential the combined effect of FV_{HR2} and inherited factor VII deficiency has been investigated in four patients with the homozygous mutation $FVII_{A294V}$. As a first result both asymptomatic patients appeared to be carrier of FV_{HR2} whereas the symptomatic patients do not carry FV_{HR2}. Furthermore both asymptomatic patients show significant increased ETP values compared to the references. The ETP values of the symptomatic patients are significantly decreased (see Fig. 3).

Discussion

The results of this study show an increased endogenous thrombin potential (ETP) for FV_{Leiden} and FV_{HR2} in presence of activated protein C. The ETP values for each three samples with homozygous FV_{Leiden} and homozygous FV_{HR2} as well as for each four samples with heterozygous FV_{Leiden} or heterozygous FV_{HR2} have been found significant above the reference values. These results can be explained as an effect of the APC resistance of FV_{Leiden} and FV_{HR2}. The ETP values of heterozygous as well as of homozygous samples have been found in the same range in each case ($p = 7\%$ for homozygous and $p = 47\%$ for heterozygous cases). This shows a similar APC resistance of FV_{HR2} compared to FV_{Leiden}.

Assuming the APC of FV_{Leiden} to be a risk factor for thrombosis, the increased thrombin generation by FV_{HR2} suggests a similar increased risk of venous thrombosis in the case of homozygous FV_{HR2}. According to our results heterozygous FV_{HR2}

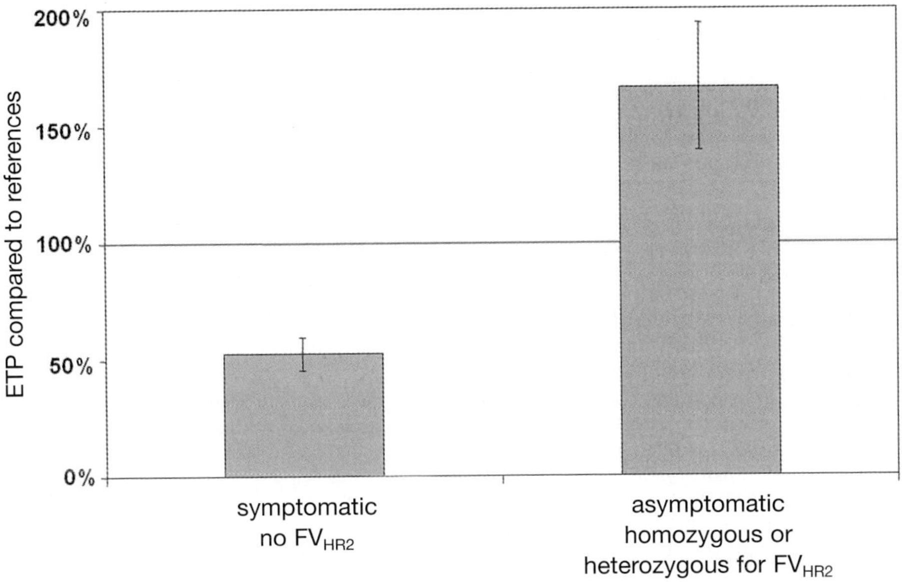

Fig. 3. Association between clinical phenotype and absence or presence of FV_{HR2} in patients homozygous for the mutation $FVII_{A294V}$

may also be a risk factor for thromboses, but due to the limited number of samples and the high statistical spread of the ETP values of the heterozygous FV_{HR2} samples this cannot be confirmed with the present data.

Additionally the measurements with samples of patients homozygous for the mutation $FVII_{A294V}$ indicate a moderating effect of FV_{HR2} to the clinical phenotype in patients with severe factor VII deficiency. Similar effects have already been reported by Nichols et al. [21] for hemophilia A and by Vianello et al. [22] for hemophilia B and can be explained by a compensation of the reduced thrombin generation caused by hemophilia A or B by an increased thrombin generation caused by the APC resistance of FV_{HR2}. The present measurements suggest a similar effect for the homozygous mutation $FVII_{A294V}$. This is reflected in the presence of FV_{HR2} in asymptomatic patients homozygous for $FVII_{A294V}$ as well as in increased ETP values of these patients.

References

1. Dahlbäck B, Carlsson M and Svensson P. Familial Thrombophilia Due to a Previously Unrecognized Mechanism Characterized by Poor Anticoagulant Response to Activated Protein C: Prediction of a Cofactor to Activated Protein C. Proc. Natl. Acad Sci. U.S.A. 1993; 90:1004-1008
2. Rosendaal FR, Koster JP, Vandenbroucke JP, et al. High risk of thrombosis in patients homozygous for factor V Leiden (activated protein C resistance). Blood 1995; 85:1504-1508
3. Ridker PM, Hennekens CH, Lindpaintner K, et al. Mutation in the Gene Coding for Coagulation Factor V and the Risk of Myocardial Infarction, Stroke, and Venous Thrombosis in Apparently Healthy Men. N. Engl. J. Med. 1995; 332:912-917

4. Koster T, Rosendaal FR, de Ronde H, et al. Venous thrombosis due to poor anticoagulant response to activated protein C: Leiden Thrombophilia Study. Lancet 1993; 342(8886-8887):1503-6
5. Bertina RM, Koeleman BPC, Koster T, et al. Mutation in blood coagulation factor V associated with resistance to activated protein C. Nature 1994; 369:64-67
6. Greengard JS, Sun X, Xu X, et al. Activated protein C resistance caused by Arg506?Gln mutation in factor Va. Lancet 1994; 343:1361-1362
7. Voorberg J, Roelse J, Koopman R, et al. Association of idiopathic venous thromboembolism with single point mutation at Arg506 of factor V. Lancet 1994; 343: 1535-1536
8. Zöller B and Dahlbäck B. Linkage between inherited resistance to activated protein C and factor V gene mutation in venous thrombosis. Lancet 1994; 343:1536-1538
9. Castaman G, Faioni EM, Tosetto A, et al. The factor V HR2 haplotype and the risk of venous thrombosis: a meta-analysis. Haematologica 2003; 88(10):1182-1189
10. Dargaud Y, Meunier S and Negrier C. Haemophilia and thrombophilia: an unexpected association! Haemophilia 2004; 10:319-326
11. Castoldi E, Brugge JM, Nicolaes DAF, Girelli D, Tans G, Rosine J: Impaired APC cofactor activity of factor V plays a major role in the APC resistance associated with the factor V Leiden (R506Q) and R2 (H1299R) mutations. Blood 2004; 103, 11:4173-4179
12. Castoldi E, Rosing J, Girelli D, Hoekema L, Lunghi B, Mingozzi F, Ferraresi P, Friso S, Corrocher R, Tans G, Bernardi F. Mutations in the R2 FV gene affect the ratio between the two FV isoforms in plasma. Thromb Haemost. 2000; 83(3):362-365
13. Bernardi F, Faioni EM, Castoldi E, Lunghi B, Castaman G, Sacchi E, Mannucci PM: A Factor V Genetic Component Differing From Factor V R506Q Contributes to the Activated Protein C Resistance Phenotype. Blood 1997; 90: 1552 - 1557
14. Herrmann FH, Salazar-Sanchez L, Jimenez-Arce G, Grimm R, Schröder W: High Prevalence of FVHR2 Polymorphism in Costarican Indians who Have no FVL. Thromb Haemost 2001; 85: 1020-1
15. Wulff K and Herrmann FH. Twenty two novel mutations of the factor VII gene in factor VII deficiency. Human Mutation 2000; 15: 489-496
16. Herrmann FH, Wulff K, Auberger K, Aumann V, Bergmann F, Bratanoff E, Franke D, Grundeis M, Kreuz W, Lenk H, Losonszy H, Maak B, Marx G, Mauz-Körholz C, Pollmann H, Serban M, Sutor A, Syrbe G, Vogel G, Weinstock N, Wenzel E, Wulff K: Molecular Biology and Clinical Manifestation of Hereditary Factor VII Deficiency. Semin Thromb Hemost 2000; 26, 4: 393-400
17. Siegemund A, Petros S, Siegemund T, Scholz U, Seyfarth H-J, Engelmann L: The endogenous thrombin potential and high levels of coagulation factor VIII, factor IX and factor XI. Blood Coagul Fibrinolysis. 2004; 15(3): 241-4
18. Siegemund T, Petros S, Siegemund A, Scholz U, Engelmann L: Thrombin generation in severe haemophilia A and B: the endogenous thrombin potential in platelet-rich plasma. Thromb Haemost. 2003; 90(5): 781-6
19. Hemker HC and Béguin S: Thrombin Generation in Plasma: Its Assessment Via the Endogenous Thrombin Potential. Thromb Haemost 1995; 74(1): 134-138
20. Castoldi E, Govers-Riemslag JWP, Pinotti M, Biondini D, Tans G, Berrettini M, Mazzucconi MG, Bernardi F, Rosine J: Coinheritance of Factor V (FV) Leiden enhances thrombin formation and is associated with a mild bleeding phenotype in patients homozygous for the FVII 9726+5G>A (FVII Lazio) mutation. Blood 2003; 102: 4014 – 4020
21. Nichols WC, Amano K, Cacheris PM, Figueiredo MS, Michaelides K, Schwaab R, Hoyer L, Kaufman RJ and Ginsburg D: Moderation of hemophilia A phenotype by the factor VR506Q mutation. Blood. 1996; 88: 1183-1187
22. Vianello F, Belvini D, Dal Bello F, Tagariello G, Zanon E, Lombardi A-M, Zerbinati P, Girolami A: Mild bleeding diathesis in a boy with combined severe haemophilia B (C10400?T) and heterozygous factor V Leiden. Haemophilia. 2001; 7: 511-514

Splice Site Mutations Effect on the *F8* mRNA Splicing

O. El-Maarri, C. Klein, J. Junen, J. Schröder, C. R. Müller, and J. Oldenburg

Introduction

Hemophilia A (HA) is caused by impaired *F8* protein activity. Various point mutations leading to either altered or truncated FVIII protein and the two major inversion hot spots, Intron 22 and Intron 1 inversions, have been reported. In addition various base changes in the Intron-Exon boundaries are reported. These are putative splice site mutations that may cause the skipping of one or more exons. The putative splice site mutations account for about 3% of identified mutations (in the *F8* gene) among hemophilia A patients.

Therefore, to further investigate if these putative splice site mutations are altering the *F8* mRNA structure, we analyzed mRNA from these patients. We report here on two interesting cases (IVS10-1 G>A and IVS14+3 A>G) where we prove that both are altering the normal *F8* mRNA and thus these base changes can be hold responsible for the hemophilia A phenotype in these patients.

Materials and Methods

Subjects

For this study we selected 30 patients that were already identified to have different putative splice site mutations in the *F8* gene (Table 1). 2.5 ml of patient's bloods were collected in PAXgene blood RNA tubes and total cellular RNA was extracted using the PAXgene Blood RNA kit according to the manufacturer's protocol (PreAnalytiX, Switzerland). For reverse transcription *F8* cDNA was divided into 4 different regions that cover all the splicing sites, exons 1–8 (region A), exons 8–14 (region B), exons 14–22 (region C) and exons 19–26 (region D) (Fig. 1). We performed reverse transcription using the Omniscript reverse transcriptase according to the manufacturer's protocol (Qiagen, Hilden, Germany).

We performed the RT-amplifications in two rounds of PCR using a nested approach. For the first PCR we used 5 µl (in total of 50 µl) from the reverse transcription. We divided each of the above 4 regions into two regions (total of 8 overlapping regions) that were amplified, by a nested PCR approach, using 5µl (in total of 50 µl) from the first RT-PCR as a template.

I. Scharrer/W. Schramm (Ed.)
36th Hemophilia Symposium Hamburg 2005

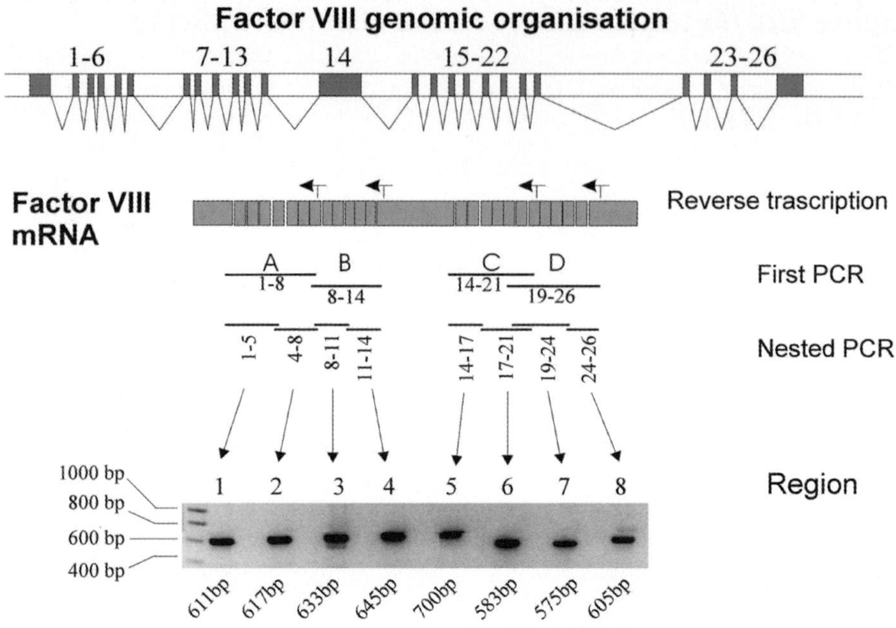

Fig. 1. Schematic diagram showing the experimental strategy

Results and Discussion

HA is caused by a variety of mutations mechanisms in the F8 gene. One group of mutations occurs within or in the vicinity of splice sites. It is not always clear whether these base exchanges are causing exon(s) skipping or alternative splicing. Web-based software tools are available to calculate the splicing probabilities of 5' and 3' splice before and after nucleotide substitution at individual positions. However, to experimentally test these changes we have previously analyzed some potential splice site mutations by RT-PCR [1, 2] (Table 1 yellow shaded cases). We were able to show that point mutations lying in or at the vicinity of a splice consensus sites caused real splicing errors in all patients studied (Fig. 2, Table 1).

In further two cases we prove here that alteration to the normal splicing take place. In the IVS14+3 a>g case we observed a smaller product than expected, the reduced size is due to the absence of the large exon 14 that code mainly for the F8-B domain (Fig. 2a). In IVS10-1 g>a a novel splicing acceptor site is generated. An abnormal sized PCR-product (smaller product) was detected. Sequencing of the RT-PCR product depicted a 36 bp deletion from nucleotide 1538 to nt 1573 of F8 cDNA, corresponding to the first 36 nucleotides of exon 11 (Fig. 2b). Both mutations are producing in frame deletions of 12 aa and 1035 aa for IVS10-1 g>a and IVS14+3 respectively.

Table 1. A list of identified putative splice site mutations in our group of hemophilia A patients. Informations regarding severity and development of inhibitor is also provided when available. The cases studied earlier and proved to be causatives are marked by yellow, the ones investigated here are shaded in red

List Number	Base	Base Change	FVIIIc	Severity	Inhibitors
1	IVS1-2	a>g	?	?	?
2	IVS1-3	c>t	?	?	?
3	IVS2+1	g>a	<1%	severe	no
4	IVS2-1	g>a	<1%	severe	no/yes
5	IVS3+5	g>a	<1%	severe	yes/no
6	IVS3-1	g>a	?	?	?
7	IVS4+1	g>a	?	?	?
8	IVS4-5	t>c	13%	mild	?
9	IVS5+1	g>t	5%	mod/severe	?
10	IVS5+5	g>c	?	?	?
11	IVS5-3	c>g	0-2%	severe	no
12	IVS6+3	a>g	1%	severe	no
13	IVS6-1	g>a	<1%	severe	?
14	IVS8+1	g>t	3% Female	moderate	?
15	IVS9+5	g>a	?	?	?
16	IVS10-1	g>a	<1%	severe	no
17	IVS11+1	g>a	?	?	?
18	IVS11+5	g>a	5%	mild/mod., severe	?
19	IVS11-2	del a	<1%	severe	?
20	IVS12+1	g>a	0-2%	severe	yes
21	IVS12+5	g>c	?	?	?
22	IVS12-3	c>g	1-2%	moderate/severe	no
23	IVS14+3	a>g	<1%	severe	no/yes
24	IVS15+1	g>a	<1%	severe	no
25	IVS16+2	t>g	<1%	severe	no
26	IVS19+2	t>c	<1%	severe	?
27	IVS20+1	g>a	?	severe	?
28	IVS21-5	g>a	2-5%	moderate/severe	no
29	IVS22+2	t>a	<1%	severe	yes
30	IVS22+5	g>t	4%	moderate/severe	no
31	IVS23+1	g>a	<1%	severe	no
32	IVS24+4	a>g	?	?	?

Conclusion

This highlights the usefulness of the mRNA analysis for routine diagnosis of such ambiguous cases including the presence of potential cryptic splice sites and clearly demonstrates the causality of the mutations which is also important for the genetic counseling of those families.

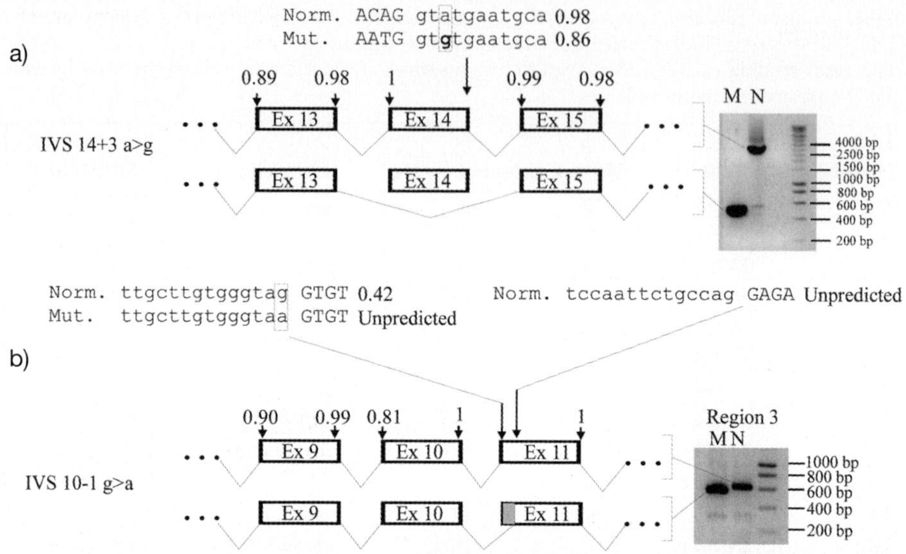

Fig. 2a, b. Schematic diagram of the exons involved in the splicing error. The position of mutation is also shown together with the change in the score for the splice sites. a) mutation involving exon 14 and b) mutation activating a new accepteor splice site at intron 10

References

1. El-Maarri O, Herbiniaux U, Graw J, Schröder J, Watzka M, Brackmann H-H, Schramm W, Hanfland P, Schwaab R, Müller CR, Oldenburg J. Detailed RNA analysis in haemophilia A patients with previously undetectable mutations, Journal of Thrombosis and Haemostasis. 2005; 3:332–339.
2. El-Maarri O, Singer H, Klein C, Watzka M, Herbiniaux U, Brackmann H, Schröder J, Graw J, Müller CR, Schramm W, Schwaab R, Haaf T, Hanfland P, Oldenburg J. Lack of F8 mRNA: a novel mechanism leading to hemophilia A. Blood, 2006;107: 2759–65.

Species-Specific Variation of VKORC1-Activity and Resistance to Warfarin

A. FREGIN, S. ROST, C. R. MÜLLER, and J. OLDENBURG

Introduction

Vitamin K serves as a cofactor for the post-translational modification by gamma-carboxylation of the Gla-proteins. Vitamin K-dependent proteins include the coagulation factors II, VII, IX, and X as well as proteins S, C and Z, illustrating the clinical importance of vitamin K-metabolism. Inhibitors of the coumarin-type reduce coagulation activity by interfering with the vitamin K 2,3-epoxide reductase enzyme complex. They are the most used oral anticoagulants for antithrombotic prophylaxis. Coumarin derivatives are also used in rodent pest control worldwide.

In humans, mutations in the VKORC1 gene lead to combined deficiency of vitamin K-dependent clotting factors type 2 (VKCFD2) or warfarin resistance. Mutations in VKORC1 were also reported for warfarin resistant strains of mice and rats.

Natural susceptibility to anticoagulants varies widely between species. Based on LD50 values house mice are about 6 times less susceptible to warfarin than brown rats. Compared to rats chicken are completely resistant against warfarin, whereas pigs *(Sus scrofa)* are extremely sensitive.

Some rodent species, e.g. *Acomys cahirinus* (Egyptian spiny mouse), were found to be relatively tolerant to anticoagulant compounds, with a great variation in response and a survival up to 698 mg/kg in a 28-day-feeding-test.

Results and Discussion

The VKOR-activities of microsomal preparations from the mouse and the highly warfarin-resistant spiny-mouse *(Acomys cahirinus)* where compared. Interestingly the basal activities of Acomys are significant lower (~25%), but are less sensitive to inhibition (Fig. 1).

Recently the VKORC1 gene was cloned. This gene is highly conserved among species. In contrast, the species-specific response to warfarin shows a wide variation. The difference of the LD50-values may therefore be result from the few amino acid-substitutions. The activity was measured after recombinant expression in HEK-293-cells.

The activity of VKORC1 was found to vary widely between species; especially the activity of the porcine protein is three times higher than the human or the rodent enzyme (Fig. 2).

I. Scharrer/W. Schramm (Ed.)
36th Hemophilia Symposium Hamburg 2005

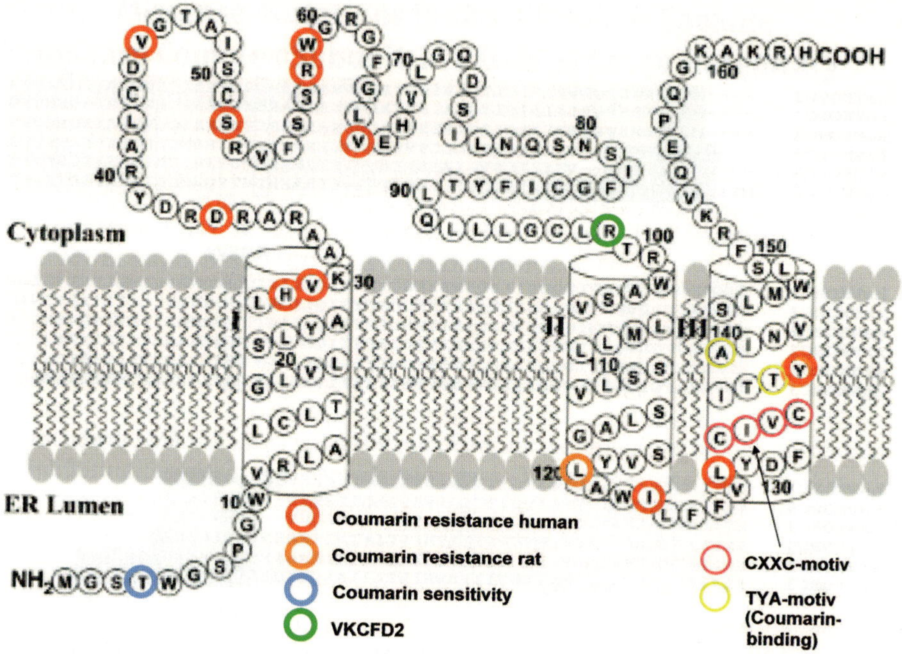

Fig. 3. Topology model of VKORC1. Localization of different mutations in the VKORC1-gene leading to coumarin resistance in man and rat, coumarin sensitivity and VKCFD2

Results and Discussion

In 10 unrelated patients with variable degrees of coumarin resistance ranging from partial to complete resistance genetic testing revealed different causative missense mutations in the VKORC1 gene (His28Gln, Asp36Tyr, Ser52Trp, Trp59Cys, Val66Met, Ile123Asn, Tyr139His) (Fig. 2, Fig. 3).

The missense mutations were scattered throughout the gene, thus indicating that not only one specific epitope seems to be critical for coumarin binding and action.

Conclusion

Mutations in VKORC1 cause coumarin resistance and are also responsible for differing dosing requirements close to the upper therapeutic range. Here we present the data in 16 patients from 14 families revealing 11 different missense mutations, six of which have not been reported previously.

Our data may contribute in identifying further functional epitopes of VKORC1 and may provide a basis for a rational design of novel anticoagulants targeting VKOR in the future.

References

1. Rost S, Fregin A, Ivaskevicius V, Conzelmann E, Hortnagel K, Pelz HJ, Lappegard K, Seifried E, Scharrer I, Tuddenham EG, Muller CR, Strom TM, Oldenburg J (2004) Mutations in VKORC1 cause warfarin resistance and multiple coagulation factor deficiency type 2. Nature 427: 537–41
2. Li T, Chang CY, Jin DY, Lin PJ, Khvorova A, Stafford DW (2004) Identification of the gene for vitamin Kepoxide reductase. Nature 427: 541–544

Establishment of an International Registry of Patients with Congenital FXIII Deficiency

V. Ivaskevicius, R. Seitz, H. P. Kohler, L. Muszbek, R. A. S. Ariens, E. Seifried, and J. Oldenburg

Introduction

FXIII deficiency is a rare autosomal recessive disorder affecting approximately 1 out of 1–3 million inhabitants. The disease is characterized by bleeding, impaired wound repair and spontaneous abortions in females. Extracellular FXIII molecule has a tetramer structure composing of two catalytic A-subunits and two B-subunits that act as a carrier molecules. Based on genotype there are two types of FXIII deficiency: A-subunit deficiency when mutation affects F13A gene and much rarely B-subunit deficiency when mutation affects F13B gene [1].

In 1993, the ETRO Working Party on factor XIII initiated a Europe-wide questionnaire on congenital FXIII deficiency with several aims:

1. establish a patient registry
2. join a study group
3. accumulate and exchange informations on symptoms, diagnostic approach, and treatment
4. stimulate research on protein and gene defects and their relation to clinical symptoms [2].

Methods

In the first questionnaire (QP1) has been requested information about patient ID, date of birth, a question for affected relatives, methods and results of diagnostic tests, symptoms (bleeding, wound healing, abortions), coexisting diseases, treatment modalities, testing for factor XIII antibodies, and genotype.

In the second questionnaire (QP2) was asked detailed data about bleeding (spontaneous and upon provocation), pregnancies and spontaneous abortions, presence of other hemorrhagic diathesis, FVIII / FIX / vWF Ristocetin cofactor values, and virus status (hepatitis B, hepatitis C, human immune deficiency virus infection).

Results and Discussion

Before the introduction of treatment severe bleeding symptoms (as judged by the attending physicians) were recognized in 55 (53%) QP1, moderate bleeding in 36

I. Scharrer/W. Schramm (Ed.)
36th Hemophilia Symposium Hamburg 2005

(34.6%) QP1, mild bleeding in 10 (9.6%) QP1 and non-bleeding in 3 (2.9%) QP1. The most common bleeding symptoms have been found to be subcutaneous (57%) and umbilical cord bleeding (56%) followed by muscle (49%), joint (36%), central nervous system (34%) and hemorrhages after surgery (40%). Naturally not every patient underwent surgery or had serious trauma. The data of the second questionnaire demonstrated the presence of bleeding upon provocation (trauma, surgery) in 67% of all cases. Impaired wound healing was recognized in 30 (28.8%)/104 QP1. Five out of 104 QP1 were expected to be heterozygous for FXIII deficiency (residual FXIII activity 33-53%). Bleeding after surgery/tooth extraction occurred in 3/5 patients, subcutaneous bleeding in 1 patient, and no bleeding was recognized in 1 patient. Spontaneous abortions have occurred in 7 of the 39 females over 18 years of age, in one of them 7, and in another patient from Hungary 8 times. The duration of the first pregnancy in the Hungarian patient was 18 weeks, while subsequently abortions occurred between 8 and 12 weeks. Successful pregnancy was possible only under substitution therapy with fresh frozen plasma (400 ml every 10 days) [3]. Antibodies against FXIII were detected in 3 patients.

Prophylactic treatment was initiated in 72 (69.2%) QP1. No treatment (fresh frozen plasma, blood transfusions, cryoprecipitate, FXIII concentrate) was required so far in 14 asymptomatic or in patients with very mild phenotype and in 1 patient with FXIII autoantibodies. The preparations used for replacement have been concentrates from placenta (31 patients), plasma (46 patients), cryoprecipitate (21 patients) and fresh frozen plasma (22 patients); the mean dosage interval was 4.1±7.2 weeks.

Hepatitis B virus (HBV) was identified in 17 (39.5%) of 43 QP2, hepatitis C virus (HCV) was detected in 13 (30.2%) / 43 QP2. Combined HBV and HCV infection was found in 11 (25.6%) patients. There were no patients with human immune deficiency virus infection (HIV).

So far the molecular defects have been analyzed in 60 (58%)/104 patients, of them 58 persons (46 unrelated families) with FXIIIA deficiency and 2 persons (1 family) with FXIIIB deficiency. In total, 35 unique mutations were identified revealing 22 (63%) missense mutations, 6 (17%) splice site mutations, 4 (11%) small deletions, 2 (6%) nonsense mutations, and 1 (3%) small insertion. A nonsense mutation in exon 14 (Arg661X) was found in 15 (14.4%)/104 individuals (9 unrelated families, 6 of them from Finland), a splice site mutation in intron 5 (IVS5-1 G>A) was identified in 11 (10.6%)/104 individuals (8 unrelated families originating from 6 European countries), a missense mutation resulting Arginine substitution by Cysteine at amino acid position 77 (Arg77Cys) was elucidated in 5 Swiss families. Eight (36%) of 22 missense mutations occurred at CpG dinucleotides thus are mutations hot-spot. In four patients with severe FXIII deficiency, the second, probably heterozygous mutation remains unknown. The F13A gene haplotype analysis of patients carrying IVS5-1 A allele demonstrated an ancient founder effect (data not shown).

In the year 2005, the ISTH FXIII subcommittee supported our initiative to enlarge the data of ETRO Working Party aiming the development of an international registry. Recently we created a new FXIII database website (www.f13-database.de) containing the information about FXIII proteins, genes, their mutation database and polymorphisms as well. This website involves also a new questionnaire for patients composing of 4 major parts including demographic, family, phenotype and genotype data). Information provided by a new questionnaire will allow better to understand the differences of diagnostic and treatment possibilities all over the world, to understand the influence of reduced FXIII activity in heterozygous relatives and finally in general will enlarge our knowledge about this rare disease. We hope that our initiative to establish a new international FXIII registry will be actively supported by the clinicians from many countries.

References

1. Ichinose A. Physiopathology and regulation of factor XIII. Thromb Haemost 2001 Jul;86(1):57-65
2. Takahashi N, Tsukamoto H, Umeyama H, Castaman G, Rodeghiero F, Ichinose A. Molecular mechanisms of type II factor XIII deficiency: novel Gly562-Arg mutation and C-terminal truncation of the A subunit cause factor XIII deficiency as characterized in a mammalian expression system. Blood 1998 Apr 15;91(8):2830–8
3. Seitz R, Duckert F, Lopaciuk S, Muszbek L, Rodeghiero F, Seligsohn U. ETRO Working Party on Factor XIII questionnaire on congenital factor XIII deficiency in Europe: status and perspectives. Study Group. Semin Thromb Hemost. 1996;22(5):415–8.
4. Boda Z, Pfliegler G, Muszbek L, Toth A, Adany R, Harsfalvi J, Papp Z, Tornai I, Rak K. Congenital factor XIII deficiency with multiple benign breast tumours and successful pregnancy with substitutive therapy. A case report. Haemostasis. 1989;19(6):348–52.

The Impact of Freezing of Plasma Samples, AB0 Blood Group and Acute-Phase Reaction on Detecting Mild Factor VIII Deficiency and Increased Factor VIII Levels as a Risk Factor for Venous Thromboembolism

J. Bach, H. Haubelt, U. Seyfert, A. Vogt, P. Hoerdt, and P. Hellstern

Introduction

Multicenter surveys have shown that there is still a wide variability in factor VIII (FVIII) levels determined in identical plasma samples by different laboratories. This may be partly due to insufficiently standardized pre-analytical conditions. Particularly, the influence of freezing and thawing on FVIII assay results has not been studied sufficiently. Whereas the impact of AB0 blood group on FVIII plasma levels has been clearly demonstrated, the significance of acute phase reaction on FVIII plasma levels in apparently healthy individuals remains to be determined.

We quantified FVIII clotting activity (FVIII:C), FVIII amidolytic activity FVIII:AM and FVIII antigen (FVIII:Ag) in 301 apparently healthy individuals (200 females and 101 males). We also determined AB0 blood group, fibrinogen antigen (FIBAg) and high sensitivity C-reactive protein (hsCRP) .

Individuals and Methods

We included 301 apparently healthy individuals (200 females, 101 males; median age, 40 years; age range, 14-66 years; 168 blood group non-0 or non-A2; 133 blood group 0 or A2). The majority of these individuals were non-donors or blood donors before their first donation or at least 8 weeks after their last donation. Subjects with any signs of infection (clinically, leukocyte count, body temperature) were excluded.

After a 30-min rest in a sitting position, blood was drawn from the antecubital vein using 21-gauge butterfly needles. Activation was minimized by light torniquet, short and moderate phlebostasis, smooth blood flow, plastic tubes from Sarstedt, Nümbrecht, Germany and gentle mixing with anticoagulant (1 part of 0.106 mmol/l unbuffered trisodium citrate to 9 parts of blood). Platelet poor plasma (PPP) was prepared by centrifugation at 3,500 x g for 10 min. Aliquots of 0.5 ml of PPP were snap-frozen in liquid nitrogen and stored at –70°C. When required for further analysis, samples were thawed at 37°C for 10 min.

The influence of freezing and thawing on FVIII plasma levels was examined in 30 further healthy individuals. FVIII:C, FVIII:AM and FVIII:Ag were determined within 6 hours after blood collection and in plasma samples which had been frozen, stored and thawed before analysis.

I. Scharrer/W. Schramm (Ed.)
36th Hemophilia Symposium Hamburg 2005

FVIII:C was determined using human FVIII-deficient plasma from Technoclone, Heidelberg, Germany and »PTT kaolin« reagent from Roche Diagnostics, Mannheim, Germany. FVIII:AM was quantified on a Dade Behring BCS analyzer using »Technochrom FVIII:C«. We measured FVIII:Ag using an »Asserachrom Factor VIII Antigen« ELISA from Stago, Asnières, France. FVIII entities were calibrated against the 5th International Standard 02/150. Fibrinogen antigen and hsCRP were determined nephelometrically using »Human Fibrinogen« antiserum and »CardioPhase hsCRP« from Dade Behring, Marburg, Germany, respectively. Fibrinogen was calibrated against the International Standard 98/612.

Data are given as means, medians, ranges, 2.5th and 97.5th percentiles. Statistical analyses included Wilcoxon's matched pairs test, the Mann-Whitney test and Spearman's rank correlation.

Results

The medians, reference ranges (2.5th and 97.5th percentiles) derived from all 301 individuals are shown in Table 1. The number of individuals with FVIII levels above 150 IU/dl and 234 U/dl, respectively, are also given in Table 1.

FVIII:C vs FVIII:AM, $p < 0.0001$; FVIII:C vs FVIII:Ag, $p < 0.0001$; FVIII:AM vs FVIII:Ag, $p = 0.099$

FVIII:C values were significantly greater than FVIII:AM and FVIII:Ag ($p < 0.0001$). In contrast, FVIII plasma levels determined amidolytically or immunologically did not differ significantly ($p = 0.099$). Both the lower and upper limits of respective FVIII reference ranges were substantially greater than reported in most previous studies. The number of healthy individuals with FVIII:C and FVIII:Ag levels above

Table 1. Reference ranges for FVIII entities, fibrinogen antigen (FIBAg) and high sensitivity C-reactive protein (hsCRP) and number of cases with high FVIII plasma levels (>150 IU/dl and 234 IU/dl, respectively), derived from 301 healthy subjects

	FVIII:C, IU/dl	FVIII:AM, IU/dl	FVIII:Ag, IU/dl	FIBAg g/l	hsCRP, mg/l
Minimum	57	58	56	1.7	0
2.5th percentile	73	68	67	1.9	0
Mean	131	120	118	2.9	2.2
Median	124	116	112	2.8	1.1
97.5th percentile	203	206	200	4.3	10
Maximum	283	254	271	5.1	23
Values above 150 IU/dl	78	40	50		
Values above 234 IU/dl	5	2	2		

Table 2. FVIII:C, FVIII:AM and FVIII:Ag in 168 individuals with blood groups non-0 or non-A2 and in 133 subjects with blood groups 0 or A2

	FVIII:C non-0 non-A2	FVIII:C 0 or A2	FVII:AM non-0 non-A2	FVIII:AM 0 or A2	FVIII:Ag non-0 non-A2	FVIII:Ag 0 or A2
Minimum	69	55	71	54	56	52
2.5th percentile	76	66	74	64	70	59
Mean	142	108	131	104	120	96
Median	136	109	126	102	117	92
97.5th percentile	257	176	221	154	193	146
Maximum	283	214	254	205	271	166

150 IU/dl was markedly higher than reported in the Leiden Thrombophilia Study (FVIII:C, 25.9% vs 11.2%; FVIII:Ag, 16.6% vs 13%; 1, 2). However, only 5 out of our 301 individuals had FVIII:C levels exceeding 234 IU/dl, which had been suggested previously as a threshold level for discriminating between patients with and without a significant risk of DVT recurrences [3].

Table 2 shows the differences in FVIII levels between blood group non-0 or non-A2 and blood group 0 or A2. FVIII:C, FVIII:AM and FVIII:Ag in subjects with blood groups non-0 or non-A2 were 27%, 20% and 24% greater than in individuals with blood groups 0 or A2 (2(A-B)/(A+B)). However, the lower limit of respective reference ranges (2.5th percentiles) were substantially higher than the 50 IU/dl reported in many papers and textbooks.

There was a strong linear correlation between FVIII:C, FVIII:AM and FVIII:Ag. However, the correlation between hsCRP and FVIII and between FIBAg and FVIII was weaker than between hsCRP and FIBAg (Table 3).

Table 3. Correlation between FVIII:C, FVIII:AM, FVIII:Ag, hsCRP and FIBAg in 301 healthy individuals

	FVIII:AM	FVIII:Ag	FIBAg	hsCRP
FVIII:C	r=0.84 p<0.0001	r=0.69 p<0.0001	r=0.28 p<0.0001	r=0.21 p<0.0001
FVIII:AM		r=0.71 p<0.0001	r=0.26 p<0.0001	r=0.18 p=0.0006
FVIII:Ag			r=0.28 p<0.0001	r=0.21 p<0.0001
FIBAg				r=0.56 p<0.0001

Table 4. FVIII:C, FVIII:AM and FVIII:Ag in 30 individuals determined in fresh plasma samples (A) and in samples frozen, stored at –70°C and thawed at 37°C for 10 min (B)

	FVIII:C A	FVIII:C B	FVII:AM A	FVIII:AM B	FVIII:Ag A	FVIII:Ag B
Minimum	86	99	92	77	72	72
Median	179	136	139	123	110	112
Maximum	239	203	215	182	156	164

FVIII:C A vs B, $p<0.0001$; FVIII:AM A vs B, $p<0.0001$; FVIII:Ag A vs B, $p = 0.655$.

When FVIII levels in individuals with hsCRP levels exceeding 5 mg/dl ($n = 36$) were compared with FVIII levels of the remaining subjects, no significant differences were observed with respect to FVIII:C ($p = 0.063$), FVIII:AM ($p = 0.098$) and FVIII:Ag ($p = 0.044$). However, individuals with hsCRP levels above 5 mg/l had significantly greater FIBAg values than the remaining subjects ($p < 0.0001$). These results suggest that FVIII plasma levels in healthy individuals are not substantially influenced by acute phase reaction.

Freezing , storage and thawing caused a substantial loss in FVIII:C (27%) and in FVIII:AM (12%). In contrast, FVIII:Ag was not influenced by freezing, storage and thawing ($p = 0.655$).

Conclusions

Despite identical calibration procedures, FVIII:C values are significantly greater than FVIII:AM and FVIII:Ag. This may be due to the fact that FVIII:C but not FVIII:AM and FVIII:Ag overestimates activated FVIII.

The lower limits of reference ranges for FVIII entities derived from frozen and thawed plasma samples are markedly greater than reported in previous studies: FVIII:C, 73 IU/dl; FVIII:AM, 68 IU/dl; FVIII:Ag, 67 IU/dl

Freezing and thawing of plasma samples reduces FVIII:C and FVIII:AM by 27% and 12%, respectively. Freezing and thawing does not influence FVIII:Ag.

Fibrinogen but not FVIII plasma levels are markedly influenced by acute phase reaction as determined by hsCRP.

Blood group non-0 or non-A2 individuals have substantially greater FVIII plasma levels than subjects with blood groups 0 or A2.

Diagnosis of mild FVIII deficiency or increased FVIII levels as a risk factor for venous thromboembolism requires carefully established references ranges and standardized pre-analytical conditions with respect to AB0 blood group and freezing/thawing of plasma samples. Before measuring FVIII, plasma samples should be frozen and thawed to obtain reliable results.

References

1. Koster T, Blann AD, Briet E, Vandenbroucke JP, Rosendaal FR (1995): Role of clotting factor VIII in effect of von Willebrand factor on occurrence of deep-vein thrombosis; The Lancet; 345; 152–5.
2. Kamphuisen PW, Eikenboom JCJ, Rosendaal FR, Koster T, Blann AD, Vos HL, Bertina RM (2001): High factor VIII antigen levels increase the risk of venous thrombosis but are not associated with polymorphisms in the von Willebrand factor and factor VIII gene; Brit J Haematol; 115; 156–8.
3. Kyrle PA, Minar E, Hirschl M, Bialonczyk C, Stain M, Schneider B, Weltermann A, Speiser W, Lechner K, Eichinger S (2000): High plasma levels of factor VIII and the risk of recurrent venous thromboembolism; N Engl J Med; 343; 457–62.

Thrombin Generation in Severely Obese Children

C. CIMENTI, H. MANGGE, B. LESCHNIK, H. HAIDL, D. ZACH, and W. MUNTEAN

Introduction

In recent years the prevalence of obesity has raised to an alarming level. Especially the increasing rate of obese children across all pediatric ages is a cause of concern. Several studies made likely a close connection between obesity and alterations in hemostasis by findings that obese subjects tend to have higher values of fibrinogen, prothrombin fragment 1 and 2 (F1 + 2), factor VII, factor VIII, von Willebrand factor (vWF), and plasminogen activator inhibitor (PAI) compared to non-obese subjects [1, 2]. These hemostatic alterations in obese patients may contribute to the development of cardiovascular disease.

Despite its undisputed importance, data on single factors or components involved in the coagulation cascade reflect only a small part of the complex hemostatic-thrombotic system and cannot replace an overall function test [3]. Therefore, we investigated the general influence of obesity in childhood on thrombin generation (TG) performing the Calibrated Automated Thrombography (CAT) representing a global test of the blood clotting system. In contrast to various conventional clotting tests, such as the partial thromboplastin time (PTT) or the prothrombin time (PT), the TG – assay is sensitive to hypercoagulable changes in the plasma [4]. Measurements of the TG represent a method to estimate the individual thrombotic risk by assessing the coagulability of blood, and – determined with platelet poor plasma – reflect the function of all plasmatic pro- and anticoagulant factors [5]. The area under the curve of generated thrombin represents the so-called »endogenous thrombin potential (ETP)« and has been shown to correlate with plasma-based hypercoagulable states [4].

In this study we compared the TG of obese children with that of healthy, normal weight, and age matched controls by means of the CAT.

Materials and Methods

Collection and Preparation of Blood

Patients were recruited from the STYrian Juvenile OBesity Study (STYJOBS) representing an attempt to focus on health related problems of obese juveniles. For this purpose children, each with a BMI greater than the 97th percentile, were examined

I. Scharrer/W. Schramm (Ed.)
36th Hemophilia Symposium Hamburg 2005

to assess the risk of preatherosclerotic lesions and metabolic disorders (such as insulin resistance, diabetes mellitus type 2, dyslipidemia, hypertension, and others) associated with juvenile obesity [6].

We examined plasma samples of the 13 most obese children from this cohort.

The study group consisted of 9 male and 4 female, aged 4.02 to 13.60 years (mean 9.62), the BMI ranged between 27.3 and 46.8 (mean 33.24). The BMI SDS ranged from 8.02 to 15.1 (mean 10.27). The control group consisted of 13 healthy, age and sex matched children. Venous blood was drawn into precitrated tubes. Plasma was separated by centrifugation at 4000 rpm for 10 minutes at room temperature and stored at –70 °.

Automated Fluorogenic Measurement of TG under Standard Conditions

TG was measured in platelet-poor plasma using a slow fluorogenic substrate (Z-Gly-Gly-Arg-AMC), purchased from Bachem, Bubendorf, Switzerland, using the Fluoroscan Ascent (Thermolabsystems OY, Helsinki, Finland) with an excitation filter at 390 nm and an emission filter at 460 nm after addition of tissue factor, phospholipids, and calcium performing the CAT, developed by Hemker's group in Maastricht [4, 5]. The measurement process lasted 40 minutes. Thrombin activity was calculated as a function of time by comparing the fluorescent signal from the thrombin-generating sample to that from a known and stable, in parallel measured standard activity.

Results

The characteristics of a typical resultant curve are shown in Figure 1 comparing an obese child with an age matched child of the control group: During the lag time no thrombin formation is detectable and the curve remains flat. After this period a steep increase up to a peak is seen. The inclination of the curve is described as time to peak. The thrombin concentration goes down again and the start tail marks the time, when the curve reaches the abscissa. The area under the curve (ETP) represents the amount of thrombin built.

Table 1. Results of TG measurement in obese children and controls

	Obese	Controls	*P* Value
Mean ETP	1948.92 ± 264.72	1421.33 ± 170.34	< 0.0001
Mean Lag time (min.)	2.26 ± 0.21	1.64 ± 0.18	< 0.0001
Mean Peak (nM)	509.42 ± 55.20	436.38 ± 48.51	< 0.001
Mean TTP (min.)	4.05 ± 0.30	3.30 ± 0.21	< 0.0001
Mean Start tail (min.)	16.33 ± 1.99	13.0 ± 1.07	< 0.0001

Values are expressed as mean ± SD
ETP = endogenous thrombin potential; TTP = time to peak

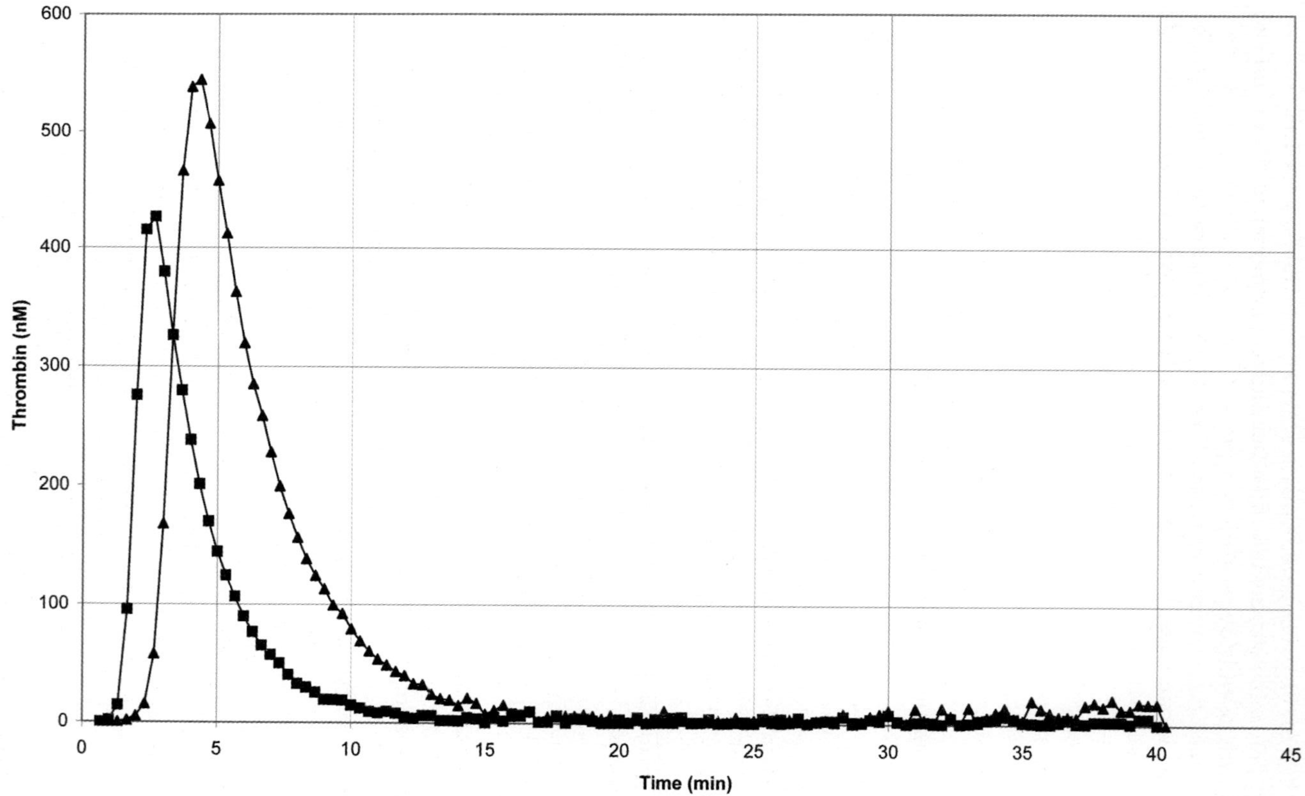

Fig. 1. TG - curves of an obese and a normal weight child.
TG in a 13.1 year old girl with a BMI of 43.10 and a BMI_{SDS} of 10.3 (▲) compared to a 13.05 year old, healthy, and normal weight girl with a BMI of 22.4 and a BMI_{SDS} of 1.14 (■)

ETP was significantly higher in obese children compared to controls. The lag time was significantly longer, and the time until the thrombin peak was reached (TTP) was prolonged in obese patients compared to controls. The thrombin peak (maximum concentration) was significantly higher in comparison to controls. The mean start tail in the obesity group was significantly higher compared to controls (Table 1).

Discussion

In this study we investigated whether differences in TG exist between obese and normal weight children. Our data show that overweight children after a significantly prolonged lag phase generate significantly higher amounts of thrombin, and that the time until the thrombin concentration approaches zero is significantly elongated in comparison to age matched, normal weight, healthy controls. Studying the metabolic and hemostatic effects of obesity in a grown-up population is often fraught with problems concerning additional risk factors like smoking, stress, and alcohol consumption. Additionally, these patients often have other co-morbidities, which manipulate the outcome directly or by their therapy. Many of these problems can be overcome by studying children who have little co-morbidities besides their obesity.

Our findings confirm the close relationship between obesity and alterations in the coagulation system. The amount of thrombin generated, the pivotal enzyme in the thrombotic-hemostatic system, represented as area under the curve (ETP), displays the individual risk of possibly being affected by thrombosis [5]. Our results are in accordance with previous papers showing that obesity is often associated with alterations in the coagulation and fibrinolytic system representing a risk factor for the development of cardiovascular disease. The fact, that elevated levels of coagulation factors i.e. FVII, FVIII, and fibrinogen are frequently detected in obese patients, could be a plausible explanation for the heightening of the ETP [1, 2, 5]. Some prospective studies have shown that increased plasma levels of fibrinogen, as well as of factors VII, and VIII indicate a risk of cardiac (i.e. ischemic heart disease, myocardial infarction) respectively vascular (i.e. arterial thrombosis) events [7, 8]. The fact that metabolic parameters exert influence on the coagulation system is confirmed by recent studies suggesting that the adipocyte itself, as a metabolically active secretory cell, is able to produce proteins like TF, contributing to atherogenesis in atherosclerotic lesions, or PAI-1, possibly explaining the high levels found in obesity [1, 8]. The association between PAI-1 antigen (PAI-1-Ag) and adiposity exists already in childhood [9]. As main physiological inhibitor of fibrinolysis in blood, elevated PAI-1 levels stand for a decreased fibrinolytic capacity and represent a risk factor for future development of atherothrombosis [10, 11, 12].

Considering all known alterations of the coagulation system in an obese population, the fact that we found a significantly prolonged lag time is surprising. This is in contrast to the observed high peaks and high ETP in obese children. We hypothesize that – using small amounts of lipidated TF as in our experiments – this prolongation of clotting time in obese patients represented as lag time in the thrombogram assay may possibly be caused by an elevation of inhibitors of coagulation such as tissue factor pathway inhibitor (TFPI). This theory is corroborated by several studies showing a correlation between TFPI levels and BMI, demonstrating that elevated TFPI levels highly depend on obesity index [13].

Our results confirm the assumption that a hypercoagulable state exists even in children with severe obesity and make likely that the observed changes in hemostatic parameters may be part of the pathomechanisms of atherosclerosis in obese patients. However, our findings with a prolonged lag phase and then increased TG show that the mechanisms of the altered TG in obese children may be more complex to explain than simply by the elevation of some clotting factors, and suggest that more work has to be done to explain the details of the observed altered TG.

References

1. Mertens I, Van Gaal LF. Obesity, haemostasis and the fibrinolytic system. Obes Rev 2002; 3: 85–101.
2. Rosito GA, D'Agostino RB, Massaro J, Lipinska I, Mittleman MA, Sutherland P, Wilson PWF, Levy D, Muller JE, Tofler GH. Association between obesity and a prothrombotic state: the Framingham Offspring Study. Thromb Haemost 2004; 91: 683–9.
3. Hemker HC, Al Dieri R, Beguin S. Thrombin generation assays: accruing clinical relevance. Curr Opin Hematol 2004; 11: 170–5.
4. Hemker HC, Giesen P, AlDieri R, Regnault V, de Smed E, Wagenvoord R, Lecompte T, Beguin S. The calibrated automated thrombogram (CAT): a universal routine test for hyper- and hypocoagulability. Pathophysiol Haemost Thromb 2002; 32: 249–53.
5. Hemker HC, Giesen P, Al Dieri R, Regnault V, de Smedt E, Wagenvoord R, Lecompte T, Beguin S. Calibrated automated thrombin generation measurement in clotting plasma. Pathophysiol Haemost Thromb 2003; 33: 4–15.
6. Pilz S, Horejsi R, Möller R, Almer G, Scharnagl G, Stojakovic T, Dimitrova R, Weihrauch G, Borkenstein M, Maerz W, Schauenstein K, Mangge H. Early atherosclerosis in obese juveniles is associated with low serum levels of adiponectin. J Clin Endocrinol Metab 2005; 90: 4792–6.
7. Martinelli I. von Willebrand factor and factor VIII as risk factors for arterial and venous thrombosis. Semin Hematol 2005; 42: 49–55.
8. Meade TW, Ruddock V, Stirling Y, Chakrabarti R, Miller GJ. Fibrinolytic activity, clotting factors, and long-term incidence of ischaemic heart disease in the Northwick Park Heart Study. Lancet 1993; 342: 1076–9.
9. Sudi KM, Gallistl S, Weinhandl G, Muntean W, Borkenstein MH. Relationship between plasminogen activator inhibitor-1 antigen, leptin, and fat mass in obese children and adolescents. Metabolism 2000; 49: 890–5.
10. Lijnen HR. Pleiotropic functions of plasminogen activator inhibitor-1. J Thromb Haemost 2005; 3: 35–45.
11. Sudi KM, Gallistl S, Trobinger M, Payerl D, Weinhandl G, Muntean W, Aigner R, Borkenstein MH. The influence of weight loss on fibrinolytic and metabolic parameters in obese children and adolescents. J Pediatr Endocrinol Metab 2001; 14: 85–94.
12. Ferguson MA, Gutin B, Owens S, Litaker M, Tracy RP, Allison J. Fat distribution and hemostatic measures in obese children. Am J Clin Nutr 1998; 67: 1136–40.
13. Vambergue A, Rugeri L, Gaveriaux V, Devos P, Martin A, Fermon C, Fontaine P, Jude B. Factor VII, tissue factor pathway inhibitor, and monocyte tissue factor in diabetes mellitus: influence of type of diabetes, obesity index, and age. Thromb Res 2001; 101: 367–75.

Subject Index

Printing: Krips bv, Meppel
Binding: Stürtz, Würzburg